Physical signs in dermatology

Commissioning Editor: Sue Hodgson
Project Development Manager: Tim Kimber
Project Manager: Scott Millar
Design Direction: Jayne Jones
Page Layout: Alan Palfreyman

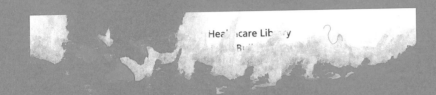

www.harcourt-international.com

Bringing you products from all Harcourt Health Sciences companies including Baillière Tindall, Churchill Livingstone, Mosby and W.B. Saunders

- ▶ **Browse** for latest information on new books, journals and electronic products

- ▶ **Search** for information on over 20 000 published titles with full product information including tables of contents and sample chapters

- ▶ **Keep up to date** with our extensive publishing programme in your field by registering with eAlert or requesting postal updates

- ▶ **Secure online ordering** with prompt delivery, as well as full contact details to order by phone, fax or post

- ▶ **News** of special features and promotions

If you are based in the following countries, please visit the country-specific site to receive full details of product availability and local ordering information

USA: www.harcourthealth.com

Canada: www.harcourtcanada.com

Australia: www.harcourt.com.au

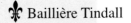 Baillière Tindall CHURCHILL LIVINGSTONE 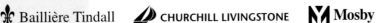 Mosby 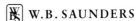 W.B. SAUNDERS

Physical signs in dermatology

Second Edition

Clifford M Lawrence MD, FRCP
Consultant Dermatologist Royal Victoria Infirmary Newcastle-upon-Tyne UK

Neil H Cox BSc, FRCP
Consultant Dermatologist Cumberland Infirmary Carlisle UK

Foreword by
Joseph L Jorizzo MD
Professor of Dermatology Wake Forest School of Medicine Winston-Salem NC USA

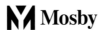 Mosby

London Edinburgh New York Philadelphia St Louis Sydney Toronto 2002

MOSBY (An imprint of Harcourt Publishers Limited)

© Harcourt Publishers Limited 2002

M is a registered trademark of Harcourt Publishers Limited

The right of Clifford M. Lawrence and Neil H. Cox to be identified as authors of this work has been asserted by them in accordance with the Copyright, Designs and Patents Act 1988

First edition published 1993

ISBN 0–7234–3184–1

British Library Cataloguing in Publication Data
A catalogue record for this book is available from the British Library

Library of Congress Cataloging in Publication Data
A catalog record for this book is available from the Library of Congress

Note
Medical knowledge is constantly changing. As new information becomes available, changes in treatment, procedures, equipment and the use of drugs become necessary. The editors/authors/contributors and the publishers have taken care to ensure that the information given in this text is accurate and up to date. However, readers are strongly advised to confirm that the information, especially with regard to drug usage, complies with the latest legislation and standards of practice.

Existing UK nomenclature is changing to the system of Recommended International Nonproprietary Names (rINNs). Until the UK names are no longer in use, these more familiar names are used in this book in preference to rINNs, details of which may be obtained from the British National Formulary.

The publisher's policy is to use **paper manufactured from sustainable forests**

Printed in China

Contents

Foreword

I am honored to have been asked by Drs. Lawrence and Cox from the United Kingdom and Harcourt Publishers Limited, to provide a few words of overview for the new edition of their outstanding introductory textbook in dermatology: Physical Signs in Dermatology. I was absolutely delighted to have been able to preview this beautifully organized, extremely well written, and spectacularly illustrated introduction to dermatology.

The authors are internationally known British dermatological educators. They have organized their book in a very useful way. They first spent considerable time giving an orientation to dermatology. They then divided our specialty into categories such as diseases that affect the color of the skin, diseases that produce scale, crust, and thicken skin, diseases that produce macular eruptions, diseases that produce blisters and vesicles, and so on. It is my belief that this is a far better introductory approach than a mechanism-oriented approach that groups diseases such as those produced by infections or by autoimmune pathogeneses. There is no question that the early learner in dermatology needs a practical approach that allows them to proceed through the differential diagnosis based on the appearance of lesions.

Harcourt Publishers Limited are rapidly becoming famous for their beautifully illustrated books. The full color photography displayed throughout the book represents a virtual atlas of dermatology. Another feature that the authors and Harcourt have brought to the mix are well-illustrated tables. Especially useful are the highlighted areas called diagnostic tips and pitfalls that appear within each chapter. There is additional value added to the learner by chapters dealing with issues such as the regional distribution of eruptions. I would also like to compliment the authors on tackling a significant percentage of our several hundred most common dermatological diseases. Because this book does this in a very reasonable way it also has value as a reference resource for physicians whose primary specialty is not dermatology. The authors and the publisher have made a valiant effort and I strongly believe that this book will be a very useful addition to the library of most physicians.

Joseph L Jorizzo
Professor and Chair
Wake Forest School of Medicine
2001

Preface

The range of clinical diagnoses that can be achieved in the skin far exceeds that for any other organ system. Clinical history and, often, additional investigations may be required to make or to refine a diagnosis, but examination of the skin is of paramount importance. Because the skin is readily visualised, and most physical signs do not need to be actively elicited, the diagnostic process appears easy. Consequently, the observation and recording of clinical features is often less systematic and analytical than for other organ systems. In fact, diagnosis is often based on assimilation of several different parameters which are observed simultaneously and whose individual features may not be consciously appreciated. Thus, subtle variations in colour, scaling, and shapes may lead to quite diverse diagnoses.

This text is primarily aimed to encourage the reader to be analytical in evaluating clinical features of dermatological conditions, to understand how these combine to lead to a diagnosis, and to convey some of the satisfaction that this understanding brings. It is not intended to be a comprehensive textbook, but most common conditions are included. Indeed, many are discussed several times when they exhibit a range of physical signs. Equally, many uncommon conditions are included when they illustrate particular diagnostic features. The signs-orientated approach may transgress traditional classifications of disorders in some respects, because physical signs are often not unique to any particular mechanism or pathogenesis. However, this format is the most helpful for conveying an understanding of the clinical features that lead to a diagnosis.

This second edition includes some signs that were not included previously. There are also many additional or substituted photographs, an expanded index, and extensive cross-referencing within and between chapters. Highlighted teaching points and pitfalls in diagnosis have been added. A larger page size and altered format have improved readability and allowed use of larger images with greater impact.

Our aim in this revised text is to enable the reader to appreciate the great range of physical signs in skin disease and promote the understanding of the diagnostic process that can be achieved by clinical observation and elicitation of physical signs. We hope that it also conveys some of the fascination of skin disease.

Clifford M Lawrence
Neil H Cox
2001

Acknowledgements

We especially wish to thank our families for their patience and support during preparation of this book; our grateful thanks to Anne, Tom, Jo, Chris and James Lawrence, and to Fi, David and Kathy Cox, for their encouragement throughout this project.

The majority of illustrations are our own but many individuals have either referred patients to us or have donated photographs to this or the first edition, including Stan Comaish, Noreen Cowley, Mike Dahl, Paul Dufton, Peter Farr, Andrew Finlay, Andrew Ilchysyn, Adrian Ive, Nick Levell, Lawrence Lever, Rona MacKie, Janet Marks, Neil Morley, Colin Munro, Raj Natarajan, Bill Paterson, Jonathan Rees, Dai Roberts, Sam Shuster, Tom Stewart, Chris Vickers, Gary White and Sandra Young. We have tried to document acknowledgements of donated photographs in the picture legends and apologise for any omissions. A few photographs are copyright of the University of Newcastle or of Durham Health Authority, and these are listed in the acknowledgements to the first edition.

Thanks also to all the team at Harcourt Health Sciences who have been involved with this project, especially Sue Hodgson, Tim Kimber and Scott Millar.

Clifford M Lawrence
Neil H Cox

1 Nomenclature: basic lesional morphology

INTRODUCTION

The teaching of undergraduate dermatology is generally brief, disease-oriented, and full of unfamiliar nomenclature. This structure is usually only helpful if an instant diagnosis can be made. When this is not possible the student must return to first principles, record a detailed history and compile an accurate description of the disorder. This chapter is an introduction to the terminology that is required to accurately describe the main types of skin lesion.

A few basic facts and principles about the different cells and tissues of the skin are required to understand the mechanism of the observed physical signs. These relate to the morphological and functional differences of the three main levels of the skin: the epidermis, dermis and subcutaneous fat (**Fig 1.1**).

EPIDERMIS

The epidermis is the outer cellular layer (approximately 0.1 mm thick) of the skin, which acts as a barrier between the body and its surroundings, preventing water loss and antigen and pathogen invasion. The epidermal cells (keratinocytes) differentiate to form a dead layer of scale (stratum corneum or horny layer) at the outer surface of the skin. Any disorder with altered scaling must therefore involve some epidermal pathology or changes in epidermal function. The epidermal thickness does not vary very much at different body sites but is thickest on the palms and soles owing to the increased thickness of the stratum corneum at these sites.

Pigment-producing melanocytes are situated within the basal layer of the epidermis; their pigment is transferred into keratinocytes and therefore extends into the outer part of the epidermis. The colour produced by melanin in the skin varies from reddish brown to blue–black, depending on the shape, clustering, number and depth of the pigment granules. Changes in the brown pigmentation of the skin are usually due to abnormalities of the

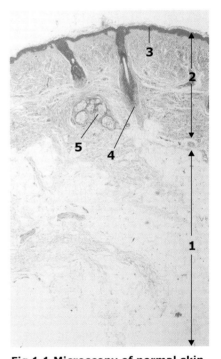

Fig 1.1 Microscopy of normal skin to show levels and structures: fat (1), dermis (2), epidermis (3), hair follicle (4), sebaceous gland (5)

basal layer melanocytes, although pigmentary change also occurs after inflammation, when pigment is lost from the epidermis and accumulates in the dermis. Dendritic Langerhans cells are also present in the epidermis. These make up part of the skin-associated lymphoid tissues (SALT) and act as the furthest outpost of the immune system.

DERMIS

The dermis is the fibrous part of the skin and principally contains collagen, which is produced by fibroblasts. Variations in skin thickness with body site (e.g. thick on the back and thin around the eyes) are due to differences in the thickness of the dermis. The junction between the dermis and epidermis is a complex structure called the basement membrane zone. Many blistering diseases are caused by abnormalities in the ultrastructure of this thin basement membrane zone. Specialised epidermal structures, such as hair follicles and sweat ducts, penetrate into the dermis and fat, but these deep hair bulbs, sebaceous glands and sweat glands are still lined by the basement membrane zone. The dermis carries the blood supply to the skin, and the haemoglobin in these vessels is the major chromophore or colour of the dermis. The epidermis, by contrast, is avascular. It follows, therefore, that abnormalities of blood vessels must be subepidermal and also that free blood in the skin must originate within the dermis or deeper tissues.

The absence of any direct epidermal blood supply means that nutrients and oxygen have to reach the epidermal cells by diffusion; similarly, inflammatory cells can only reach the epidermis from the blood vessels via the dermis, even if the site of an inflammatory stimulus is the epidermis. The dermis acts as a barrier against physical trauma and provides support for cutaneous blood vessels, nerves and lymphatics and the overlying epidermis. The fibrous or leathery nature of the dermis means that lesions in the subcutaneous fat may be difficult to see or feel through it.

SUBCUTANEOUS FAT

Fat forms an insulating layer and acts as a site for energy storage. Inflammation in the fatty layer (panniculitis) produces diffuse swelling deep within the skin.

FUNDAMENTALS OF DIAGNOSIS

Physical signs are a consequence of the normal or abnormal structure of the skin. Identifying a combination of physical signs leads to a differential diagnosis. An exact diagnosis may be achieved by combining these findings with the additional information obtained from the history and investigation; these aspects are, however, not the purpose of this book.

Accurate use of nomenclature enables the observed physical signs to be recorded succinctly. In practice, a full description of a lesion often requires combined use of some of these terms, for example 'crusted nodule' or 'telangiectatic plaque'. The remainder of this chapter outlines the terms used to describe the features of the main types of skin lesions.

Macules

The macule (**Fig 1.2**) is a discrete flat lesion. It is not palpably raised above adjacent normal skin but is distinguished by a change in colour. A large macule (diameter greater than 15–20 mm) can be called a 'patch,' but this term is also sometimes confusingly applied to thin plaques.

DIAGNOSTIC TIPS AND PITFALLS

● Surface scaling indicates the presence of epidermal involvement in the pathological process

DIAGNOSTIC TIPS AND PITFALLS

● Absent scaling indicates that the disease is entirely dermal or deeper in origin

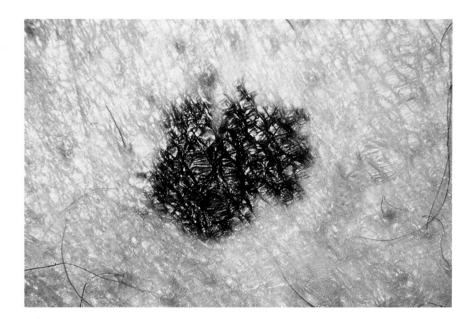

Fig 1.2 Lentigo. A typical example of a macule in which there is an increased number of melanocytes in the basal layer of the epidermis; colour is altered, but there is no scaling and no change in skin thickness. This dark lentigo with an irregular stellate shape is typical of lesions that develop in some patients having photochemotherapy

Most macules are darker red or brown compared with the normal skin. Diseases involving pigment loss often result in macular lesions. Fine scale associated with pigment loss is a useful physical sign because it indicates associated altered keratinocyte function as well as the colour change. Macules may be sharply demarcated from the normal skin or may have an indistinct border. Slightly depressed flat lesions should be termed atrophic macules. Thus, in describing a macular lesion, it is diagnostically useful to comment on the colour, shape and characteristics of the border, presence of scaling and presence of atrophy. Examples include:

Lentigo

Lentigos, flat tan-coloured epidermal macules, are due to a localised increase in number of basal epidermal melanocytes.

Purpura

A purpura is a good example of a dermal macule and is caused by extravasation of blood from capillary vessels without epidermal change.

Papules and nodules

Papules and nodules (**Fig 1.3**) are discrete lesions that are usually visibly raised above the skin surface and which mainly originate in the dermis. However, some nodules lie deep to the dermis (e.g. lipoma), therefore producing a less sharply defined raised area (*see* Fig 9.8). Others, even though they are situated in the dermis, can sometimes produce indentation of the skin rather than a raised lesion (e.g. dermatofibroma).

The term used depends arbitrarily on the size of the lesion, and there is no generally agreed definition. A papule is usually smaller than 5–10 mm in diameter. Lesions between 5 and 10 mm in diameter will be called large papules or small nodules, and those larger than 10 mm in diameter are usually referred to as nodules. The arbitrary size differential between papules and nodules and the change in size with time mean that it is best to document the actual size. Other useful characteristics to note include colour, morphology and surface changes (*see* Chapter 9).

DIAGNOSTIC TIPS AND PITFALLS

- Disorders producing a brown pigment change are likely to be related to the melanocytes of the basal epidermis

3

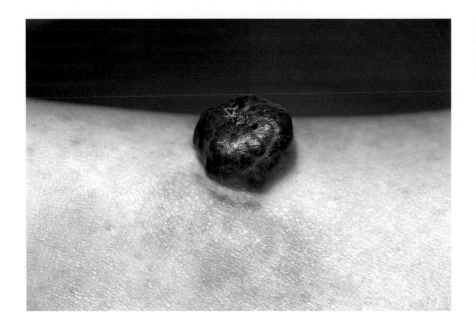

Fig 1.3 Nodular melanoma.
A nodular melanoma of this size is
unusual, but this shows a deeply
pigmented and ulcerated nodule

Examples of papules and nodules:

Benign compound naevus ('mole')

A compound naevus is a good example of a pigmented papule caused by a collection of melanocytes in the dermis and at the junction of the dermis and epidermis.

Nodular melanoma

A nodular melanoma is an aggressive type of malignant melanoma, which forms as malignant melanocytes both invade into the dermis and grow out above the skin surface (**Fig 1.1**).

Plaques

Plaques (**Fig 1.4**) are areas of raised or texturally altered skin with a flat top. Scaling is usually present. The diameter of a plaque is much greater than the degree of elevation above the skin. Examples include:

Psoriasis

Lesions of stable plaque psoriasis are a characteristic example of scaly plaques.

Morphoea

Areas of hardened or sclerotic morphoea are often called plaques. These lesions are not scaly, but there is a textural change. The flat, pigmented and atrophic or depressed lesions of resolved morphoea (*see* Fig 11.37) are by contrast best described as atrophic macules.

Weals

The weal (**Fig 1.5**) is a transient swelling of the skin due to dermal fluid. Patients often refer to weals as blisters, but the fluid content is dispersed within the dermal tissue and does not form a localised collection, so that the

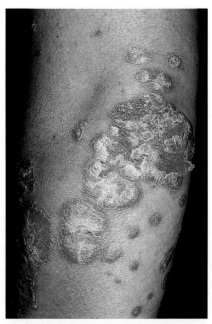

Fig 1.4 Psoriasis plaques. These show multiple discrete plaques becoming confluent. The individual lesions are palpably thickened

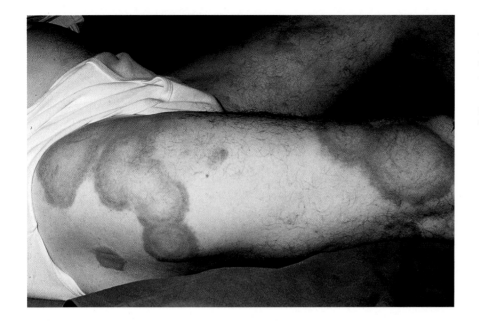

Fig 1.5 Weal. Weals may be of various shapes, but all are palpable, discrete collections of extravasated fluid. The centre of a weal is often white due to extreme skin oedema, but the early phase and the surrounding flare are red due to vasodilatation

lesion cannot burst and leak fluid. Weals can be of various sizes and shapes, and thus form papules, nodules or plaques.

A weal has the following specific features:

- An individual lesion lasts less than 24 hours. New lesions may come and go, but any one lesion will disappear after minutes or hours, leaving little or no visible residual abnormality.
- Severe attacks may leave residual purpura.
- The swelling is due to dermal fluid, and this produces a sharply defined border.
- There is no epidermal component, so there is no associated scale or surface change.
- The pink or red colour is due to vasodilation. However, if a lot of fluid accumulates quickly, the dermal vessels are compressed, and the weal often becomes white (i.e. as is seen after rapid intradermal injection of local anaesthetic).
- The surrounding flare or border of non-palpable, red colour is due to vasodilatation, e.g. urticaria.

If the same pathological process occurs deeper than the dermis, this results in a poorly defined, more diffuse swelling known as angio-oedema. Compared with typical urticarial weals, angio-oedema lasts several days, and there is no associated flare.

Examples of weals include:

Idiopathic urticaria

This reaction can occur for a variety of reasons, but usually, no cause is found. Patients develop multiple raised itchy red weals. The individual lesions only last for less than 24 hours, but new lesions occur at other sites, and the attack may last many days if not prevented by taking antihistamines (**Fig 1.5**).

Hereditary angio-oedema

Tissue inflammation occurs spontaneously and in an uncontrolled fashion with hereditary angio-oedema due to an inherited deficiency of C1 esterase inhibitor. Patients develop massive swelling at any body site after minor trauma. The swelling is disfiguring at any site but potentially life-threatening if it occurs near the airway.

DIAGNOSTIC TIPS AND PITFALLS

- Blood vessels in the dermis are more easily damaged, causing purpura, if the surrounding collagen is abnormal

DIAGNOSTIC TIPS AND PITFALLS

- Lesions in the fat layer may be difficult to see or feel through the fibrous dermis

Vesicles and bullae

Vesicles and bullae (**Figs 1.6** and **1.7**) are terms used to describe different sizes of blister. Blisters contain fluid, so that if the blister is pricked or breaks, the contents run out and the blister collapses. Blisters may form within or just below the epidermis depending on the disease process (*see* Fig 13.4).

In general, the term vesicle is used to describe a small (i.e. 5 mm diameter) blister and bulla a large blister (i.e. >5–10 mm in diameter). The precise cut-off point varies between authors, and it is more important to record the actual size. Bullae may form from a single expanding vesicle, from a large bulla at the outset or by coalescence of adjacent vesicles. Many blistering eruptions produce both large and small blisters—i.e. both bullae and vesicles. In practice, most dermatologists use the term vesicle to describe tiny blisters a few millimetres in diameter, and these generally occur as multiple lesions.

When describing blisters, it is often helpful to record the size range of the majority of lesions, e.g. 'tense blisters mainly 10–20 mm in diameter', and note whether blisters are unilocular, as in pemphigoid (**Fig 1.6**), or multilocular as in eczema (**Fig 1.7**).

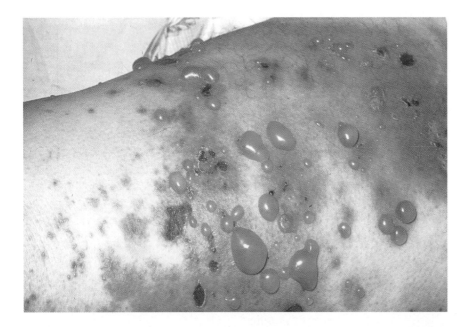

Fig 1.6 Pemphigoid. Classic unilocular blisters. Note that the blisters are tense, a sign that the level of split is subepidermal

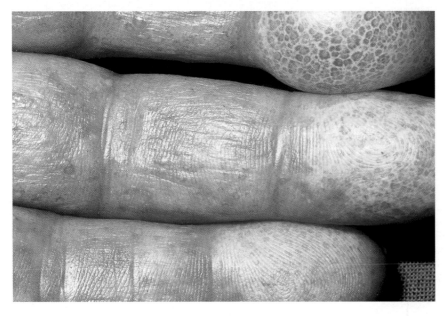

Fig 1.7 Eczema. A large blister formed by coalescence of many small intra-epidermal blisters (vesicles), with some epidermal structures being maintained and therefore forming multilocular blisters

Examples include:

Bullous pemphigoid

This immuno-bullous disease produces subepidermal blisters. Pemphigoid blisters usually contain tense clear fluid and are unilocular. Because the blister base sits on the underlying dermis, blood may occasionally leak into the blister, producing a blood-filled blister.

Acute eczema

In eczema, the blisters are usually small and hence called vesicles. They are characteristically multilocular because all the blisters are confined within the epidermis.

Pustules

Pustules (**Fig 1.8**) are an epidermal or upper dermal accumulation of pus, a breakdown product of polymorphonuclear leucocytes. They are clinically turbid and yellow or green in colour. Deeper collections of pus present as a palpable nodule called an abscess, but the pus content is not visible through the skin.

Some pustules form by infiltration of polymorphs from the outset, e.g. in acne, whereas others start as vesicles and gradually accumulate pus cells. Thus, there may be a stage between a clear vesicle and a turbid pustule during which the vesicle contains cloudy fluid and is known as a vesicopustule.

The most important morphological feature of a pustular eruption is whether the pustules do or do not arise from the pilosebaceous (i.e. hair) follicles. Examples include:

Pustular psoriasis

Pustules in this type of psoriasis form within the epidermis due to rapid and extensive migration of polymorphonuclear leucocytes into the epidermis. The pustules may be much closer together than occurs in disorders characterised by follicular pustules, and the pustules often merge together to produce lesions of various sizes.

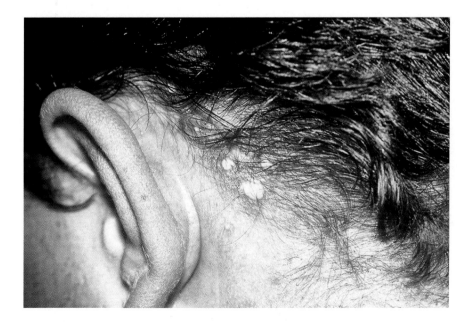

Fig 1.8 Pustule. These follicular pustules exhibits the typical yellow–green colour. The hair within the lesion identifies it as being of follicular origin

Acne

In acne, lesions are caused by inflammation around the sebaceous glands due to infection of the sebaceous gland secretion by a bacterium called *Propionibacterium acnes*. The pustules are therefore restricted to hair follicles.

Ulcers, erosions, excoriations and fissures

The terms ulcer, erosion, excoriation and fissure describe different morphologies of breaks in the integrity of the skin surface. Examples include:

Erosion: de-roofed bullous pemphigoid blister

When the roof of a blister is removed, the underlying dermis is exposed producing superficial surface loss involving the epidermis only.

Ulcer: venous leg ulcer

The full thickness skin loss of a varicose ulcer produces an ulcer that extends into the dermis (Fig 1.9).

Fissure: angular cheilitis

A fissure is a small, deep, but narrow ulcer with a slit or cleft shape; the split at the corner of the mouth produced by angular stomatitis is a good example (Fig 1.10).

Excoriation: atopic eczema or scabies

Excoriation is a common consequence of scratching an itchy rash such as caused by scabies or atopic eczema. Severe scratching may result in an erosion or an ulcer (*see* Chapter 12) and implies that the cause of the lesion is external, due to a scratch. Excoriations are usually multiple and are often oval or linear. Areas that the patient cannot reach (e.g. the mid-back) will be free from excoriation (*see* Fig 15.5).

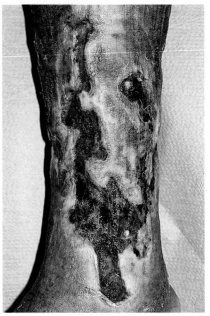

Fig 1.9 Leg ulcer. This large chronic leg ulcer is showing signs of healing, with islands and projections of epithelialised skin growing over the ulcer producing the odd geographical pattern

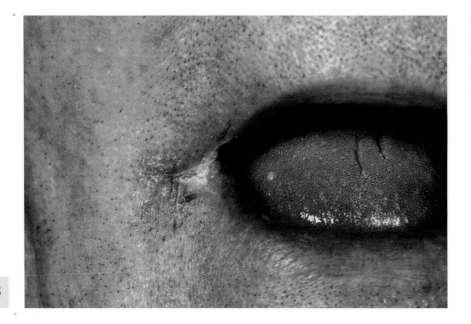

Fig 1.10 Angular cheilitis. A common example of fissures, this disorder is usually due to badly fitting dentures causing deep creases at the angles of the mouth, often with secondary yeast infection

Scale and crust

The terms scale and crust (**Figs 1.11–1.13**) are often confused, probably because they usually occur together. Scale is flaking of the skin surface due to increased loss from the stratum corneum. The presence of scaling implies an abnormality in stratum corneum formation or damage to the epidermis. This may be due to an increased rate of keratin production (e.g. psoriasis), qualitatively abnormal keratin (e.g. psoriasis and pityriasis rubra pilaris), damage to the epidermis (e.g. a fungal infection) or decreased rate of stratum corneum shedding (e.g. X-linked ichthyosis (**Fig 1.11**). Hyperkeratosis, in which there is a thickening of the stratum corneum, should be distinguished from scaling, e.g. keratoacanthoma (**Fig 1.12**).

Crust is a dried exudate of blood or serous fluid on the skin or lesion surface and is commonly known as a scab. Crusting and scaling occur together in lesions where there is exudation and increased and/or abnormal keratinisation, e.g. squamous cell carcinoma and Bowen's disease.

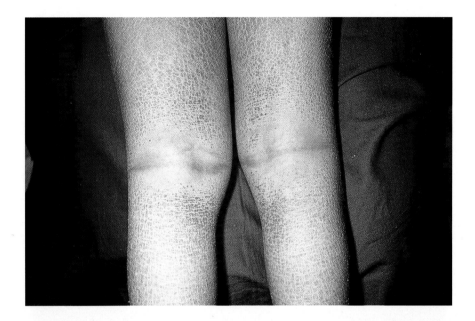

Fig 1.11 Ichthyosis. A good example of scaling, in this case due to an X-linked defect of steroid sulphatase. It gives rise to the typical pattern of large dirty brown scales and popliteal sparing

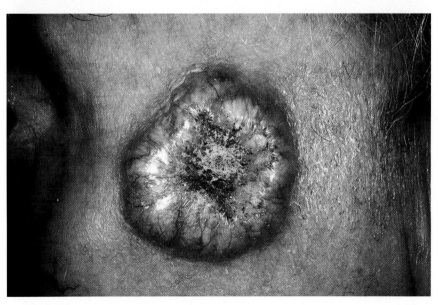

Fig 1.12 Kerato-acanthoma. This tumour is a classic example of hyperkeratosis. The mass of keratin is morphologically different from the thin sheets that form scale and is much harder than a crust

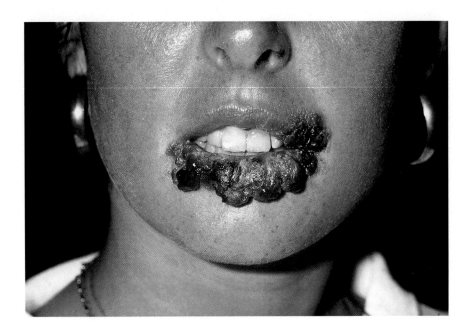

Fig 1.13 Impetigo. Dried serous exudate due to superficial staphylococcal infection causes formation of crusts

Examples of scale and crust include:

Psoriasis

Chronic plaque psoriasis produces abnormal and excess keratin. The keratin may build up on the top of the plaque but, unlike hyperkeratosis affecting otherwise normal skin (e.g. on a walker's heel), the thickened stratum corneum is poorly attached and forms large white flakes on the skin.

Impetigo

The crust that forms in impetigo (**Fig 1.13**) is caused by a serous exudate provoked by a bacterial infection of the skin. The water content of the exudate dries, leaving behind the crust.

Atrophy

Atrophy (**Fig 1.14**) is loss of skin substance, producing thinning. It may be epidermal, dermal or a combination of both. Pure dermal atrophy results from loss of collagen. Thus, there is a loss of substance producing a depressed surface and greater transparency of the skin. In some atrophic diseases, the body reacts by producing scar tissue. However, scaring and atrophy are not the same and should not be confused. An example of atrophy includes:

Dermal atrophy due to the application of topical corticosteroids

Regular use of potent topical steroids may produce damage and ultimately loss of the dermal collagen. The skin becomes thinner and transparent, and blood vessels easily burst when traumatised because they are not adequately supported by collagen.

Sclerosis

Sclerotic skin feels firm and indurated, and the change may be more palpable than visible. In some instances, such as scar tissue, the affected skin is white

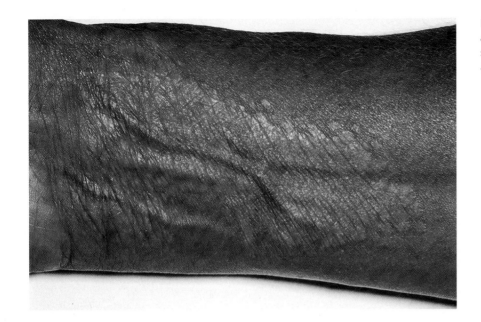

Fig 1.14 Lichen sclerosus et atrophicus. An example of atrophic skin, in which there is easy wrinkling and increased visibility of vessels

and shiny, with loss of skin surface ridges and markings. Sclerosis occurs as a result of an increase in the amount of dermal collagen (e.g. morphoea), expansion of the collagen by ground substance material (e.g. mucin) or altered quality of collagen (e.g. the increased cross-linking between individual collagen fibres, which occurs in insulin-dependent diabetes).

An example of sclerosis includes:

Morphoea

Morphoea causes inflammation of the dermis, which then becomes hardened. Because the skin loses some of its mobility, it appears to be thickened, whereas it is actually just tethered to the underlying structures.

Erythema, telangiectasia, purpura, petechiae and ecchymosis

The terms erythema, telangiectasia (**Fig 1.15**), purpura and petechiae all describe changes related to blood vessels and therefore all occur in the dermis. An ecchymosis or bruise is a deeper process, which may affect the dermis along with underlying tissues.

- Erythema is diffuse redness due to increased visibility of intravascular blood, resulting from vasodilatation and/or increased blood flow. The vessels involved are deep in the skin and of narrow bore, so the individual vessels are not visible.
- Telangiectasia refers to individually visible dilated vessels near the skin surface (**Fig 1.15**).
- Purpura is visible blood that has leaked out of blood vessels, usually into the dermis; if this occurs as tiny pinpoint spots, it is called petechiae; if there is a large area of extravasated blood in deeper tissues, e.g. fat and muscle, it is called an ecchymosis or bruise.

These changes, and how to distinguish between them, are discussed further in Chapter 17.

Poikiloderma

Poikiloderma (**Fig 1.16**) is the combination of atrophy, pigmentation (with a blotchy or reticulate pattern) and telangiectasia. This constellation of signs occurs in several rare disorders. An example includes:

Poikiloderma atrophicans vasculare

Poikiloderma atrophicaus vasculare is a type of pre-lymphomatous skin change that shows the characteristic features of atrophy, pigmentation and telangiectasia.

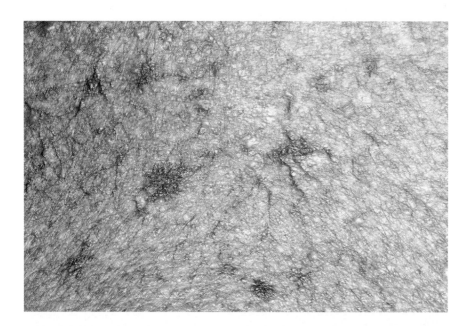

Fig 1.15 Telangiectasia. Small dilated superficial vessels form telangiectasia, in this case due to increased circulating corticosteroids in a patient with ectopic adrenocorticotrophic hormone secretion

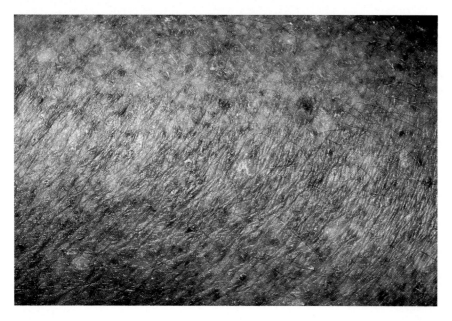

Fig 1.16 Poikiloderma vasculare atrophicans. This process, involving skin atrophy (indicated by the fine surface wrinkling), variable pigmentation and telangiectasia, is visible on the skin of this patient with poikiloderma vasculare atrophicans

2 Shapes and patterns of lesions

INTRODUCTION

The variety of shapes and patterns of lesions that the skin can produce is a demonstration of the complexity of this organ. Fascinating patterns develop when lesions follow the skin developmental lines, vascular supply, innervation or lymphatic drainage. Correct recording of the shape of lesions is important and may lead directly to the diagnosis or cause of a reaction pattern in the skin. This chapter illustrates the more important shapes and patterns of lesions and lists some of the disorders that may produce these different morphologies.

In all of these examples, it is important to consider the effect of time. An annular lesion for example may arise *de novo* (e.g. purpura annularis telangiectoides), be formed by gradual radial movement of an active edge (e.g. ringworm or urticaria), evolve by central clearing of a discoid lesion (e.g. some psoriasis) or be an apparent coalescence of small individual lesions (e.g. granuloma annulare).

13

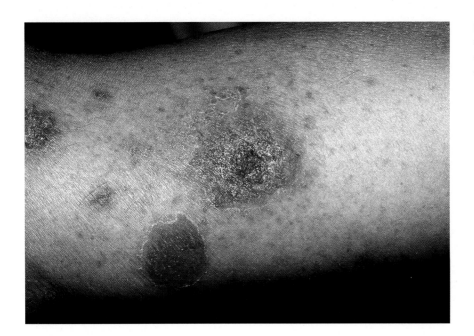

Fig 2.1 Discoid eczema. A discoid or nummular lesion is approximately circular, fairly sharply demarcated and uniform across its surface

MAIN SHAPES AND PATTERNS

Discoid or nummular

Discoid or nummular describes a filled circle or 'coin-shaped' lesion. Examples include discoid eczema (**Fig 2.1**) and psoriasis. It can be useful to further qualify the shape, for example, larger lesions of Bowen's disease often have a rather irregular or 'geographical' outline rather than being a neat disc shape, and lesions of discoid eczema are generally not quite as 'neat' or well defined at the periphery as those of psoriasis.

Figurate

The rather vague term of figurate implies a degree of patterning (as in 'figurate erythemas') that does not quite amount to the shape of a ring (annular), arc (arcuate) or interlocking circle (polycyclic). Because of its vagueness, it is not a very useful descriptive term.

Annular

Annular describes a ring or empty circle shape. This is a fairly common pattern that occurs in several inflammatory dermatoses (**Figs 2.2–2.4** and **Table 2.1**). It is diagnostically important to qualify the description of annular lesions, particularly with regard to scaling and evolution. For example, urticaria causes lesions that are non-scaling and come and go from day to day, erythema annulare centrifugum lesions often have a 'trailing edge' of scaling and may vary over several weeks, and ringworm lesions are diffusely scaly with marginal accentuation and slow radial expansion.

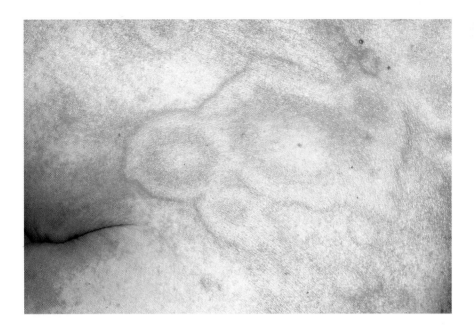

Fig 2.2 Urticaria. Lesions of urticaria are often circular or annular. Note that annular is not the same as a target (*see* 2.5); because of this, urticaria and erythema multiforme are often confused by non-dermatologists

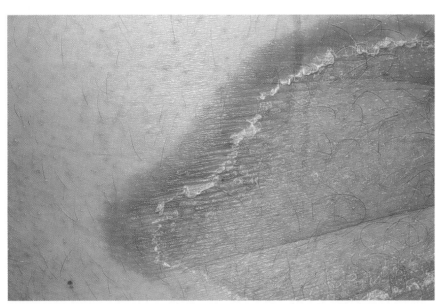

Fig 2.3 Erythema annulare centrifugum. Lesions in this disorder slowly migrate and often have some marginal scale (described as a 'trailing edge'). The speed and pattern of evolution and the presence or absence of scaling are both diagnostically useful when describing annular lesions

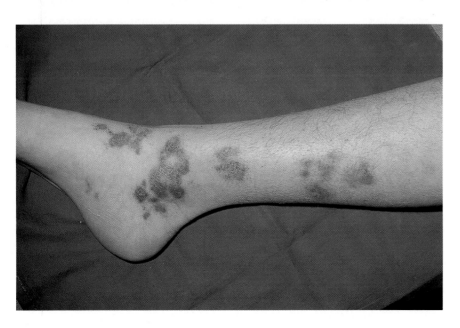

Fig 2.4 Purpura annularis telangiectoides. A benign eruption, that may be confused with vasculitis. Fixed annular lesions are typical

Table 2.1 Examples of annular lesions

Typically annular	Often include annular component
With scale	
Ringworm (15.19)	Psoriasis (2.7)
Pigmented purpuric dermatoses	Seborrhoeic eczema (2.9)
Erythema annulare centrifugum (2.3)	Pityriasis rosea (herald patch)
	Impetigo
	Subacute cutaneous lupus erythematosus (2.8)
	Mycosis fungoides
Without scale	
Granuloma annulare (11.29)	Urticaria (2.2)
Jessners lymphocytic infiltrate	Erythema multiforme (2.5)
'Annular erythemas'	Lichen planus
Erythema annularis telangiectoides (2.4)	Sarcoidosis
Serum sickness	

Target

Target refers to an arrangement of concentric rings (also known as iris or bull's eye lesions). This is a frequently misinterpreted sign, because target lesions are often thought to be synonymous with erythema multiforme. In fact, targets can occur in vasculitic disorders and sometimes in conditions such as lupus erythematosus or urticaria; conversely, histologically typical erythema multiforme can often produce lesions that are not typical target lesions. The most typical target lesions of erythema multiforme are often those on the palms (**Fig 2.5**), occurring as a reaction to herpes simplex virus infection. A similar term is cockade, or 'en cocarde,' which means like a rosette. In practice, target is used in the description of rashes whereas en cocarde is applied to an unusual, but static, variant of a benign pigmented naevus (*see* Fig 9.28).

DIAGNOSTIC TIPS AND PITFALLS

- The terms annular and target are often confused—a target lesion consists of multiple concentric circles, not a single ring

- The pattern and speed of evolution of annular lesions and the presence or absence of scaling are important diagnostic features

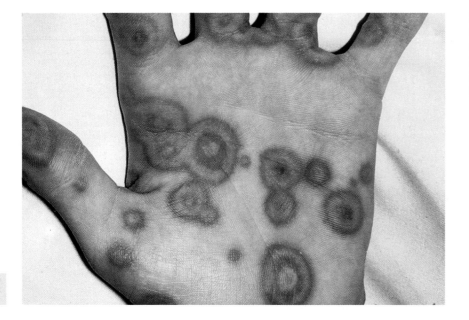

Fig 2.5 Erythema multiforme. True target lesions are typical of erythema multiforme; classic targets (as shown here) are most common in erythema multiforme triggered by herpes simplex infection

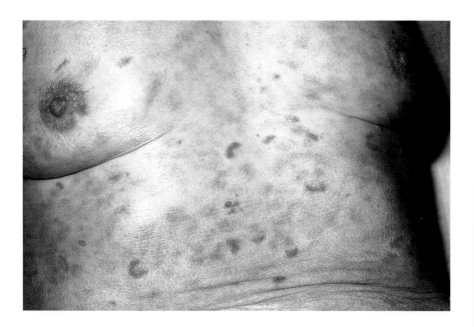

Fig 2.6 Lupus erythematosus. This disorder can cause lesions that have an urticarial appearance, often forming arcuate lesions

Arcuate and circinate

Arcuate refers to curved lesions with the appearance of a part, or arc, of a circle. Examples include lupus erythematosus (**Fig 2.6**) and urticaria.

Another related term is circinate, which means circular. It could therefore be applied to annular lesions, but in practice is often used to describe lesions with the appearance of incomplete circles, e.g. penile lesions of Reiter's syndrome (*see* Fig 5.32) and many urticarial lesions.

Polycyclic

Polycyclic describes interlocking or coalesced, unfilled circles. Such eruptions are usually formed by enlargement of annular lesions that meet, coalesce and enlarge further as a single lesion, e.g. psoriasis (**Fig 2.7**) or dermatophyte infection (ringworm). The active rim of a circle does not usually spread into a previously clear centre of an adjacent circle, although rings do occasionally appear to cross over into each other, e.g. in subacute cutaneous lupus erythematosus (**Fig 2.8**).

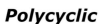

Fig 2.7 Psoriasis. Individual plaques of psoriasis often expand outwards, with central clearing; when several lesions merge, the centres remain resistant to involvement, and the series of fused peripheral parts of the rings form this polycyclic appearance

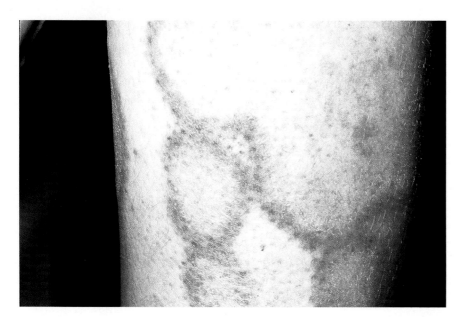

Fig 2.8 Lupus erythematosus (subacute cutaneous type). In rare cases, expanding rings appear to interlock (as shown here) rather than having the central resistance to involvement shown in 2.7

Gyrate

Strictly, gyrate means spiralled, coiled or winding in shape. Dermatologists use it to describe circles within a circle, rather like a wood-grain pattern. The rash classically associated with this pattern of involvement is erythema gyratum repens, a distinctive skin disease associated with systemic malignancy.

Petaloid

The term petaloid is similar to polycyclic, but refers to interlocking filled circles rather than the fusion of ring-shaped lesions. The typical example is the rather flower-shaped lesions that may occur on the chest or back in seborrhoeic dermatitis (**Fig 2.9**).

Whorled

A whorled pattern describes roughly concentric parts of circles or spirals, with a whirled or stirred appearance. Lesions with this distribution are often naevoid and follow a developmental pattern defined by the lines of Blaschko (**Fig 2.10**); it is not uncommon to see the combination of whorled areas on the trunk, streaky linear areas on the limbs (**Fig 2.11**) and an approximately midline cut-off point between affected and unaffected sides. In fact, lesions with this pattern may show some tendency to cross the midline, especially on the back. A typical example is an epidermal naevus.

Stellate

Stellate means star-shaped and is a relatively uncommon pattern. Most skin lesions develop radial spread in a more or less uniform fashion. Examples

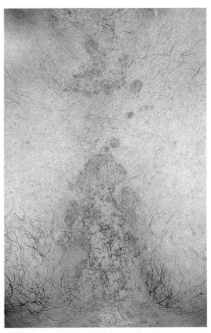

Fig 2.9 Seborrhoeic eczema. Fused discoid lesions form a petaloid pattern equivalent to the polycyclic pattern formed by fused annular lesions.

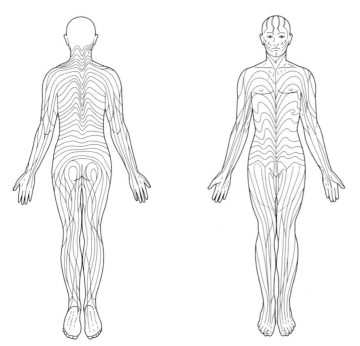

Fig 2.10 Blaschko's lines. Many congenital naevoid skin conditions have this pattern, which is whorled on the trunk (*see also* 4. 19) but linear or streaky on the limbs

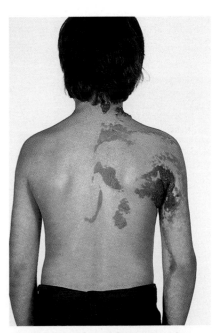

Fig 2.11 Epidermal naevus. An example of a naevoid condition that follows Blaschko's lines

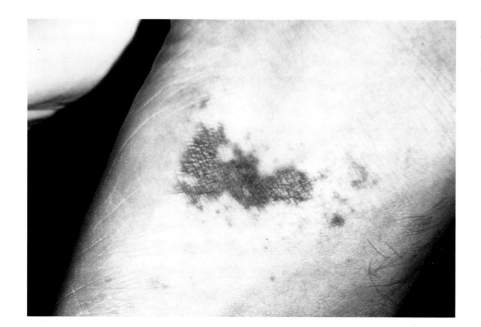

Fig 2.12 Meningococcal infection. The skin lesions of meningococcal septicaemia are typically irregular in outline, often with a stellate shape

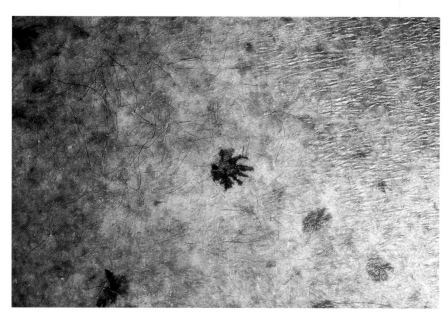

Fig 2.13 PUVA lentigines. The melanocytic proliferation, which can occur in patients exposed to PUVA therapy, e.g. for psoriasis, often has a stellate pattern

Fig 2.14 Digitate dermatosis. This disorder is one of many variants of a group of disorders known as parapsoriasis. This clinical pattern is so characteristic that the digitate (digit-like) morphology is now used to name the condition

include the vascular lesions of meningococcaemia (**Fig 2.12**), and psoralen ultraviolet A (PUVA) lentigines (**Fig 2.13**), which occur in patients having photochemotherapy.

Oval and digitate

Oval lesions are often seen in the skin. They may arise in conjunction with discoid lesions in many exanthematous rashes. They are especially common on the trunk, where they tend to be uniformly aligned with long axes following dermatomal lines, so that they are oriented downwards and laterally from the midline of the back. When many lesions are present, a fir-tree pattern is produced, typically seen in pityriasis rosea (*see* Fig 7.21).

Digitate lesions are more extreme elongated ovals, long and thin or finger shaped. Lesions with this shape typically occur in the disorder digitate dermatosis (**Fig 2.14**), which is one of the patterns of 'chronic superficial dermatitis' or 'parapsoriasis.'

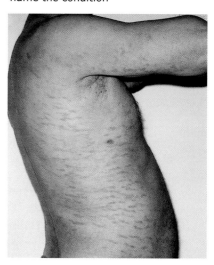

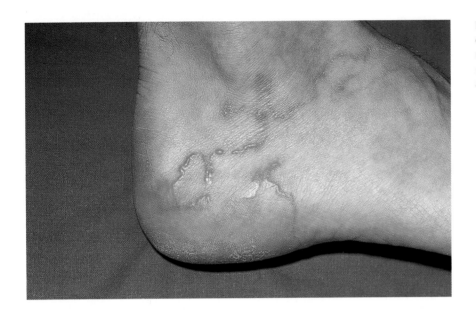

Fig 2.15 Larva migrans. The larvae of the hookworm create a bizarre but readily recognisable serpiginous (snake-like) pattern in the skin; they are acquired on tropical beaches

Serpiginous, rippled and gyrate

The term serpiginous describes a wavy, angulated or 'snake-like' line. The track left by the various forms of larva migrans (**Fig 2.15**) is a good example. The burrows of the scabies mite (*see* Figs 15.12 and 15.13) are a more common, although shorter, version of the same pattern and may be more linear than angulated.

Rashes that consist of several essentially parallel wavy lines may be described as rippled or gyrate. In practice, the term gyrate is used for a very rare paraneoplastic rash in which the pattern is likened to the grain of wood (known as erythema gyratum repens). Eruptions that have a rippled appearance (similar to a beach after the tide has receded) include macular amyloid (*see* Fig 3.16) and atopic dirty neck (*see* Fig 3.15).

Linear

Many lesions occur in lines and are termed linear. Examples are listed in **Table 2.2** according to the mechanism. Some of these have particular diagnostic significance and are described below.

Koebner's phenomenon

Koebner's phenomenon occurs in a variety of dermatoses and describes the apparent triggering effect of trauma in initiating new lesions. The trauma can range from a small scratch or burn to a surgical scar. This tendency is found in a variety of disorders and is most noticeable during the actively increasing phases of the causative disorder. There is typically a 7–10 day interval between the trauma and visible skin lesions developing, e.g. in lichen nitidus (**Fig 2.16**). Some authors include viral warts in the list of disorders that can show Koebener's phenomenon, but we prefer to think of a viral wart as a direct inoculation of the infective agent into damaged skin. It occurs when there are pre-existing warts locally, and there may have been an obvious scratch, damage from shaving or penetrating injury. However, injuries such as solar or thermal burns, which may elicit Koebner's phenomenon in disorders such as psoriasis (**Fig 2.17**), do not cause spread of warts. Keloid scars are also probably best considered as a different mechanism, as they are not associated with rash at other sites. Some disorders, such as sarcoidosis, have a tendency to affect pre-existing scars, but this is not the same as Koebner's phenomenon as the affected scars may be old (**Fig 2.18**).

Table 2.2 Examples of linear lesions

Determinant of pattern	Examples
Blood vessels	Thrombophlebitis, Mondor's disease (linear thrombophlebitis on the trunk) Eczema related to varicose veins Temporal arteritis
Lymphatics	Lymphangitis (2.19) Sporotrichosis, fish tank granulomas (2.20)
Dermatome	Herpes zoster (2.21), zosteriform naevus, zosteriform Darier's disease, zosteriform metastases
Nerve trunks	Leprosy (thickened cutaneous nerves)
Developmental and Blaschko's lines	Pigmentary demarcation line (6.32), linea nigra Epidermal naevi (2.11) Incontinentia pigmenti (3.29, 3.30), hypomelanosis of Ito (3.28) Linear psoriasis, linear lichen planus, lichen striatus
Skin stretching	Striae due to growth spurt (on lower back) (6.35)
Infestation	Scabies (15.12), larva migrans (2.15)

External injury
   Plants
   Allergens
   Chemical
   Thermal
   Physical
	Phytophotodermatitis (13.3)
	 Elastoplast, nail varnish (neck) (15.40), necklace, waistbands, etc.
	 Caustics, e.g. phenol
	 Burns
	 To normal skin
	 Keloid scar, bruising, dermatitis artefacta (15.47), amniotic constriction bands
	 To abnormal skin
	 Purpura (cryoglobulinaemia, amyloid (17.24), vasculitis (2.39))
	 Blisters (epidermolysis bullosa, porphyrias)
	 Inoculation
	 Warts, molluscum contagiosum
	 Koebner's phenomenon
	 Psoriasis, lichen planus (8.22), lichen nitidus (2.16), vitiligo
	 Other
	 Scar sarcoid (2.18)

Other determinants	Linear scleroderma (limb, central forehead) (11.37) Senear–Caro ridge (on hands in psoriasis) (7.47) Dermatomyositis (dorsum fingers) (17.9)

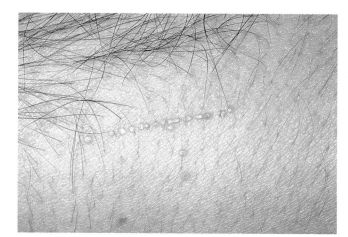

Fig 2.16 Lichen nitidus. This is one of a variety of disorders where lesions can be triggered in sites of minor injury (Koebner's phenomenon), causing linear lesions made up of a row of small confluent papules

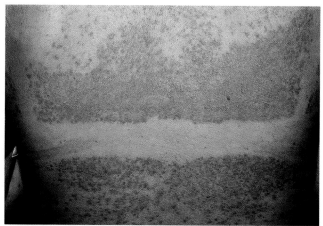

Fig 2.17 Psoriasis koebnerised into an area of sunburn. This young woman developed psoriasis localised to an area where she had been sun-burnt on her back. The skin protected by her bikini was not affected

21

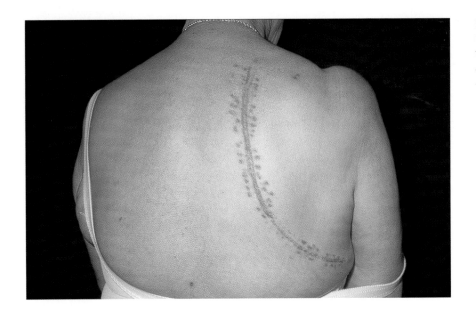

Fig 2.18 Scar sarcoid. The mechanism of this process is different to that of the Koebner phenomenon, as sarcoidosis may affect scars that are many years old

Lymphatics

Bacterial infections can produce red lines because of inflammation around lymphatic vessels that run between the lesion and the local draining lymph nodes (**Fig 2.19**). Infection within lymphatics may also cause a series of nodules at discrete intervals along lymphatics, occurring because of linear spread of infection, even though there is no clinically apparent line connecting the nodules. This pattern is known as sporotrichoid spread because it is typically seen in sporotrichosis, but in the UK, it is much more commonly due to atypical mycobacteria from infected tropical fish tanks (**Fig 2.20**).

Dermatomal

Although having a linear pattern on the trunk and limbs, lesions that have a nerve dermatome distribution on the face, neck or sacrum are not linear, and it is more exact to term the distribution dermatomal. The classic example is the eruption of herpes zoster (**Fig 2.21**), although the visible lesions may

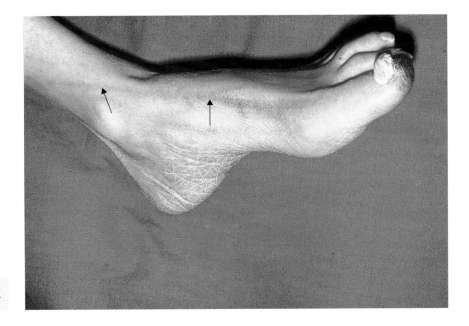

Fig 2.19 Lymphangitis. Spreading infection from a gangrenous toe in a diabetic patient has followed the path of the lymphatic system, producing linear lesions (arrowed)

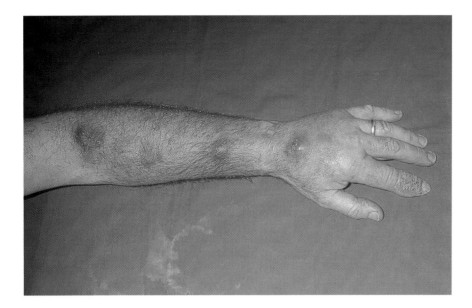

Fig 2.20 Mycobacterial infection (fish tank granulomas). This is a less obvious example of linearity. The spread of infection causes localised swellings along the line of lymphatic vessels from the portal of entry in the finger (a pattern known as sporotrichoid spread, after the infection in which it is commonly recognised)

affect just small parts of the skin within the affected dermatome. This distribution is so typical of herpes zoster that other disorders with the same distribution may be termed zosteriform (e.g. zosteriform naevus, zosteriform Darier's disease, zosteriform metastases).

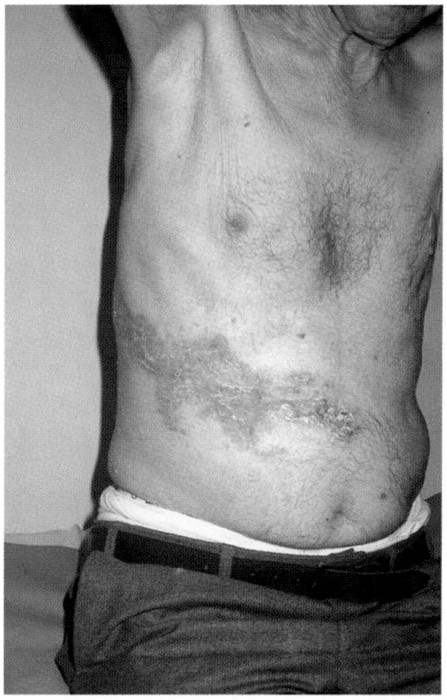

Reticulate, livedo and cribriform

Reticulate, livedo and cribriform describe three types of net-like patterning that are usually seen in rashes, patterning of erythema and scarring, respectively.

Reticulate (retiform) describes a lace-like appearance, which may be used to describe the overall appearance of an eruption or close-up features of individual lesions. Wickham's striae in lichen planus, which are most easily seen on the buccal mucosa, are a good example of this pattern (**Fig 2.22**). Rashes that may have a reticulate pattern include those caused by Rothmund–Thomsen syndrome, dyskeratosis congenita and confluent and reticulated papillomatosis of Gougerot–Carteaud (*see* Fig 3.7).

Fig 2.21 Herpes zoster. The prototype zosteriform lesion following the pattern of the skin dermatomes

Fig 2.22 Oral lichen planus. A classic example of a reticulate pattern

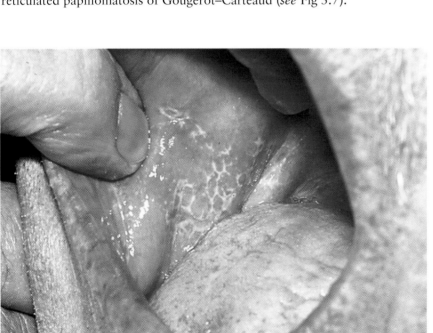

Livedo is a type of reticulate eruption that follows the vascular supply to the skin (*see* Fig 6.22) and shows a characteristic spacing of lesions due to the underlying vascular supply. The eruption follows the lines of the low flow 'watershed' areas between the higher flow deep arteriolar blood supply. Examples include polyarteritis nodosa and erythema ab igne (**Fig 2.23** and *see also* Table 17.6).

Cribriform is used to describe a similar pattern, although the appearance is more like that of a colander than of a net. The term is generally limited to description of a characteristic pattern of strand-like scarring seen in pyoderma gangrenosum (**Fig 2.24**).

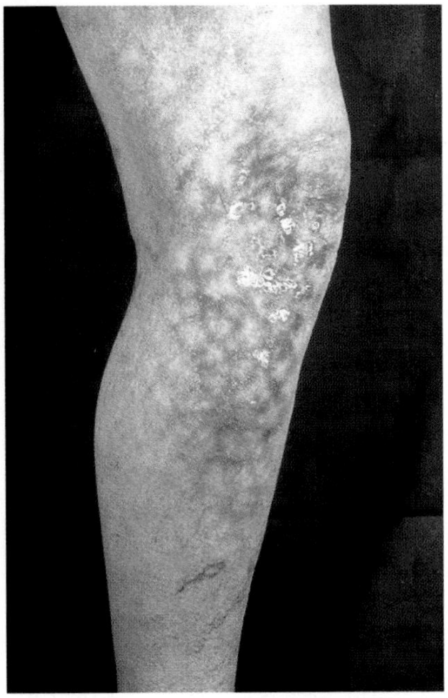

ARRANGEMENTS OF MULTIPLE LESIONS

Terms that have a useful descriptive purpose include grouped, satellite, disseminated, scattered, exanthematous, morbilliform, scarlatiniform and confluent.

Grouped

Where multiple discrete lesions occur in localised areas, they are described as grouped lesions. There are a variety of causes of this arrangement (**Table 2.3**). Reactions to insect bites (**Fig 2.25**) are a typical cause. An area of closely grouped vesicular or small ulcerated lesions may be termed herpetiform, after the typical pattern of herpes simplex virus infection (**Fig 2.26**).

A particularly close grouping of nodules is known as agminated ('grouped together'), e.g. agminate Spitz naevus (**Fig 2.27**).

Satellite

Satellite also describes grouped lesions, but with the implication that there is an initial, generally larger, lesion with adjacent lesions that have spread from this. Such an appearance can occur in some angiomas, but the most common

Fig 2.23 Livedo in erythema ab igne. The whole of a rash may have a reticulate pattern, rather than just the individual lesions of an eruption as shown in 2.22 (*see also* 6.23)

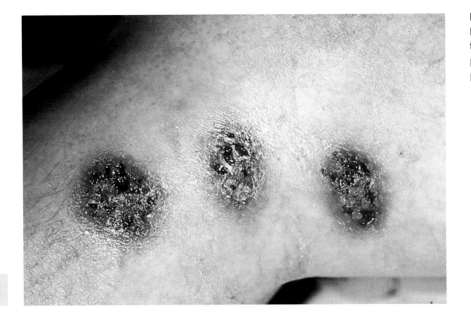

Fig 2.24 Pyoderma gangrenosum. Lesions of this ulcerative disorder typically heal with a cribriform pattern, in which small holes perforate the scar

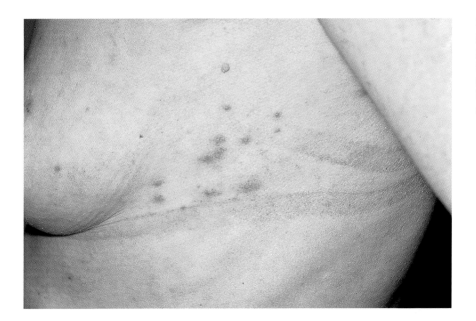

Fig 2.25 Insect bites. Fleas that get trapped under clothing may produce bites that are limited by tight areas. This woman allowed her dog to sit on her knee, and grouped flea bites were confined within the tight areas of her bra

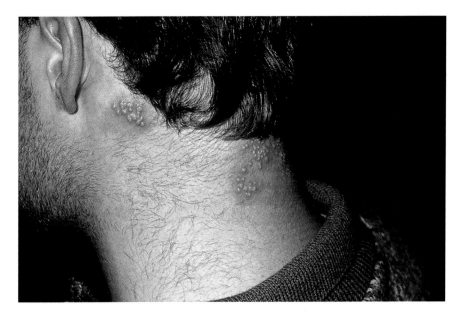

Fig 2.26 Herpes simplex. The prototype of herpetiform lesions. Closely grouped, small vesicopustules on the neck of a rugby player (a variant known as scrumpox). *See also* 14.12

Fig 2.27 Spitz naevus. Usually solitary lesions, these benign childhood naevi can be multiple, with either a disseminated pattern or the grouped agminate pattern shown here (*see also* 4.4 and 4.5)

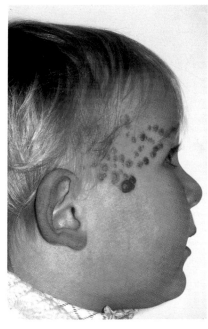

Table 2.3 Examples of grouped lesions

Mechanism	Examples
Infective	Wart (7.54), molluscum contagiosum, impetigo (7.4), herpes viruses (2.26), cowpox
External	Insect bites, including papular urticaria (2.25) Lichenification (lichen simplex)
Vascular/lymphatic	Lymphangioma circumscriptum (9.70) Metastatic carcinoma
Naevoid	Localised neurofibromas, naevus spilus (9.27) Unilateral naevoid telangiectasia
Neoplastic	Leiomyoma Syringomata (eyelids) (9.61)
Inflammatory dermatoses	Lichen planus (8.22), dermatitis herpetiformis (15.3), linear IgA disease/chronic bullous disease of childhood, bullous

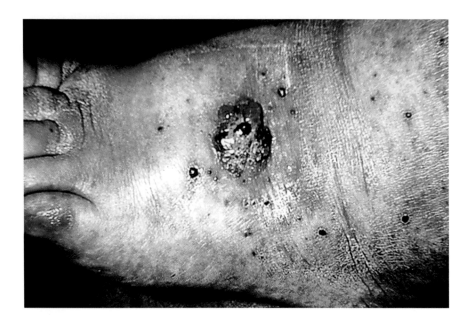

Fig 2.28 Satellite lesions. Small lesions arising around a larger central lesion, in this case due to local cutaneous metastases from a neglected primary malignant melanoma

lesions with this pattern are those in which there is local spread of a malignant tumour (**Fig 2.28**). In chronic bullous disease of childhood, blisters may occur in rings (annular) or groups (likened to a cluster of jewels) but sometimes surround a larger central blister and therefore suggest a satellite pattern.

Scattered and disseminated

Scattered and disseminated are terms used to describe multiple lesions at various parts of the skin but without any of the other specific distribution patterns. Disseminated is best used for multiple small, uniformly distributed lesions. Scattered is a better term for widespread discrete lesions with a less uniform pattern. These can be further qualified as localised, regional or generalised. Sometimes, additional features that help in differential diagnosis can be recognised—for example, small infected lesions centred around hair follicles might be described as 'scattered follicular pustules on the legs.' Accurate combinations of these descriptive terms narrows the list of differential diagnoses.

Exanthematous

Exanthematous is a term used to describe multiple red and/or scaly lesions, which are generally predominant on the trunk and which often have some degree of patterning similar to the fir-tree pattern of pityriasis rosea (*see* Fig 7.21) although not as distinct. Infections and drug eruptions are the usual causes. Where possible, it can be helpful to be more specific and describe exanthematous reactions in terms of their resemblance to the classic appearance of either measles (*see* Fig 10.4) (i.e. morbilliform—blotchy pinkish brown lesions) or scarlet fever (i.e. scarlatiniform—tiny red papules or petechiae).

Confluent

Confluence refers to lesions of any type and severity when they merge to cover a wider area. Examples include confluent scaly macules of pityriasis versicolor, a superficial yeast infection, or confluent plaques of psoriasis.

Table 2.4 Some causes of erythroderma

Cause	Approximate frequency
Eczema (atopic, contact allergies, seborrhoeic)	40%
Psoriasis	30%
Drug eruptions (sulphonamides, anticonvulsants, allopurinol, penicillins)	15%
Cutaneous lymphomas, Sézary syndrome	10%
Others, e.g. pityriasis rubra pilaris, some forms of ichthyosis, infestations, dermatophytosis, pemphigoid	5%

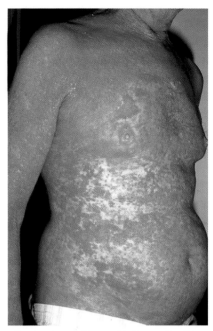

Fig 2.29 Confluent lesions. In this case due to adverse reaction to a thiazide diuretic. This patient subsequently developed total erythroderma related to a different diuretic

Erythroderma is a term used when there is total or virtually total redness of the skin surface. It implies confluence of lesions over a wide part of the skin (**Fig 2.29**) and is not the same as multiple large plaques of erythema. Causes of erythroderma are listed in **Table 2.4**.

OTHER USEFUL PATTERNS

Symmetry and asymmetry

A noticeable degree of symmetry or asymmetry of a rash can be a helpful clue to the aetiology. Most endogenous or systemic disorders produce a more or less symmetrical rash, whereas an asymmetrical rash suggests the possibility of an exogenous cause, such as a skin infection. Classic examples of a symmetrical eruption include psoriasis, atopic dermatitis, viral exanthemata and vitiligo.

There are, however, many exceptions to this concept. Distribution of a contact dermatitis is determined mainly by the distribution of exposure. For example, hand dermatitis due to the irritant effect of exogenous detergents is usually symmetrical in people who have both hands in water; however, it is often asymmetrical in hairdressers because the dominant hand holds scissors and is relatively dry, whereas wet hair is held between the fingers of the non-dominant hand. Conversely, systemic reactions to ingested drugs may produce strikingly symmetrical cutaneous signs, but a fixed drug eruption (*see* Figs 3.10 and 3.11) that recurs at the same place every time the causative drug is ingested is usually asymmetrical.

Photosensitive

An acute photosensitivity pattern is initially confined to light-exposed areas (**Figs 2.30** and **2.31**), generally the face, nape and V of the neck and dorsum of the hands and arms. Classically, there is sparing of skin creases and naturally shaded sites, such as below the eyebrows, behind the ears and under the chin. Sparing may also occur under jewellery, e.g. watchstraps. The natural position of the hands, except during deliberate sunbathing, is for the thumb to be uppermost and the fingers to be slightly flexed, so photosensitive rashes are relatively less prominent on the ulnar border of the hand and distally on the fingers. Some causes are listed in **Table 2.5**. The pattern of a photosensitivity eruption may be indistinguishable from a reaction to an airborne contact allergen, especially once the eruption is established, as the regions of sparing tend to be lost. However, involvement of the typically light-shielded areas in the acute stage of an eruption is suggestive of contact allergy rather than photosensitivity; in some cases, airborne agents may become ingrained in skin creases, and the exposed areas between the creases are relatively spared (*see* Fig 2.41).

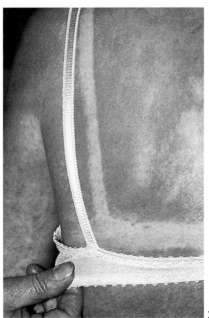

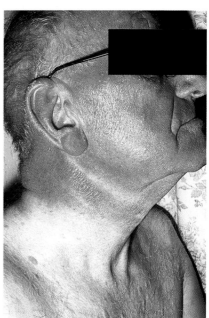

Fig 2.30, 2.31 Drug-induced photosensitivity. Clothing shields the skin from sunlight (2.30). In this case, sunlight readily passed through a thin blouse but not the thicker bra strap in a patient who was photosensitive to a thiazide diuretic. 2.31 shows classic sparing of naturally shielded areas, especially the skin creases and covered areas of skin, in a man with acute photosensitivity due to an oral hypoglycaemic drug

2.30   2.31

Table 2.5 Causes of rash with photosensitive distribution

Cause	Examples
Idiopathic	Photosensitive eczema/actinic reticuloid, solar urticaria, polymorphic light eruption, photo-aggravated rashes (lupus erythematosus, dermatomyositis) (17.8, 17.9)
Genodermatoses	Xeroderma pigmentosum, congenital poikilodermas (17.7)
Metabolic	Pellagra, porphyria cutanea tarda (13.39)
Drugs	Systemic: thiazides, nalidixic acid, sulphonamides, non-steroidal anti-inflammatory drugs, sulphonylureas, tetracyclines, phenothiazines, quinine
	External: tar, perfumes, furocoumarins (plants)
Other	Sunburn (may be prominent in patients with decreased melanin, e.g. those with vitiligo)

Fig 2.32 Venous eczema. The typical lower leg involvement and marked pigmentation around a long-standing leg ulcer

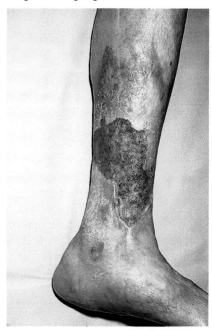

Photosensitivity can occur through thin clothing (**Fig 2.30**) and gradually loses the sharp borders and areas of sparing. Some topical applications, such as perfumes or tanning agents, may cause photosensitivity, and in these cases the pattern of eruption depends both an the areas of application and on sun exposure.

Gravitational

Some patterns of rash suggest that the major aetiological component is venous pathology, e.g. 'stasis' eczema (**Fig 2.32**). However, the appearance of many other eruptions may be influenced by a gravitational component that alters the features. For example, it is common to show purpura in eczema or exanthemata of the lower leg (*see* Fig 10.7), even when capillary leakage is not a visible part of the same process occurring at other body areas in the same patient. Most vasculitic disorders produce their most obvious effects in the lower legs (*see also* Chapter 17). Dermatitis related to varicose veins typically affects the lower leg over the medial perforating veins or, in more severely affected patients, in a circumferential pattern. However, lines of dermatitis following the line of a lower leg varicose vein may also be seen.

UNUSUAL SHAPES

Patterns due to exogenous agents and effects of clothing

Linear, angulated or geometrical shapes

It is worth carefully considering external causes if lesions are linear, square, perfect circles or oddly shaped, especially if there is an erosive or ulcerated component. These are generally caused by some external factor, and, in the absence of co-existing skin disease, when the patient does not offer a plausible explanation, deliberate injury should be suspected. Causes include:

- Accidental physical damage to normal skin, e.g. thermal burn (**Fig 2.33**).
- Accidental damage to abnormally fragile skin, e.g. in bullous disorders or amyloidosis (*see* Fig 17.24).
- Deliberate self-induced lesions (dermatitis artefacta) (*see* Figs 15.46 and 15.47).
- Non-accidental injury (**Fig 2.34**). Note, however, that several dermatological disorders may be confused with battering and sexual abuse (**Figs 2.35** and **2.36** and **Table 2.6**).
- Idiosyncratic damage such as reactions to adhesive dressing plasters (**Fig 2.37**).
- Unusual patterns of reaction to external agents (**Figs 2.38** and **2.41**).

Scars and trauma

Trauma, usually in the form of minor scratches, has been discussed as a cause of Koebner's phenomenon. However, established scars can also give rise to skin lesions in the following instances:

- Sarcoidosis, which often affects previous scars (*see* Fig 2.18)
- Pigmentation of scars, which may occur in a variety of disorders, especially Nelson's syndrome (pigmentation due to increased adrenocorticotrophic hormone concentrations after adrenalectomy for treatment of Cushing's syndrome).
- Disorders, such as morphoea, which have been reported to localise to previous radiotherapy areas.

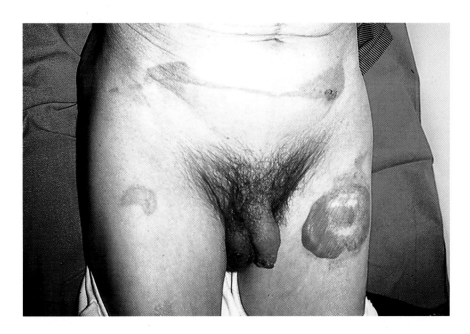

Fig 2.33 Thermal burn. Unusual shapes of lesions suggest external causes

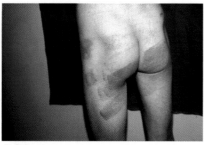

2.34

Fig 2.34–2.36 Child abuse and differential diagnosis. Strap marks (2.34). Note the uniformity of the bands of erythema, the distribution affecting the buttocks and the sparing of the natal cleft (*photo courtesy of Dr WD Paterson*). A linear epidermal naevus is shown in 2.35. This may be confused with warts. Lichen sclerosus et atrophicus (2.36) may be confused with scarring following sexual abuse

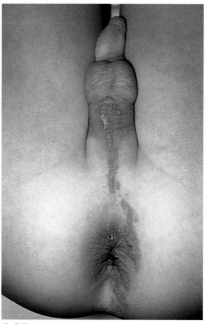

2.35

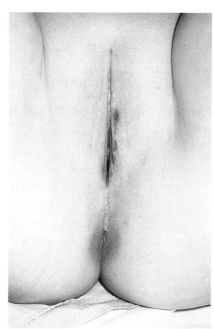

2.36

Table 2.6 Skin diseases that may be confused with child abuse

Disease	Apparent injury
Lichen sclerosus of vulva (2.36)	Sexual abuse
Localised vulval pemphigoid	Sexual abuse
Mongolian spot (6.13)	Bruising due to battering
Growth ('whiplash') striae (6.35)	Whip marks
Accidental bruising (also haematological disease)	Battering
Linear epidermal naevus affecting genital region (2.35)	Warts related to sexual abuse
Molluscum contagiosum in genital area (a common site normally)	Warts related to sexual abuse
Dermatitis artefacta (15.46)	Battering, burns, etc.
Plant contact dermatitis (13.3) or phytophotocontact	Lash injury or burns reaction (linear blisters, weals, pigmentation)
Pityriasis lichenoides acuta (17.38)	Cigarette burns
Epidermolysis bullosa	Burns and scalds
Ehlers–Danlos syndrome (easy bruising, stretched scars, fragile skin) (11.12, 11.13)	Battering
Napkin rashes (5.26–5.29) of various causes	Sexual abuse (NB some are due to neglect)
Genital psoriasis	Sexual abuse
Hypersensitivity to aluminium (causes nodules at vaccination sites on upper arm or buttocks)	Blunt injury

Injury may be a source of innoculation of infection (e.g. warts, fish tank granulomas). Some infections related to injury are less easy to explain, such as:

- Streptococcal cellulitis and necrotising fasciitis, which are well documented to occur after blunt non-penetrating injury.
- Varicella, which may localise around recent vaccination sites.

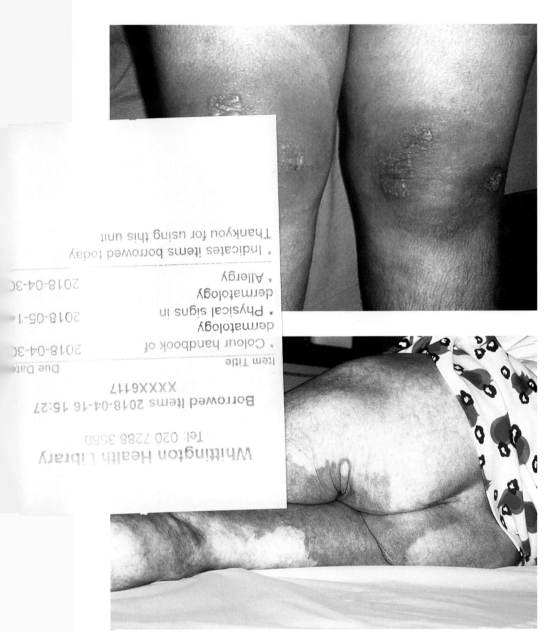

Fig 2.37 Adhesive plaster allergy. Unusual shapes of lesions suggest external causes

Fig 2.38 Dorbanex/ co-danthromer rash. This patient had taken a laxative containing danthron, which is converted into dithranol by gut bacteria. Subsequent faecal soiling was accompanied by staining of the skin of the buttocks and posterior aspect of the legs (from Cox NH & Vickers CFH (1984) *Clin Exp Dermatol* **9**: 624–625, *courtesy of Blackwell Scientific Publications*

Distributions related to clothing

In addition to the sparing effects of clothing discussed with regard to photo-sensitivity (*see* above), clothing may also influence distributions of skin lesions in other ways, for example:

- Exanthemata may appear to localise specifically to areas under garments or may selectively spare such areas (typically under tight areas of clothing such as shoulder or brassiere straps and waistbands).
- Vasculitis may be localised or exaggerated by areas of pressure such as the elasticated portion of a sock or wristwatch straps (**Fig 2.39**).
- Insect bites are commonly localised to exposed skin but are also limited by tight areas of clothing; cat flea bites are often most prominent just above the tops of socks (*see* Fig 2.25).
- Allergic reactions to specific constituents of clothing may produce odd patterns of localisation (**Fig 2.40**).
- Sunburn is a cause of Koebner's phenomenon (*see* Fig 2.17) and can therefore determine the distribution of rashes such as psoriasis.

31

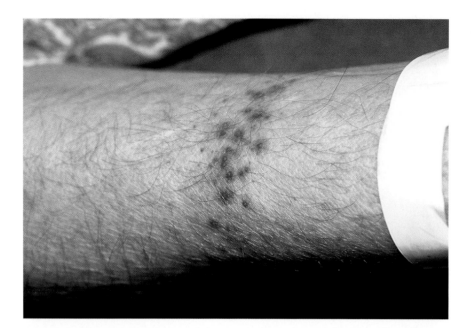

Fig 2.39 Vasculitis. Localisation to site of pressure from a wrist watch strap

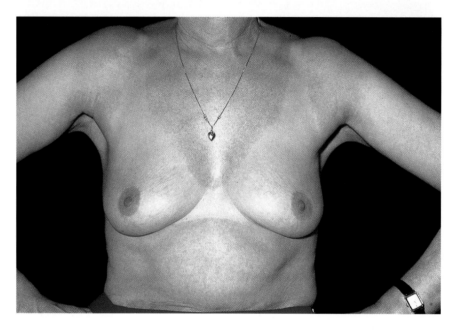

Fig 2.40 Allergic contact dermatitis to clothing. This patient was allergic to the blue dye in her dress. She developed widespread rash at all sites except those covered by her underwear (*photo courtesy of Dr Colin Munro*)

Regions of sparing and anatomical demarcations

Some rashes typically involve certain parts of the body (*see* Chapter 5), but there are also various patterns of sparing that can be a useful aid to diagnosis. The physical signs can be striking, and some examples are illustrated.

Creases

Eczema due to external irritants or photosensitivity may spare crease areas. In babies with nappy rash, irritant stool and urine constituents classically spare the deep creases (*see* Figs 5.26–5.29); conversely, candida infection classically involves the creases (although in practice, both causes are often combined). Clothing dermatitis around the axilla affects the anterior and posterior axillary folds but spares the vault of the axilla; by contrast, deodorant dermatitis primarily affects the axillary vault.

Endogenous disorders may also spare creases. This is seen in some patients with eczema but is most prominent as the so-called 'deckchair sign' in a disorder known as papuloerythroderma. Whether this disorder is distinct from a papular eczema in elderly men is uncertain, but the pattern is notable; it consists of sheets of confluent papules with a striking sparing of the back and abdominal creases, reminiscent of the areas that would be spared from sunburn in individuals sunbathing in a deckchair (**Fig 2.42**).

Islands

Sparing can present as small islands within large areas of erythema, although it is uncertain why these occur. The classic example is a condition called pityriasis rubra pilaris (**Fig 2.43**), in which small white islands are found within large orange–red plaques or erythroderma.

Central back

The central back is spared in conditions where scratch or rubbing are important as a cause of the physical signs (*see* Figs 15.5 and 15.6). It is therefore common to find less excoriation on the back than the limbs in widespread eczema, and the central back may be completely spared in patients with systemic causes of itch in whom the cutaneous signs are purely determined by the areas that are able to be reached and scratched. In primary biliary cirrhosis, in which excoriation and rubbing is associated with hyperpigmentation, this sparing of the back has been termed the butterfly sign, but it is not specific to this disorder. Loss of the butterfly sign occurs because a means to scratch can always be found by an inventive subject.

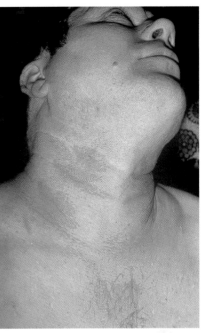

Fig 2.41 Airborne contact sensitivity to balsam in sawdust. Dust has been more ingrained in the skin creases around the collar line

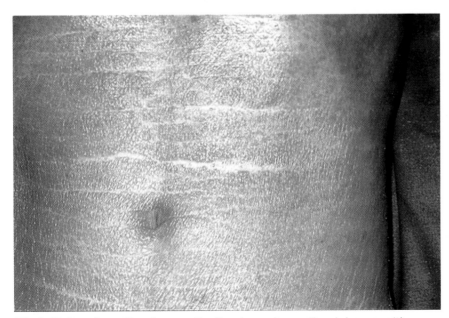

Fig 2.42 Papuloerythroderma. Confluent papules on the abdomen, with sparing of creases in the pattern of the 'deckchair sign'

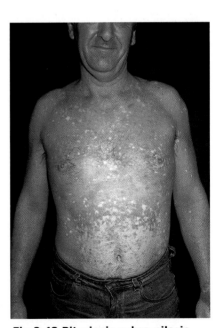

Fig 2.43 Pityriasis rubra pilaris. This uncommon disorder has several variants, including a pattern of almost universal orange–red erythema with small islands of pale spared skin

33

Perioral region

In rosacea and the related disorder perioral dermatitis, there is characteristically a band of sparing around the mouth (**Fig 2.44**). In this region, eczematous processes such as atopic dermatitis, lip licking or contact allergy to toothpastes may involve the skin up to the vermilion border.

Anatomical factors

Some eruptions spare areas for specific anatomical reasons. Good examples include:

- Relapsing polychondritis—this is an inflammatory disorder of collagen, which may affect the ear, nose, conjunctivae, trachea and bronchi. It typically affects the ear but spares the non-cartilaginous ear lobe (**Fig 2.45**).
- The trigeminal trophic syndrome—owing to altered sensation, patients with this condition pick at the skin of the sidewall of the nose or paranasal skin, leading to ulceration. However, due to cross-over of innervation, the tip of the nose is characteristically spared (**Fig 2.46**, *see also* Fig 12.37)

Wallace's line is an interesting line of demarcation between the skin of the sole and of the upper part of the foot (**Fig 2.47**). The reason why some rashes cut-off at this point is not clearly defined and may be related to blood or lymphatic vessels rather than a sharp difference in skin thickness. The importance is that it is distinct from either a sparing effect (e.g. photosensitivity affecting the dorsum of the foot but sparing the covered sole) or a causative effect such as allergy to constituents of shoes.

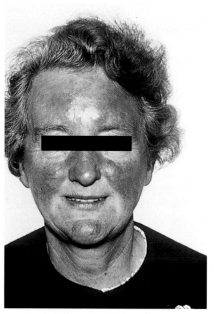

Fig 2.44 Rosacea. The region of skin around eyes and mouth is typically spared. In a classic example, the overall distribution of eruption is said to be in the shape of a Maltese cross involving the forehead, cheeks and chin

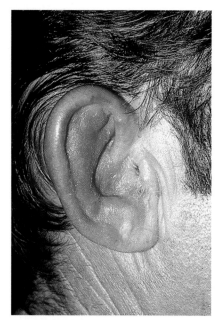

Fig 2.45 Relapsing polychondritis. Sparing of the ear lobe occurs because the inflammation of collagen is directed at the cartilaginous part of the ear

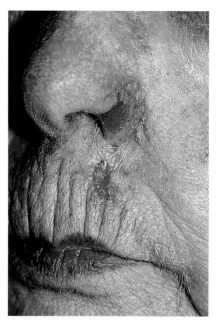

Fig 2.46 Trigeminal trophic syndrome. Sparing of the nasal tip is characteristic due to cross-innervation from the normal side of the face

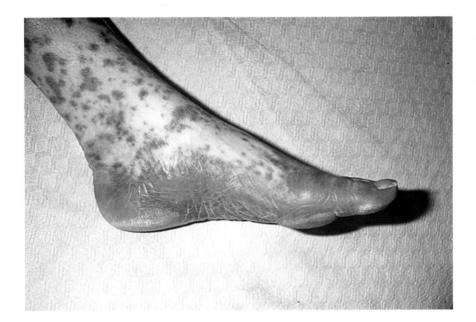

Fig 2.47 Wallace's line. This is a common line of functional demarcation on the border of the foot, which may limit the extent of an eruption, in this case of erythema multiforme

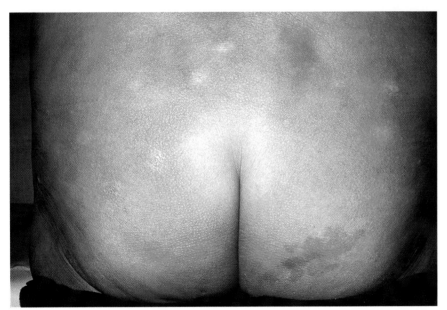

Fig 2.48 Localisation of absent tanning due to hypoxia. This patient lay on her back on the base unit of a UVA sunbed and failed to tan at pressure points on the sacrum and each scapula. This effect depends on the wavelength and does not occur with UVB (the burning component of natural sunlight). The shape may resemble a butterfly (from Cox NH (1992) *BMJ*, **305**: 1236)

External factors

There are many examples of specific localisation of eruption that can be explained by external factors such as chemical contact, but patterns of sparing are also of interest, and two examples are described:

- Compression of the skin causes transient hypoxia, which is usually not apparent. However, tanning by long-wavelength ultraviolet radiation does not occur if the skin is hypoxic at the time of irradiation, so patients who lie on a UVA sunbed may have areas of skin that will not tan (**Fig 2.48**); this only occurs with the type of bed that has lamps underneath the subject, as there is no direct skin pressure with the canopy type of bed.

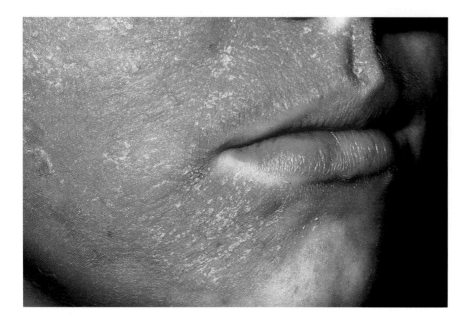

Fig 2.49 Dermatitis artefacta. This patient had a uniform area of intense inflammation on the cheek, with sharp borders and a thin rim of sparing at the angles of the mouth, vermilion border of the lip and eyelid margin. The overall picture was of dermatitis artefacta, and the distribution of the sparing suggested that the eyes and mouth were squeezed tightly shut during application of an irritant chemical

- Although many facial rashes tend to spare the lower eyelid, e.g. rosacea, when the eyelids are involved, there is virtually always involvement of the border of the lid. Examples include atopic dermatitis, reactions to eye-drops, discoid lupus erythematosus and causes of blepharitis. Even allergic reactions to cosmetics that may not actually be applied to the lid margin tend to spread to this area. Similarly, most rashes around the mouth extend to the vermilion border, although sparing of this region is a feature of rosacea and a similar disorder known as perioral dermatitis. A band of sparing at both of these sites is therefore unusual except in rosacea but can occur in dermatitis artefacta due to irritant chemicals (**Fig 2.49**).

3

Colours, hyperpigmentation and hypopigmentation

INTRODUCTION

Skin colour is the net result of different pigments, the thickness and quality of the structures between the pigment and the observer, and the light it is viewed in. The main pigments are melanin (shades of brown), haemoglobin (red to purple depending on state of oxygenation) and carotenoids (yellows); the fibrous dermis contributes a white colour. Two different types of melanin exist: eumelanin produces the black and brown colours and phaeomelanin produces red and yellow shades.

Subtle melanin or deeper pigmentation that is obscured by the red colour of intravascular blood may be revealed by diascopy (**Fig 3.1**). This technique involves pressing on the skin with a clear glass or plastic strip to express intravascular blood pigment and to allow subtle shades of yellow and brown to be seen.

Dark pigments such as those found in a carbon tattoo, deep angioma or blue naevus appear more blue if deeply situated within the skin. The blue colour is the result of an optical phenomenon called the Tyndall effect. This phenomenon also explains the blue colour of the sky, the bluish colour of cigarette smoke and the bright blue colour of some fresh-water lakes that contain suspended clay particles. Professor Tyndall was the first to show how the different wavelength components of white light are scattered by suspended particles. The shorter blue wavelengths are scattered more than the longer red wave lengths, which presumably bend around small particles. Some of the scattered blue light reaches the observer's eye. Altered refractile properties caused by changes in epidermal thickness can exert important

DIAGNOSTIC TIPS AND PITFALLS

- Vascularity of lesions may obscure melanin pigmentation, which can be revealed by diascopy

- Loss of blood pigment without loss of melanin causes hypopigmentation, which is not visible using Wood's light

- Epidermal pigment disturbance is exaggerated, but dermal pigment disturbance is obscured under Wood's light

37

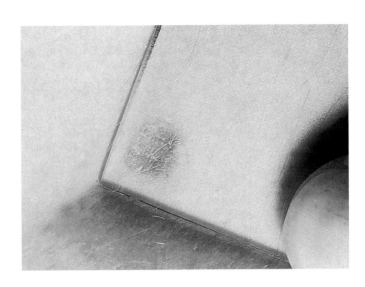

Fig 3.1 Diascopy. This technique compresses intravascular blood out of skin lesions to demonstrate other colour changes, or to demonstrate extravasated blood. It is usually performed using a glass microscope slide or, with a greater degree of safety, with a stiff strip of colourless plastic. In this case, diascopy of a rather vascular nodule reveals the faint pigmentation of a Spitz naevus.

effects, causing, for example, Wickham's striae (*see* Fig 4.16), which appear as white reticulate streaks on the violet–purple background of lichen planus lesions. This same principle can be used in conjunction with magnification in epiluminescent microscopy (dermatoscopy) for the assessment of pigmented lesions (**Fig 4.17**).

Surface scale may obscure features present beneath the scale. These features are seen more clearly if oil is rubbed on the skin. Oil application replaces the air–keratin interfaces that occur in scaly dermatoses with oil–keratin interfaces. An oil–keratin interface does not reflect as much light as an air–keratin interface. As a result, the surface looks less white because there is less reflected light, and structures beneath the scale can be seen more easily because the stratum corneum is more transparent. A similar effect can be achieved by the application of water, but it is more transient because of evaporation.

The emphasis in this chapter is on brown and yellow colours and hypopigmentation. The importance of red colours in differential diagnosis is discussed in relation to erythema (*see* Chapter 17), and the importance of colours of papules and nodules is addressed in Chapter 9.

ASSESSMENT OF COLOUR

The important principles of colour assessment are:

- Colour can be judged only in a good light.
- Some colours may be enhanced by special techniques, such as diascopy (**Fig. 3.1**), application of oil or changing the light source (*see* Wood's light, p. 63–66).
- Record shades of colour. They may give important diagnostic clues, for example, the beefy red of erysipelas compared with the red–brown colour of seborrhoeic dermatitis.
- Record interlesional and intralesional variations. For example, variation of colours within a solitary lesion is typical of malignant melanoma (*see* Fig 9.38–9.44); multiple plaques of different shades of red and brown, especially if apparently superimposed on each other, are strongly suggestive of mycosis fungoides (*see* Fig 8.6), a cutaneous lymphoma.
- Note associated features. For example, a café au lait patch in neurofibromatosis (*see* Fig 9.18) may be the same colour as post-inflammatory pigmentation but has a sharp border rather than an indistinct edge. Similarly, the white lesions of vitiligo have a sharp border and smooth surface compared with the less distinct edge and fine scale of pityriasis alba.

Table 3.1 Colours of lesions

Colour	Examples
Black	Melanin, e.g. some naevi, melanoma (9.38–9.44) Exogenous pigments, e.g. tattoos, pencil/ink Exogenous chemicals, e.g. silver nitrate, gold salts (3.18)
Blue–grey	Deep blood, e.g. angiomas (9.69) Deep melanin, e.g. blue naevus (9.33) Inflammatory, e.g. orf (3.33) Drugs, e.g. phenothiazines, minocycline (3.12, Table 3.5)
Dark brown	Melanin near surface, e.g. melanocytic naevi (9.23–9.25) Exogenous pigments, e.g. dithranol staining
Pale brown	Melanin near surface, e.g. lentigo (9.14), freckles (9.12)
Muddy brown	Melanin in superficial dermis, e.g. post-inflammatory pigmentation (3.14)
Purple	Vascular lesions, e.g. angiomas (9.68), Other disorders where telangiectasia is a prominent feature, e.g. lupus pernio (chronic sarcoidosis) (5.3), dermatomyositis (17.8)
Dusky blue	Reduced haemoglobin, e.g. poor arterial supply Cyanosis Methaemoglobinaemia
Violaceous and lilac	Lichen planus (8.22) Edge of plaques of morphoea (8.27) Connective tissue disorders, e.g. dermatomyositis (17.8)
Pink–red	Many exanthemata and common disorders, such as psoriasis
Red–brown	Inflammatory, e.g. seborrhoeic eczema (2.9), secondary syphilis Haemosiderin, e.g. pigmented purpuric dermatoses (17.25)
Scarlet–red	Lesions with strong arterial supply, e.g. pyogenic granuloma (9.65), spider naevus (17.17) Altered haemoglobin, e.g. carbon monoxide poisoning
Orange	Haemosiderin, e.g. lichen aureus Inflammatory, e.g. pityriasis rubra pilaris
Yellow–white/yellow–pink	Xanthomatous disorders (3.35)
Yellow–orange	Carotenaemia (ingested carotene, myxoedema) (3.34)
Yellow–green	Jaundice
Green	Exogenous pigment, e.g. copper salts
White–ivory	Lichen sclerosus, morphoea (3.32)
White (or pale pink, depending on vascularity)	*See* Table 3.8

Examples of different colours are given in **Table 3.1**, and colours that different pigments can cause are listed in **Table 3.2**. Colours of nodules are discussed further in Chapter 9.

HYPERPIGMENTATION: MELANIN AND BROWN COLOURS

Hyperpigmentation can be usefully divided into three groups:

- Generalised or widespread increase in pigmentation (**Table 3.3**).
- Localised hyperpigmentation (**Tables 3.4** and **3.5**).
- Hyperpigmentation with skin thickening or hyperkeratosis (*see* **Tables 3.4** and **3.6**).

Table 3.2 Skin colour changes caused by various pigments

Pigment	Colour produced	Example
Eumelanin	Brown	Suntan, acquired naevus (9.23)
	Black	Malignant melanoma (9.38–9.44)
	Blue	Blue naevus (9.33), Mongolian spot (6.13)
	Blue–brown	Drug-induced, e.g. chlorpromazine
Phaeomelanin	Red–brown	Ginger hair
Haemosiderin	Red–brown	Capillaropathy (17.25), venous stasis (2.32)
Drug pigments	Slate-grey	Amiodarone
	Blue	Minocycline (3.12)
	Yellow/brown/grey	Mepacrine (19.69)
Heavy metals	Grey	Silver (argyria)
	Blue–grey	Gold (chryiasis)
Tattoos	Blue–black	Carbon, including coal
	Red	Mercuric sulphate
	Blue	Cobalt aluminate
	Green	Chromium oxides
	Yellow	Cadmium sulphide
	Brown	Iron oxide

Table 3.3 Causes of generalised or widespread brown colour of skin

Genetic, congenital	Racial
Nutritional and metabolic	Wilson's disease, haemochromatosis, some porphyrias, liver disease (especially primary biliary cirrhosis), pellagra and malabsorption
Endocrine	Addison's disease (3.2–3.5), tumours producing adrenocorticotrophic hormone or melanocyte stimulating hormone (see below), Cushing's syndrome, Nelson's syndrome
Physical and inflammatory	Ultraviolet exposure (suntan), scleroderma/diffuse morphoea
Malignant neoplasms	Metastatic melanoma Tumours producing adrenocorticotrophic hormone or melanocyte stimulating hormone (oat cell carcinoma of bronchus)
Drugs and chemicals	Arsenic, busulphan

As usual, no classification is perfect, and there are some areas of overlap between these groups. For example, ordinary suntan may be localised or generalised, depending on exposure, and is associated with epidermal thickening (although this is not usually clinically obvious). Furthermore, many causes of generalised pigmentation are not uniform but rather blotchy or irregularly distributed. Discrete pigmented lesions are discussed in Chapter 9.

Generalised or widespread increase in pigmentation (Table 3.3)

The degree of skin pigmentation varies depending on recent exposure to sunlight, which can usually be determined by the presence of spared areas under clothing, etc. Pathological causes of generalised or widespread pigmentation are often systemic diseases, and their evaluation may require a detailed medical evaluation. Many drugs may also cause pigmentation, either

Table 3.4 Causes of discrete brown areas of skin*

Genetic, congenital and naevoid	Regional variation, especially dark-skinned races **Small brown patches** Lentigines and freckles in syndromes, e.g. neurofibromatosis (Crowe's sign, 9.19) Peutz—Jeghers syndrome, xeroderma pigmentosum **Large brown macular areas** Albright–McCune syndrome, i.e. polyostotic fibrous dysplasia with hyperpigmentation and precocious puberty Zosteriform reticulate hyperpigmentation Becker's naevus **Reticulate pigmentation** Dowling–Degos disease (reticulate pigmentation of the flexures) **Streaky and whorled pigmented patches** Pigmentation in epidermal naevi (2.11) Incontinentia pigmenti Ichthyoses (1.11, 7.5) Atopic 'dirty neck' (3.15)
Nutritional, metabolic and endocrine	Chloasma (6.28) Linea nigra (6.29, 6.30) Kwashiorkor Pellagra—especially exposed skin, Acanthosis nigricans—insulin-resistance type
Infections	Exanthemata may have a brownish colour, e.g. measles, secondary syphilis, cutaneous infections, e.g. pityriasis versicolor Confluent and reticulate papillomatosis
Physical and inflammatory	Burns, trauma, erythema ab igne (2.23) Post-inflammatory especially lichen planus, drugs, lichen simplex, chronic pruritus (3.14) Poikiloderma of Civatte
Vascular	Chronic purpuric disorders (haemosiderin) Gravitational pigmentation (2.32) Poikiloderma vasculare atrophicans (1.16)
Localised benign lesions	Naevi, lentigines, freckles, seborrhoeic warts, plane warts, dermatofibroma, mastocytoma, many others (*see* Chapter 9)
Malignant neoplasms	Melanoma (9.38–9.44), Acanthosis nigricans with internal malignancy
Drugs and chemicals	*See* Table 3.5

*Includes smooth and scaling disorders. *See also* Table 3.5.

Table 3.5 Pigmentation due to drugs and medicaments

Route of administration	Type of agent or mechanism	Examples
Topical	Photosensitisers Staining	Psoralens (3.8) Silver nitrate (9.49), potassium permanganate, Dithranol (anthralin; dithranol staining of perineal skin also occurs after faecal excretion of ingested co-danthrusate)
Systemic	Photosensitisers Cytotoxic agents Fixed drug eruption Others	Psoralens, amiodarone, phenothiazines Bleomycin, busulphan, cyclophosphamide, 5-fluorouracil Sulphonamides phenolphthalein, codeine Minocycline (3.12), mepacrine (19.69) chloroquine

generalised or localised in pattern (**Table 3.5**). Associated skin findings that may be helpful include:

- **Prominent distribution of photosensitivity**—Notably seen in pellagra, including a pigmented band around the neck (Casal's necklace).
- **Pruritus**—Occurs in primary biliary cirrhosis, chronic renal failure, pellagra and many others. A notable pattern is sparing of the mid-back (the 'butterfly sign' (*see* Figs 15.5 and 15.6)), which occurs because the skin signs are at least partially due to chronic rubbing and because the centre of the back cannot be reached.
- **Scaling or crusting**—Chronic infestation (e.g. crusted scabies), chronic renal failure, haemochromatosis, pellagra.
- **Palmar keratoses**—Chronic arsenic ingestion causes generalised hyperpigmentation with scattered drop-like hypopigmented patches, palmar keratoses and squamous cell carcinomas (*see* Fig 7.48).
- **Hypertrichosis**—Cushing's disease, porphyria cutanea tarda (*see* Fig 18.9).
- **Induration of skin**—Scleroderma/diffuse morphoea, POEMS syndrome (Polyneuropathy, Organomegaly, Endocrinopathy, M-protein, Skin changes).
- **Palmar crease and buccal pigmentation**—Addison's disease (**Figs 3.2–3.5**).
- **Nail changes**—e.g. pigmentation of nail beds associated with cytotoxic drug therapy, leuconychia associated with chronic renal or hepatic disease.

Localised hyperpigmentation

Many disorders cause localised pigmentation (**Table 3.4**). Some of these, especially the localised benign lesions and some causes of lentigines (*see* Chapter 9), are covered in other parts of this book. Drug-induced pigmentation and other patterns are briefly discussed below.

Unusual patterns of pigmentation

In neonates or early childhood, pigmented areas are often in a naevoid distribution, such as the whorled pattern of epidermal naevi (*see* Figs 2.10 and 2.11).

Patterned pigmentation may reflect the distribution of underlying blood vessels, for example the reticulate patterning seen in erythema ab igne, a form of thermal damage that predominantly affects the legs of elderly patients.

Reticulate patterns of pigmentation occur in Dowling–Degos disease (**Fig 3.6**), confluent and reticulate papillomatosis (**Fig 3.7**) and a variety of rare inherited dyschromic conditions.

A more rippled pattern of pigmentation occurs in macular amyloid (*see* Fig 3.16).

Pigmentation with a streaky pattern occurs secondary to phytophotodermatitis. Psoralen chemicals in some plants and fruits cause a phototoxic reaction, with inflammation, blistering and residual hyperpigmentation. This usually occurs where a relevant plant has brushed against exposed skin or where fruit juice (such as lime juice, **Fig 3.8**) has dribbled on to the skin. The streaky lesions may erroneously suggest a diagnosis of lymphangitis. Drug-induced pigmentation (*see* below) may also be streaky or bizarre in pattern.

Spotty pigmentation on the hands occurs in Peutz–Jegher's syndrome (*see* Fig 9.15) associated with periorbital and perioral lentigines and buccal pigmentation), and blotchy macular pigmentation of the palms may occur in Laugier–Hunziker syndrome (*see* Fig 19.72, with buccal pigmentation and longitudinal melanonychia).

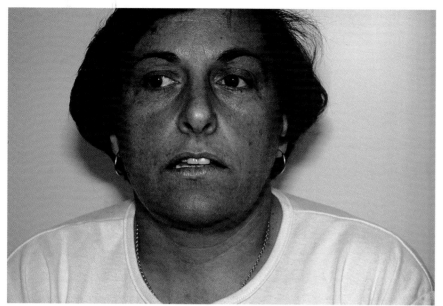

Figs 3.2

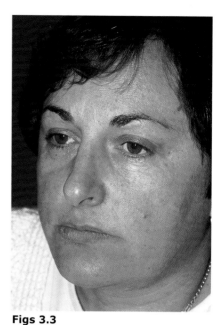

Figs 3.3

Figs 3.2, 3.3 Addison's disease.
Diffuse pigmentation at diagnosis
(3.2) and improvement 5 months
after treatment (3.3). The patient's
hair had not darkened and was the
same colour 3 years later

Drug-induced pigmentation

Drugs may cause diffuse or localised pigmentation (**Table 3.5**). Systemic or topical drugs may be implicated, and the pigmentation may affect nails or mucosae as well as the skin. Drug-induced pigmentation may assume bizarre formations, such as the streaky 'flagellate' pattern caused by some cytotoxic agents (notably bleomycin, **Fig 3.9**) or the macular discoid lesions of a recurrent fixed drug eruption (**Figs 3.10** and **3.11**). Pigmentation due to minocycline (**Fig 3.12**) may occur as a diffuse pattern on the face or may localise either to old scars or to acne lesions.

Pregnancy

Pregnancy stimulates melanin pigmentation, causing darkening of areolae, development of a linea nigra (*see* Fig 6.29) and the exaggeration of chloasma

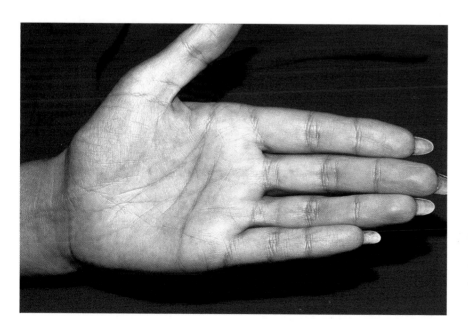

Fig 3.4 Addison's disease. Palmar crease pigmentation. Compare with normal palm crease pigmentation (*see* 6.31)

Fig 3.5 Addison's disease. Buccal pigmentation. Compare with the buccal pigmentation in Laugier–Hunziker syndrome (*see* 19.73)

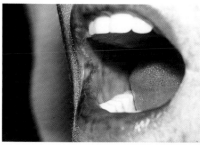

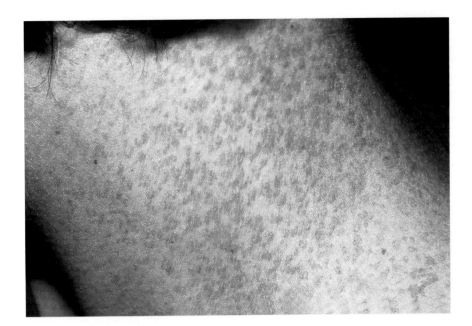

Fig 3.6 Dowling–Degos disease.
Patient shows a typical rather reticulate pattern of flexural pigmentation

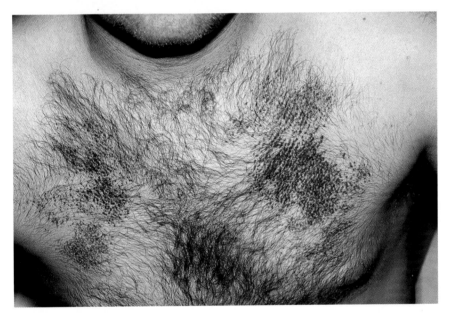

Fig 3.7 Confluent and reticulate papillomatosis. Brown pigmented rather greasy scaling on the chest wall. Biopsy confirmed the presence of yeast hyphae in the stratum corneum, and the pigmentation disappeared after topical ketoconazole therapy

(*see* Fig 6.28). Pigmentary demarcation lines (*see* Fig 6.32) are often exaggerated during pregnancy.

Poikiloderma of Civatte

Poikiloderma of Civatte is a pigmentary disorder of debated aetiology. It may be due to perfume agents as it occurs mainly on the sides of the neck, especially in women; it is less uniform in pigmentation than chloasma, and telangiectasia is a feature.

Post-inflammatory pigmentation

Post-inflammatory pigmentation can occur as a result of many chronic itchy disorders where scratching or rubbing occurs, particularly in racially pigmented skin. It is a notable feature of eruptions in which the inflammatory process damages the basal layer of the epidermis, where melanocytes are normally situated. As a consequence of this, pigment granules drop into the upper dermis, where they are engulfed by macrophages. The fine dusting of

DIAGNOSTIC TIPS AND PITFALLS

- Streaky hyperpigmentation is usually due to an external cause (e.g. photosensitising chemicals) or some drugs

- In patients with patchy pigment disturbance and scaling, consider infection as a cause (e.g. pityriasis versicolor)

- Localised discord hyperpigmented patches, especially on the penis, may be due to an old fixed drug eruption dermal pigment looks slightly blue–brown rather than a pure brown, as noted earlier. As inflammation subsides and dermal melanin increases, an initially red lesion therefore becomes rather violaceous and then fades to a muddy brown (**Fig 3.14**). Lichen planus is a good example of this sequence, and residual pigmentation is also a typical feature of fixed drug eruptions in which a systemic drug taken intermittently produces inflammation at the same skin site on each exposure (**Figs 3.10** and **3.11**). Discoid lupus erythematosus, phytophotodermatitis and discoid eczema may also cause prominent post-inflammatory pigmentation.

In some conditions, post-inflammatory epidermal pigmentation occurs. This is potentially amenable to topical treatment.

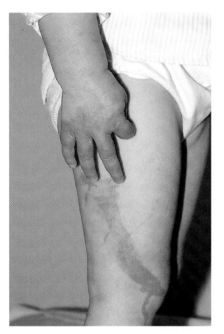

Fig 3.8 Pigmentation due to phytophotodermatitis. Citrus fruit juice had dribbled from this child's hand down the leg. Many cases are due to brushing against plants of the hogweed family, producing a typical streaky pattern of post-inflammatory pigmentation

Fig 3.9 Flagellate pattern of inflammation. This occurs secondary to systemic bleomycin therapy. Pigmentation occurs subsequently (Courtesy of Dr GM White)

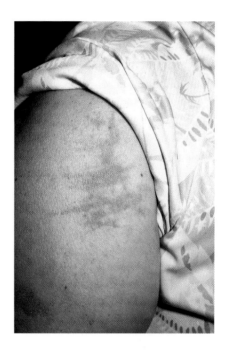

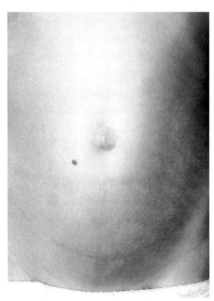

Fig 3.10   **Fig 3.11**

Fig 3.10, 3.11 Fixed drug eruption. Example of an unusually large fixed drug eruption, showing residual hyperpigmentation (3.10) and erythematous phase after challenge with the causative sulphonamide antibiotic (3.11) (*see also* 5.33)

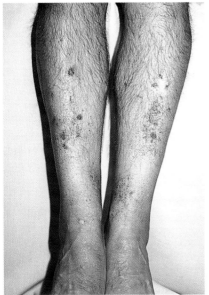

Fig 3.12

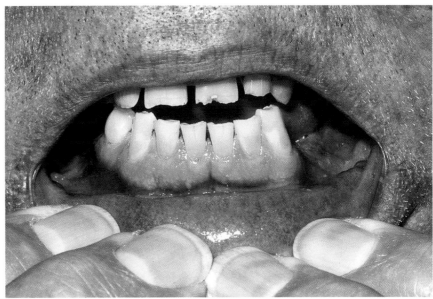

Fig 3.13

Fig 3.12, 3.13 Pigmentation due to minocycline. Pigmentation is a greyish blue or black colour. It may be diffuse, spotty or localised to scars (3.12). Teeth and nails are affected at any age (3.13)

Iron deposition

Patients with frequent minor leakage of blood from small vessels, e.g. in capillaropathy, develop pigmentation that is typically a golden-brown colour (lichen aureus). This typically occurs on the lower legs; the pigment has the appearance of a dusting or small granules when viewed closely and is often associated with a scattering of tiny red spots representing more recent extravasation. Similar leakage occurs in patients with venous disease, but it is also associated with an increase in melanin, the two pigments accounting for the hyperpigmentation that is common in association with chronic venous leg ulcers.

Hyperpigmentation with skin thickening or hyperkeratosis (Table 3.4)

Congenital and inherited conditions

Hyperkeratosis associated with hyperpigmentation is a typical feature of some localised congenital lesions, e.g. epidermal naevi, and as a localised or generalised pattern in inherited disorders such as some ichthyoses. The latter may be associated with pigmentation that is often a dirty brown colour; this can be seen in lamellar ichthyosis (*see* Fig 7.8), X-linked ichthyosis (*see* Fig 7.9) and hyperkeratotic atopic dermatitis, where it is known as atopic 'dirty neck' (**Fig 3.15**).

Effects of rubbing the skin

As in generalised pruritus, localised scratching and rubbing may produce hyperpigmentation, for example in lichen simplex—especially of the lower leg—or in patients with notalgia paraesthetica (a localised area of pruritus to one side of the spine in the scapular region). A localised rippled pattern of pigmentation, reminiscent of sand after the tide has receded, occurs in macular amyloid (**Fig 3.16**), a disorder in which the amyloid deposition is believed to be secondary to chronic rubbing of the skin.

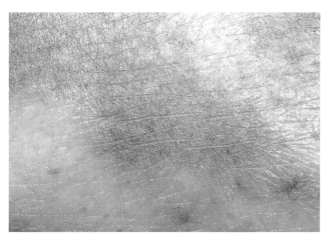

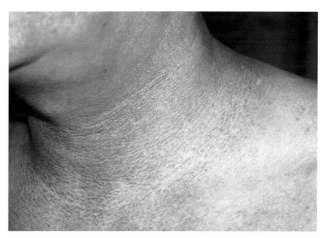

Fig 3.14 Post-inflammatory pigmentation.
Pigmentation has a typical muddy-brown colour, due to
melanin deposition in the upper dermis (*see also* 6.40)

Fig 3.15 Atopic dirty neck. Typical rippled pattern of
pigmentation associated with hyperkeratosis

Acanthosis nigricans

Acanthosis nigricans (**Fig 3.17**) is a disorder in which pigmentation is most
noticeable in flexural areas and around the nape of the neck. Although the
classic form of the disorder presents in association with an internal tumour,
especially adenocarcinoma of the stomach, a much more common, although
less severe version of the disorder occurs in insulin-resistant states (**Table 3.6**,
see also Fig 11.23). In one study, 85% of black obese adults and 75% of white
obese adults had acanthosis nigricans; its presence was a reliable cutaneous
marker for hyperinsulinaemia in these subjects. This has been termed the
HAIR-AN syndrome (HyperAndrogenism Insulin Resistance Acanthosis
Nigricans).

Infections

Scaling is a feature of many of the infective causes of pigmentation, including
both systemic infections such as measles and external skin infections such as
pityriasis versicolor, which is discussed in the section on hypopigmentation
below.

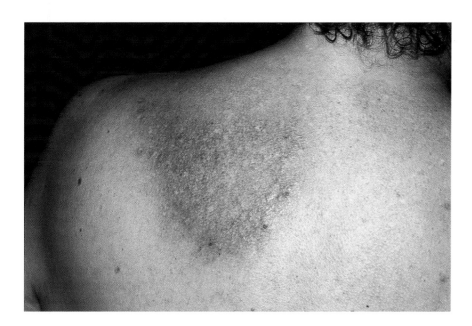

Fig 3.16 Macular amyloid. Rippled
pattern of pigmentation is seen in
macular amyloid, usually on the
upper back, as in this case

Table 3.6 Comparison of benign and malignant forms of acanthosis nigricans

Feature	Malignant	Benign
Flexural change	Severe	Mild
Pigmentation	Pronounced	Mild
Generalised wartiness	Yes	No
Palm changes	'Tripe palms'	No
Mucous membranes	Warty changes visible on the gingival margin	None
Body habitus	Thin	Obese or hyper-androgenic in female
Cause	Tumour, usually adenocarcinoma of stomach	Insulin resistance, associated with obesity, polycystic ovaries

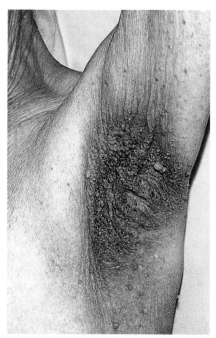

Fig 3.17 Acanthosis nigricans due to malignant disease. This shows the typical distribution of pigmentation in the axilla and the gross warty changes that occur in malignant acanthosis nigricans. Similar warty changes are seen on eyelids; thickening and exaggeration of epidermal ridges cause the appearance known as 'tripe palms' (see 11.23)

BLUE–BLACK LESIONS (TABLE 3.7)

Lesions that appear blue–black are generally those in which melanin pigment is present in large amounts, densely packed and deeply situated within the skin. However, some topical agents may cause black discoloration of the skin.

External causes

Black dermographism and metals

Black dermographism is due to deposits of gold on the skin in the vicinity of gold jewellery, usually rings. It is due to the abrasive effects of other chemicals that are handled (**Fig 3.18**). The name is a misnomer as there is no weal

Table 3.7 Causes of blue, grey and black areas of skin*

Genetic, congenital naevoid	Mongolian spot (sacral area, especially in Asian people) (6.13) Naevi of Ota and Ito (especially in Japanese people) (9.17)
Nutritional, metabolic and endocrine	Alkaptonuria Ochronosis Macular amyloid (3.16)
Physical and inflammatory	Erythema dyschromicum perstans (ashy dermatosis) Pigmented contact dermatitis (Riehl's melanosis) Tattoo pigments, ink
Vascular	Acrocyanosis
Localised benign lesions	*See* Chapter 9
Malignant neoplasms	*See* Chapter 9
Drugs and chemicals	**Systemic** Metals, e.g. mercury, silver (argyria), bismuth, lead or gold (chrysoderma) Sun-exposed areas, e.g. chlorpromazine, amiodarone Antimalarials, e.g. mepacrine, chloroquine, hydroxychloroquine (look at the nails (19.69), sclerae and palate for other areas of pigment change) Antibiotics: minocycline (may localise to scars, may affect teeth at any age (3.12) **Topical** Gold salts ('black dermographism,' 3.18),

*See also **Table 3.4**.

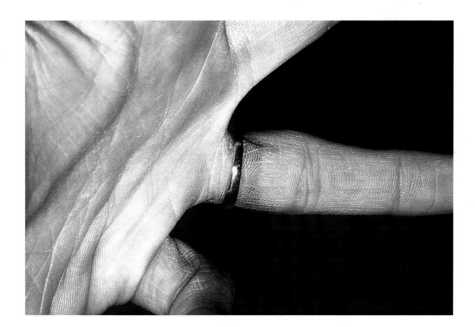

Fig 3.18 Black discoloration of the skin due to gold salts. This is known as black dermographism, although wealing is not actually a feature. It may occur, as in this case, due to the action of abrasive chemicals on a gold ring or simply due to gold rubbing on the skin. The discoloration can be removed by gentle cleaning of the affected skin

or symptomatic component. The diagnosis is made by the localisation of the skin pigment to the shape of the piece of jewellery—usually a ring.

Ingested metals such as gold or silver may cause generalised pigmentation. Localised pigmentation has been reported on earlobes owing to earrings that have become buried under the skin surface.

Others

External agents such as silver nitrate may cause black discoloration of the skin (*see* Fig 9.49). Tattoo pigmentation usually causes no diagnostic difficulty, but implantation of small amounts of coal into the skin of miners may cause confusion if a history is not provided. These deposits may occur either in scars after injury or in a 'buckshot' pattern ('blast tattoo') after underground explosions.

Melanocytic lesions

Mongolian spot is a type of birthmark—usually on the lumbar region—which occurs primarily in Asian children (*see* Chapter 6). Naevus of Ota (*see* Fig 9.17) and naevus of Ito are blue–black macules of the face and upper trunk, which occur mainly in Japanese people.

Other localised blue–black or very dark lesions include some angiomas, blue naevi, occasional dermatofibromas and malignant melanoma. These are discussed in Chapter 9. Drug-induced pigmentation is often complex, involving both a drug (or its metabolites) and increased melanin (e.g. minocycline pigmentation).

HYPOPIGMENTATION (TABLE 3.8)

Apparent pigment loss

Pale or white areas of skin are usually the result of loss of melanin pigment but may be due to altered blood flow or changes in the dermal connective tissue. Digital ischaemia due to Raynaud's phenomenon and arterial disease

Table 3.8 Causes of white areas of skin

Genetic, congenital and naevoid	Localised	Piebaldism (3.24) Waardenburg's syndrome Tuberous sclerosis Ataxia telangiectasia and other syndromes
	Generalised	Albinism Phenylketonuria Vitiligo (3.21, 3.22)
Idiopathic Nutritional, metabolic and endocrine	Localised	Note the association of vitiligo with thyroid disease, Addison's disease, pernicious anaemia, diabetes mellitus, multiglandular insufficiency syndrome and hypoparathyroidism
	Generalised	Hypopituitarism
Infections	Localised	Pityriasis versicolor (7.14) Spirochaete infections (syphilis, yaws and pinta) Leprosy (tuberculoid and lepromatous)
Physical and inflammatory	Localised	Burns trauma, scars Sarcoidosis Lupus erythematosus Morphoea (3.32, 8.27), lichen sclerosus (7.39) Post-inflammatory hypopigmentation, psoriasis and eczema (3.27), guttate hypomelanosis
Vascular	Localised	Arterial insufficiency—distal limb (17.43), around vascular lesions—steal effect (17.12), tissue fluid effect—in urticaria (*see* Chapter 16) Transient vasoconstriction, e.g. white dermographism (16.9)
	Generalised	Anaemia
Localised lesions	Benign	Halo naevi (9.34)
	Malignant	Melanoma—as part of the wide variation in pigment shades (9.40) Mycosis fungoides—a rare variant
Drugs and chemicals	Iatrogenic	**Topical** Hydroquinone, monobenzyl ether of hydroquinone, topical and intralesional corticosteroids **Systemic** Physostigmine, thiotepa, chloroquine, arsenic **Phototoxic reactions to systemic agents** Tetracyclines and chlorothiazides
	Industrial	*See* Table 3.9

causing pallor are covered in Chapter 17. This section describes causes of localised pale areas of skin that are not caused by epidermal pigment loss but may be confused with this.

Naevus anaemicus

Naevus anaemicus is a rare congenital condition that is characterised by a patch of pale skin. It can occur at any site but seems to be most common on the trunk (**Fig 3.19**). The pale area may be over 20 cm in diameter and has a characteristic irregular border with multiple pale satellite areas beyond the main lesion. During Wood's light examination, the pale area becomes invisible because the overlying epidermal pigment is normal. Excluding the blood from the adjacent normal skin by diascopy shows that the naevus anaemicus is the same colour as normal skin (**Fig 3.20**), consistent with the idea that the pale appearance is due to vasoconstriction of the affected skin. The vasoconstriction is caused by an abnormal sensitivity to circulating catecholamines.

The same colour change occurs in a disorder termed white dermographism. This is a transient vasoconstrictive process, which is common in inflamed skin after scratching and therefore has a linear or streaky pattern. In itself, it causes no symptoms (*see* Fig 16.9).

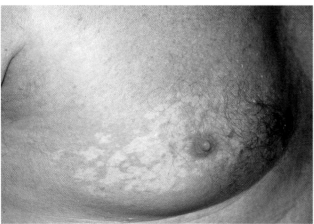

Fig 3.19

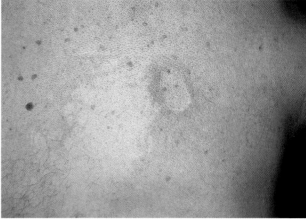

Fig 3.20

Fig 3.19, 3.20 Naevus anaemicus. (3.19) This appears as a large area of pale skin usually on the chest, with adjacent but separated similar pale areas likened to the leaves of a maiden hair fern. Despite the hypopigmented appearance, the pale colour is actually due to vasoconstriction, so that if the surrounding normal skin is blanched (3.20), no colour difference can be distinguished between the two areas (in this case, the photo was taken immediately after pressure applied by a thumb). Under Wood's light examination, the pale colour disappears, because the colour difference is due to the difference in blood flow and not due to absence of melanin from the pale areas

Morphoea

Morphoea (**Fig 3.32**) and other types of sclerotic skin (*see* Chapter 11) may appear white. The associated sclerosis or hardening of the skin is characteristic and enables the diagnosis to be made (*see* Fig 11.36).

Lichen sclerosus

Lichen sclerosus et atrophicus produces white patches around the genital and perianal skin and at other sites, where the lesions are small, ivory-white areas with surface change, slight sclerosis and follicular plugging (*see* Figs 7.39, 8.28, 8.29, 11.4 and 11.5).

Generalised pigment loss

Oculocutaneous albinism

In this group of inherited disorders, melanocytes are present, but melanin production is abnormal due to different enzyme defects. In the more common complete or tyrosinase-negative form of albinism, there is a complete absence of pigment from the hair, skin and eyes. In this type, photophobia, rotatory nystagmus, pink irises and a pronounced red reflex result. Associated refraction defects are commonly severe. By contrast, albinos who are tyrosinase-positive develop some pigment in later life and thus may have blue irises, pigmented patches, naevi and freckles and yellowish brown hair.

Phenylketonuria

Phenylketonuria is characterised by fair skin and hair, photosensitivity, mental retardation and extrapyramidal signs. It is caused by the absence of a liver enzyme known as phenylalanine hydroxylase, which converts phenylalanine to tyrosine; the latter is a precursor of melanin, and lack of tyrosine therefore causes deficient melanisation. The condition is identified at birth using the

Guthrie test. The neurological symptoms can be avoided by a phenylalanine-depleted diet, thus avoiding the toxic effects of excessive levels.

Hypopituitarism

Absence of melanocyte-stimulating hormone and adrenocorticotrophic hormone leads to generalised hypopigmentation, so the skin appears pale yellow. The skin is also soft and 'infantile' to touch. Secondary sexual hair is absent.

Patchy pigment loss without surface change

There are many causes of patchy pigment loss, and some are listed in **Table 3.8**. More important causes are discussed below.

Vitiligo

Vitiligo is a common cause of pigment loss and is due to the disappearance of melanocytes from the skin. Pigment loss is patchy but generally symmetrical **Fig 3.21**, although unilateral or segmental variants occur (**Fig 3.22**). The lesions are scattered, discrete, multiple, sharply circumscribed and usually several centimetres in diameter. There is a predisposition for the wrists, axillae, neck, face, nipples, ankles and genitalia, although generalised pigment loss may occasionally occur. A useful physical sign is that hairs within lesions are also usually depigmented, although this should not be confused with the sparing or white hair regrowth that may occur in alopecia areata (*see* Fig 18.20).

Repigmentation of vitiligo can occur from follicular melanocytes, causing small spots of pigment to appear in white areas. Perilesional areas show hyperpigmentation. Occasionally, shades of colour intermediate between the white areas and the normal skin occur ('trichrome' vitiligo). Vitiligo may be present at injury sites (*see* Table 8.3) and is indistinguishable from chemically induced leucoderma (*see* below).

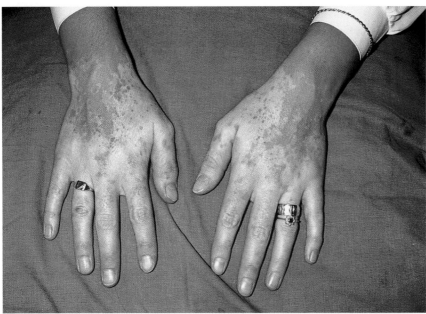

Fig 3.21

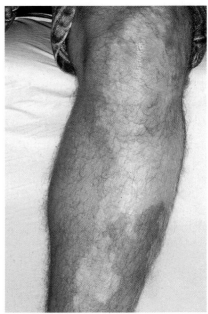

Fig 3.22

Fig 3.21, 3.22 Vitiligo. (3.21) Symmetrical depigmentation of the hands and follicular repigmentation in vitiligo. Melanocytes within hair follicles may be spared in this disorder and are a focus for repigmentation. In the patient shown, gradual follicular repigmentation has caused small spots of different shades of brown within symmetrical vitiligo on the hands. (3.22) Hairs in areas of vitiligo also lose pigment

Other diseases associated with vitiligo include thyroid disease, Addison's disease, pernicious anaemia, diabetes mellitus, multiglandular insufficiency syndrome and hypoparathyroidism.

Chemical depigmentation (leucoderma)

Iatrogenic—Topical hydroquinone can be used therapeutically to produce temporary lightening of black skin, although the hypopigmentation is often patchy and thus cosmetically unacceptable. The hypopigmentation produced by the monobenzyl ether of hydroquinone is permanent. This agent is occasionally used to depigment areas of residual unaffected skin that is cosmetically embarrassing in racially pigmented individuals with widespread vitiligo. Other therapeutic agents reported to cause depigmentation include physostigmine and thiotepa. Chloroquine causes hair and, exceptionally, associated skin pigment loss. Arsenic produces multiple small raindrop-like hypopigmented areas years after ingestion. Temporary hypopigmentation with topical and intralesional corticosteroids is uncommon but should always be remembered when treating people with black skin. Phototoxic reactions to tetracyclines and chlorothiazides may result in hypopigmentation.

Corticosteroids, especially intralesional and soft-tissue depot injections, may cause hypopigmentation that lasts for several months. This may appear as a localised pale area (**Fig 3.23**) or as streaking following the line of lymphatics. There may be associated atrophy.

Industrial—The chemicals used in industry that cause depigmentation are virtually all substituted phenols. Some of the major causes are listed in **Table 3.9**. Chemical depigmentation occurs principally on the backs of the hands as scattered spots of white skin. Distant sites may also be affected, and the final appearance may be clinically and histologically indistinguishable from vitiligo. Contact dermatitis may precede whitening but is not necessary for the development of pigment loss, as depigmentation is a toxic, rather than an allergic, phenomenon.

Piebaldism

In the autosomal dominant disorder of piebaldism, melanocytes are absent from the white patches, which are usually solitary or few in number. Changes are present at birth and remain constant throughout adult life. Depigmented areas on the face are usually associated with a streak of white hair (*see* Fig 18.44). White patches also occur on the limbs (**Fig 3.24**) and trunk, sometimes with pigmented patches in the white areas.

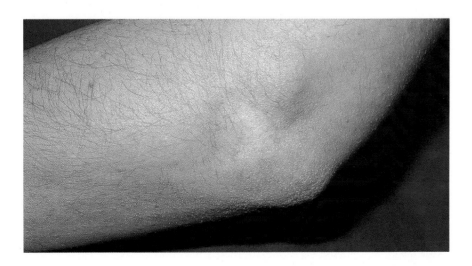

Fig 3.23 Effects of steroids. Depot steroid injections may cause depigmentation locally after injection for tennis elbow

Table 3.9 Major chemical causes of industrial depigmentation

Chemical	Industrial use
Hydroquinone p-tertiary butyl phenol (PTBP)	Photographic developer Manufacture of PTBP formaldehyde resin* Ingredient of deodorants, antioxidants, neoprene adhesives, inks, varnish, oil, antiseptic detergents (see below), etc.
Monobenzyl ether of hydroquinone Phenolic germicidal agents in detergents, e.g. PTBP, p-tertiary amylphenol, chlorophene, p-cresol, etc.	Antioxidant in rubber articles Ingredients of germicidal or antiseptic detergents

*Patch testing with PTBP formaldehyde resin may produce localised hypopigmentation due to residual free PTBP in the resin.

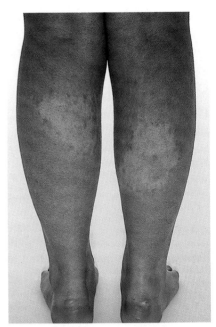

Fig 3.24 Piebaldism. Cutaneous depigmentation may be the only clinical finding in 10–20% of cases. Lesions are commonly bilateral and symmetrical and chalk-white in colour, with hyperpigmented areas bordering the white areas, as shown here (same patient as in 18.44)

Naevus depigmentosus

Naevus depigmentosus is a congenital lesion, in which the absence of pigment is probably due to abnormal melanosomes within the melanocytes. It is sharply demarcated, often with a rather geographical outline (**Fig 3.25**).

Ash leaf macules

Elongated oval-shaped areas of white skin oriented transversely on the trunk are one of the first signs of tuberous sclerosis and are present in 90% of affected people (**Fig 3.26**). Other shaped white areas, including thumb print, confetti and segmental-shaped patches, also occur. The white patches contain melanocytes, but these contain fewer and smaller melanosomes. Hence, the patches are not completely white, unlike vitiligo, and so in white skin may only be identified by ultraviolet light examination of the skin (*see* pp 63–66). If these white patches are present in hair-bearing areas, localised loss of hair pigment, or poliosis, occurs. Such patches may occur anywhere but are most obvious on the scalp, eyebrows and eyelashes. Poliosis can result from other conditions, including alopecia areata, vitiligo, piebaldism and rare syndromes such as Waardenburg's syndrome.

Post-inflammatory hypopigmentation

Temporary hypopigmentation after eczema and psoriasis and other inflammatory dermatoses is common in both white and black skin (**Fig 3.27**).

Idiopathic guttate hypomelanosis

Idiopathic guttate hypomelanosis is an extremely common appearance, seen in approximately 50% of normal adults, both black and white. Typical lesions are depigmented round or angular macules 5 mm in diameter on sun-exposed skin. The size of the macules does not increase with time, although the number of lesions increases with age. The cause is unknown.

Infections

Small, multiple hypopigmented macules may be an early feature of lepromatous leprosy.

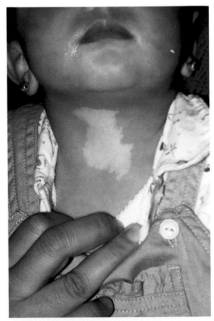

Fig 3.25 Naevus depigmentosus. Lesion showing absent pigment with a geographical border

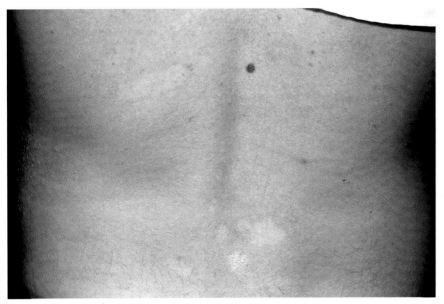

Fig 3.26 Ash leaf macules. Long oval-shaped areas of white skin are one of the first signs of tuberous sclerosis to appear and are present in 90% of affected patients. In white skin, the macules may sometimes only be identified by UV-light examination in a darkened room (daughter of patient shown in 19.56)

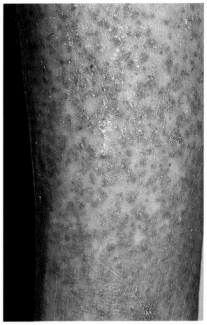

Fig 3.27 Post-inflammatory hypopigmentation. This is common in white and black skin after inflammatory dermatoses. In this patient, there is post-inflammatory hypopigmentation after eczema on the shin, with follicular repigmentation.

Pinta (caused by *Treponema carateum*), yaws (caused by *Treponema pertenue*) and secondary syphilis can all produce hypopigmented macules. In secondary syphilis, the so-called 'necklace of Venus,' comprising round or oval hypopigmented macules on the lateral neck of women, is said to be pathognomonic. Wood's light examination may be necessary to detect the changes.

Whorled and reticulate pigment loss ('marbled cake skin')

Whorled, streaky and segmental depigmentation that appears to follow Blaschko's lines (*see* Fig 2.10) occurs in some cases of naevus depigmentosus, in incontinentia pigmenti and in hypomelanosis of Ito (**Fig 3.28**).

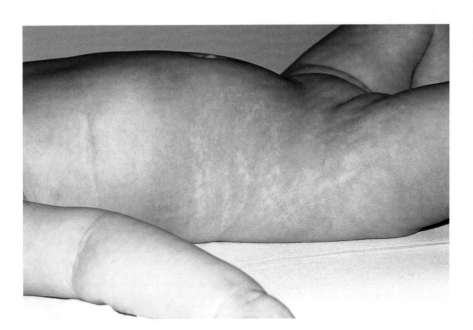

Fig 3.28 Hypomelanosis of Ito. Lesions have a swirled pattern, following Blaschko's lines (*see also* 2.10)

Incontinentia pigmenti is an uncommon, sex-linked, dominant dermatosis that affects girls; pregnancies with male fetuses usually result in spontaneous abortion. Affected babies have linear blisters (**Fig 3.29**), which resolve spontaneously by approximately 6 months of age, leaving irregular, streaky hypopigmentation and hyperpigmentation. In adult life, affected women can be identified by the presence of apparently hypopigmented streaky patches in which no hair follicles or sweat glands occur. These streaks are best seen on the backs of the calves (**Fig 3.30**). Loss of skin colour may be due to loss of hair follicles rather than pigment abnormalities, because histologically, they contain the same amount of pigment as the adjacent normal skin.

Patchy pigment loss with surface change

Pityriasis versicolor

In black or tanned skin, scattered white scaly patches appear (*see* Figs 7.14 and 7.15). This is discussed on pp. 75 and 122.

Pityriasis alba

Pityriasis alba usually presents on the face of children as slightly scaly hypopigmented patched with an indistinct border. It occurs in any race, but is most easily seen in people with black skin (**Fig 3.31**). It is a form of mild atopic eczema with associated post-inflammatory hypopigmentation.

Tuberculoid leprosy

In tuberculoid leprosy, lesions appear as few or solitary reddish plaques with a hypopigmented centre. Occasionally hypopigmented, but never totally depigmented, macules occur. The important feature to look for is loss of pinprick and fine touch sensation in the visibly altered skin, and palpable nerves radiating from the lesion. Nerves at distant sites may also be enlarged. Enlarged, purely sensory nerves are sometimes biopsied, including the greater auricular nerve in the neck and the sural nerve at the ankle.

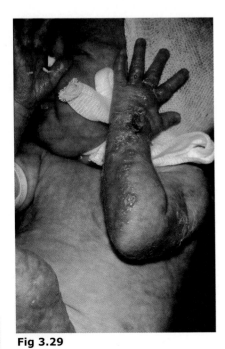

Fig 3.29

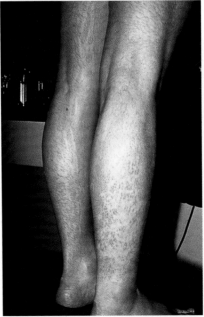

Fig 3.30

Fig 3.29, 3.30 Incontinentia pigmenti in a child (3.29). Linear, vesicular and crusted lesions on the limbs and trunk usually appear in the first few weeks of life. These resolve spontaneously at 4–6 months of age. Hyperpigmented streaks have been noted from 2 years of age. **Incontinentia pigmenti in an adult (3.30).** White hairless streaks, seen best on the limbs, are the predominant cutaneous abnormality in adult females with incontinentia pigment. Hair and sweating are absent in the white lesions (*photo courtesy of Dr Celia Moss*)

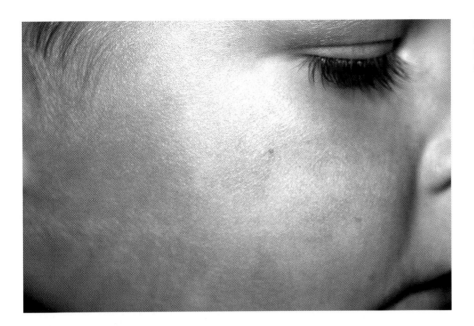

Fig 3.31 Pityriasis alba. Mild atopic eczema with associated post-inflammatory hypopigmentation on the face

Patchy pigment loss with thinning or thickening of the skin

Patchy pigment loss with thinning or thickening of the skin occurs in radio-dermatitis (*see* Figs 11.9 and 18.30), morphoea (**Fig 3.17**, *see also* Figs 8.27 and 11.36), lichen sclerosus et atrophicus (*see* Figs 8.28, 8.29, 11.4 and 11.5) and burns and scalds. These are discussed in Chapter 11.

RED/PURPLE COLOURS

Red/purple colours are the hallmark of lesions that have increased vascularity, inflammation or extravasation of blood into the skin. They are discussed separately in Chapter 17. Some inflammatory processes typically have a violaceous or purple component, such as lichen planus, dermatomyositis or orf (**Fig 3.33**).

DIAGNOSTIC TIPS AND PITFALLS

- Hairs in areas of vitiligo are usually white; regrowth of hair in alopecia areata may also be white, but the underlying skin colour is normal

- Jaundice and carotenaemia can be distinguished by examining the sclerae

- Not all blue–black pigmentation is due to melanoma

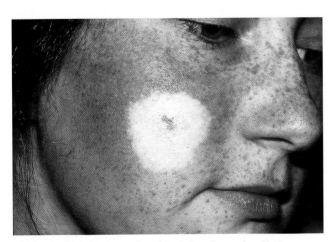

Fig 3.32 Morphoea. The skin is hard or sclerotic to touch, and the central area is white (*see also* 8.27)

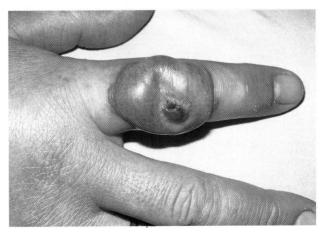

Fig 3.33 Inflammatory disorders. These usually cause a red or purple colour in skin, but lesions of orf often appear dusky blue

YELLOW COLOURS

Diffuse patterns of yellow colour

Jaundice

Jaundice produces a slightly greenish shade of yellow colour, most easily seen over the white sclerae in the early stages as, in the skin, it is masked by other pigments. Small green dots of bile emanating from sweat ducts have also been described.

Carotenaemia

Increased levels of carotene in blood may occur due to excessive ingestion, secondary to other conditions such as hypothyroidism or as an isolated metabolic abnormality. The yellow colour of carotenaemia is most readily seen on the palms (**Fig 3.34**) and around the axillary folds, but not in the sclerae—this distribution is explained by its excretion in sweat.

Localised yellow lesions

Xanthomas

Xanthomatous disorders may occur in different clinical patterns but are unified by their yellowish colour and are therefore described in this chapter. Types of xanthoma are described in **Table 3.10**, with the Fredricksen classification of hyperlipidaemia summarised in **Table 3.11**. Some examples are shown in **Figs 3.35–3.36**.

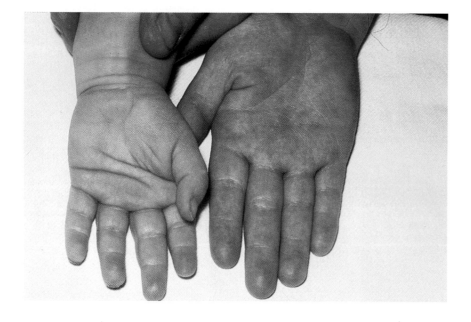

Fig 3.34 Carotenaemia.
Yellow–orange pigmentation due to carotenaemia, compared with the colour of a normal palm

Table 3.10 Types of xanthoma

Type of xanthoma	Clinical appearance	Underlying causes
Xanthelasma	Creamy yellow papules and plaques around the eyelids	Approximately 25% have hyperlipidaemia, usually hypercholesterolaemia in hyperlipoproteniaemia of Fredricksen types IIa or IIb (see below)
Tendon	Subcutaneous lumps on tendons and ligaments	Hyperlipoproteinaemia, Fredricksen types IIa, IIb or III, associated with diabetes mellitus, hypothyroidism, obstructive liver disease, cerebrotendinous xanthomatosis (plasma lipid levels may be normal)
Tuberous	Yellow papules and tumours, especially on pressure areas	Hyperlipoproteinaemia, Fredricksen types IIa, IIb or III
Plane	Yellowish macular or just palpable plaques present at various sites	Hyperlipoproteinaemia of Fredricksen type III, associated with diabetes mellitus Palmar crease plane xanthomas (xanthoma palmaris) are characteristic of type III dysbetalipoproteinaemia
Eruptive	Multiple yellow papules that come and go, sometimes itchy on the buttocks shoulders and extensor surfaces	Hyperlipoproteinaemia, Fredricksen types I, (IV) or V Associated with diabetes mellitus, pancreatitis, hypothyroidism (secondary hypertriglyceridaemia)
Diffuse plane xanthoma	Yellow or orange macules and palpable plaques	Associated with multiple myeloma, paraproteinaemia, acquired C1 esterase inhibitor deficiency (lipid levels are normal)

Table 3.11 Fredricksen classification of hyperlipoproteinaemia

Type	Lipid abnormality	Clinical appearances
Type I	Increased triglycerides levels in chylomicrons, due to deficiency of lipoprotein lipase or apoC-II deficiency	Eruptive xanthomas
Type IIa	Increased low-density lipoprotein (LDL) concentration	Xanthelasma Tendinous Xanthoma
Type IIb	Increased LDL and very-low-density lipoprotein concentration (VLDL). These occur in familial hypercholesterolaemia, familial combined hyperlipidaemia (may also present with type IV phenotype), polygenic hypercholesterolaemia	Xanthomas are usually tendon or xanthelasma; also plane xanthomas of fingerwebs and pressure areas in homozygous familial hypercholesterolaemia
Type III	Increased cholesterol and triglyceride concentrations, hyperbetalipoproteinaemia, due to deficient apoE	Combination of plane and tuberous xanthomas is diagnostic, may cause combination of eruptive and tuberous xanthomas
Type IV	Mild hypertriglyceridaemia, increased VLDL concentration without chylomicrons, due to various causes.	Most are asymptomatic
Type V	Increased VLDL concentration and chylomicrons, molecular defect uncertain.	Eruptive xanthomas

Juvenile xanthogranuloma

These lesions occur mainly in children—often on the face or scalp—and may be solitary or multiple (**Fig 3.37**). Rarely, but importantly, they may be associated with neurofibromatosis.

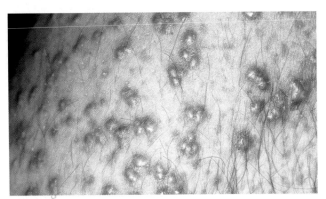

Fig 3.35

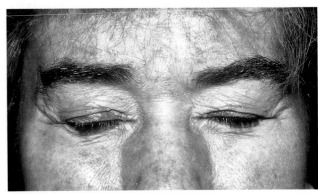

Fig 3.36

Fig 3.35, 3.36 Xanthomatous disorders. These may present as solitary nodules or papules, multiple papules, sheets of confluent papules or lesions localised to eyelids, palmar creases or over tendons. However, a unifying feature is the yellowish colour. (3.35) Eruptive xanthomata in a man who had a triglyceride concentration of 33.3 mmol/l (normal range 0.45–1.8) and a cholesterol concentration of 12.5 mmol/l (normal range <5.2). (3.36) Xanthelasma in a woman with normal fasting lipid concentrations.

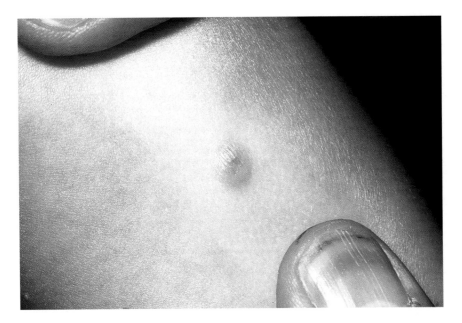

Fig 3.37 Juvenile xanthogranuloma. These yellow lesions are found mainly in children and are usually solitary or few in number. They do not signify the presence of hyperlipidaemia

4 Elicitation of physical signs

INTRODUCTION

Although most physical signs in dermatology are visual, many signs can be actively elicited. As with examination of any other organ system, experience dictates when to use special techniques to look for a specific feature, such as using Wood's light to demonstrate fluorescence of dermatophyte fungi or when there is a need to examine mucous membranes, hair, nails or teeth. Basic aspects of examination of the skin and simple techniques that can be helpful in making a diagnosis are considered in this chapter.

VISUAL INSPECTION OF THE SKIN

Examination of the skin requires a good light, preferably daylight. It is useful to have an additional light source so that side lighting can be used, as this may help to identify textural changes in the skin (*see* Chapter 11). A magnifying lens can be valuable for some purposes, notably examination of small lesions, capillary vessels (especially nailfold changes in connective tissue disorders (*see* Chapter 19)) and surface texture.

Do not forget that the first part of visual inspection is of the patient as a whole, which may reveal relevant associated features such as anaemia, jaundice or rheumatological or joint disease. An impression of degree of itch and of general malaise can also be gained. Details of clothing, dressings (**Fig 4.1**), cosmetic usage and evidence of cigarette smoking can all be useful in some situations. Formal examination of other organ systems may be required.

Simple techniques to assist in recording the results of inspection include:

- Measurement, tracing or photography to record the size and shape of lesions (for example, to record healing of wounds and ulcers).
- Marking the margin of lesions to demonstrate enlargement or resolution (for example, demonstrating the day-to-day variation in lesions of urticaria, **Figs 4.2** and **4.3**.

AIDS TO INSPECTION

Diascopy

Pressing a glass slide or, more safely, a colourless translucent plastic strip on to the skin forces blood out of surface vessels. Other colours in the skin are thus less obscured by the red colour of intravascular blood and can be visualised. This technique is also useful in the identification of purpura, as blood outside vessels will not disappear. Faint melanin pigmentation can be obscured by redness but is made visible by diascopy (**Figs 4.4** and **4.5**), and brownish translucent areas known as apple-jelly nodules are characteristic of lupus vulgaris (**Fig 4.6**). Stretching the skin with the fingertips is a less satisfactory method to blanch the skin, as it is too crude to visualise small lesions, but may be adequate. Occasionally, even blunt fingertip pressure can be used to demonstrate the non-vascular pigmentation of the skin (*see* Fig 3.20), but this only decreases blood flow very briefly and does not allow relaxed examination of the appearances. However, it is important to recognise that 'blanching with pressure' is common to any disorder in which vasodilation is a feature, and any erythematous rash will therefore blanch on pressure.

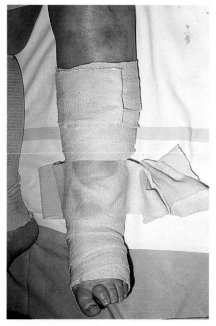

Fig 4.1 Inspection starts before the skin lesion is visible. The blue–green staining of this bandage over a leg ulcer strongly suggests pseudomonas infection

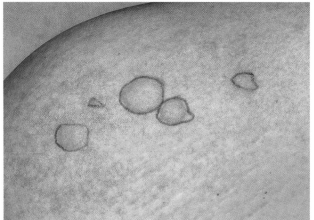

Fig 4.2

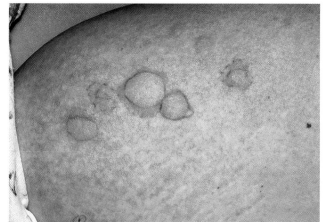

Fig 4.3

Figs 4.2, 4.3. Urticaria. The margin of lesions was marked with ink (solid line) when initially examined (4.2), and again after 30 minutes (dotted line (4.3)) showing asymmetrical expansion of the lesions. Small unmarked weals at the upper part of the figure have become more prominent, being little more than erythematous patches at baseline

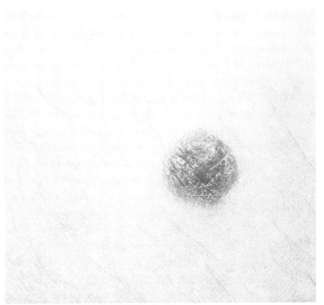

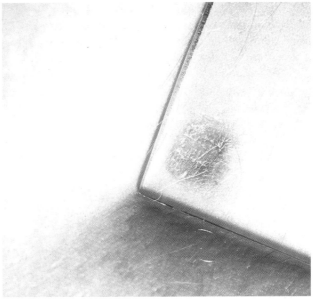

Fig 4.4

Fig 4.5

Figs 4.4, 4.5 Diascopy. Diascopy enables faint brown melanin pigment to be seen in this Spitz naevus (4.4). These lesions have a characteristically prominent vascular component, so faint pigmentation is obscured by the bright red colour of haemoglobin (4.5)

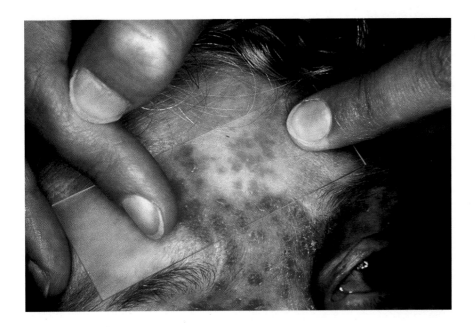

Fig 4.6 Diascopy of lupus vulgaris. This shows granulomatous apple-jelly nodules.

Wood's light

Examination of the skin using longwave ultraviolet (UV) light needs to be performed in a dark room, preferably without any other sources of fluorescence. It is used mainly in examination of pigmentary disorders and some cutaneous infections. It accentuates epidermal pigmentation and therefore exaggerates the difference between normal skin and depigmented areas, e.g. vitiligo, piebaldism and chemical leucoderma. By contrast, dermal pigmentation disorders with normal overlying epidermal pigmentation are obscured; thus post-inflammatory pigmentation is less obvious under Wood's light than it is in visible light. Similarly, naevus anaemicus (*see* Fig 3.19), a pale area of skin with normal melanin content but abnormal vasoconstriction, may be obvious in normal lighting but becomes invisible under Wood's light.

This technique is also used to demonstrate fluorescence in several infective disorders, such as some types of scalp ringworm (green–blue), pityriasis versicolor (yellow, **Figs 4.7** and **4.8**) and erythrasma (coral pink, **Figs 4.9** and **4.10** *see also* Fig 5.13). It may also be used in the clinic as a screening test for urinary porphyrins (seen best in acidified urine, but sometimes visible in routine urine samples, (**Figs 4.11** and **4.12**). In addition, it has been used to examine clothing in an unusual disorder known as chromhidrosis, in which coloured apocrine sweat fluoresces (**Fig 4.13**).

Limitations of the technique in inexperienced hands are the difficulties in recognition of non-pathological fluorescence due to clothing fibres or some oils (pale blue–green fluorescence) or of simple reflection of violet light from scaling dermatoses. White medical coats or white shirts are best avoided when using Wood's light, since these usually fluoresce very brightly due to optical brighteners added to detergents (**Figs 4.14** and **4.15**), and this may obscure the less prominent fungal fluorescence. Topical therapies can cause confusion, for example tetracyclines fluoresce yellow–green.

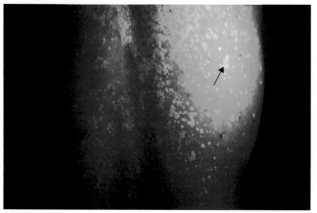

Fig 4.7

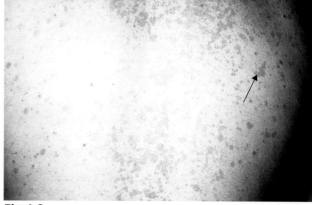

Fig 4.8

Figs 4.7, 4.8 Wood's light examination of pityriasis versicolor. Yellow fluorescence (4.7), although the lesions are a pale brown colour in normal lighting (4.8). An individual large lesion is identified (arrow) to demonstrate this point

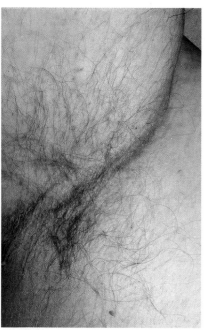

Figs 4.9, 4.10 Use of Wood's light to identify erythrasma. The erythrasma fluoresces coral pink (4.9). The chemical producing the fluorescence is a water-soluble porphyrin. This is why negative results may be obtained if the patient has previously washed the affected area. In this case, the extent of fluorescence is less than the extent of the pigmentation, probably representing incomplete removal of the porphyrin from the apex of the axillary vault (4.10).

Fig 4.9

Fig 4.10

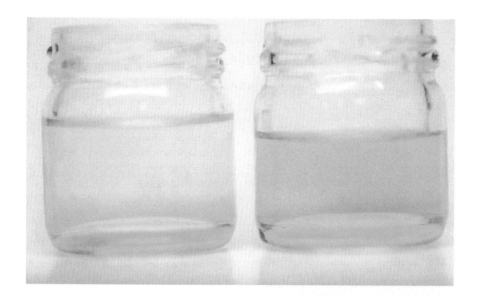

Fig 4.11 Porphyria cutanea tarda.
The urine from a patient with this
condition has a slightly darker colour
than that of the control sample

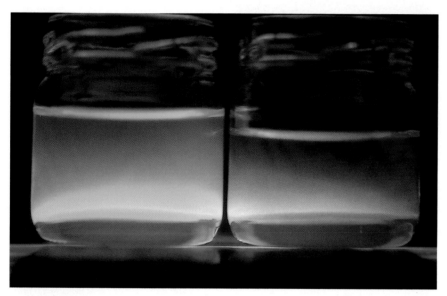

Fig 4.12 Porphyria cutanea tarda.
Same urine samples as in Fig 4.11,
showing pink fluorescence of the
affected urine under Wood's light.

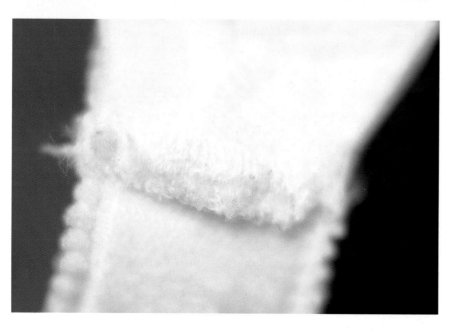

Fig 4.13 Chromhidrosis. This
patient described her clothing as
turning green. Faint green
discoloration of seams of underwear
was accentuated under Wood's light
(shown), and skin biopsy revealed
that lipofuscins in her apocrine glands
also autofluoresced

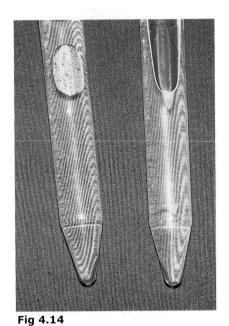

Fig 4.14

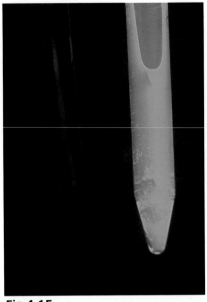

Fig 4.15

Figs 4.14, 4.15 Optical brighteners in detergents. These fluoresce with a blue colour under Wood's light. In, 4.14 the tube on the left contains water only, and that on the right a dilute solution of a household washing powder. Under Wood's light (4.15), the tube of water is invisible, whereas the detergent fluoresces vivid blue. This is the explanation for washed clothing looking 'whiter than white,' but it is a distraction when performing Wood's light examination

Wood's light can be utilised in conjunction with the external application of fluorescent chemicals such as fluorescein to identify the burrows of the scabies mite. Fluorescein is applied topically and the excess wiped off; the curvilinear burrows can then be viewed under Wood's light. Fluorescein has also been used in trials of topical agents to determine sites of application.

Oil

Application of oil or water to the skin replaces air between scales with the applied liquid and therefore alters the reflective properties of the multiple air–keratin interfaces in the stratum corneum, making it more translucent, by reducing reflection from keratin. The classic situation where this is helpful is in the identification of the presence of Wickham's striae in lesions of lichen planus (**Fig 4.16**). The same technique is used in dermatoscopy (or epiluminescent microscopy), a surface magnification technique that can help in diagnosis of pigmented lesions (**Fig 4.17**). It can also help in the visualisation of the burrows of scabies mites. The same effect can be achieved by wetting the skin but is much more transient.

Ink

Fountain pen blue–black ink can be used for mycological examination of fungi and pityrosporum yeasts in skin scrapings (**Fig 4.43**). Details of clinical mycology are discussed later. Ink can also be used to outline the burrows of scabies mites (in a similar manner to the use of fluorescein) but can be viewed without the need for a UV light source.

Other chemicals

Functional sweat glands can be identified by the use of Minor's starch–iodine test. Anhydrous iodine, which is yellow, and starch in oil are applied to the skin. The water content of sweat causes the formation of a black reaction product, which is visible as small dots at the site of the sweat duct orifices (**Figs 4.18** and **4.19**). Localised abnormalities of sweating can be identified using this technique or other chemicals such as o-phthalaldehyde, or ferric chloride-tannic acid (*see* Fig 6.1).

DIAGNOSTIC TIPS AND PITFALLS

- Erythema may obscure other colours but can be reduced or removed by stretching the skin or by direct pressure, ideally with a translucent glass or plastic strip so that the residual colours can be visualised

- Wood's light accentuates epidermal pigmentary disorders but conceals dermal and vascular lesions

- In using Wood's light to examine the skin for dermatophyte or yeast infection, be aware that only certain species will fluoresce; a negative examination therefore does not exclude fungal disease

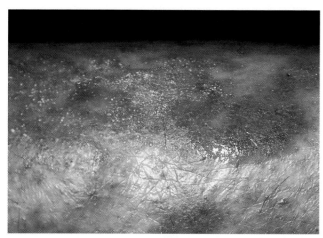

Fig 4.16 Application of oil to the skin. This decreases reflection from the skin surface and prevents reflected light obscuring underlying details such as these fine white reticulate Wickham's striae in lichen planus. Water can be used in the same way, but the effect is brief as the water rapidly evaporates

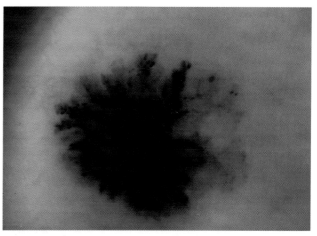

Fig 4.17 Dermatoscopy (epiluminescent microscopy). Dermatoscope view of malignant melanoma

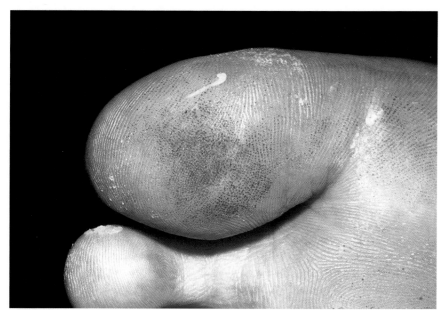

Fig 4.18

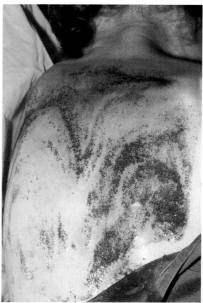

Fig 4.19

Figs 4.18, 4.19 Starch–iodine test. Plantar surface of the hallux, in a patient with hyperhydrosis, treated with iodine in alcohol and then corn starch in oil. Black dots at the orifices of the sweat ducts can be seen, where water has allowed the formation of a black reaction product between the starch and iodine (4.18). In 4.19, the same test used in a patient with hypohidrotic ectodermal dysplasia clearly shows absent sweating in a pattern that follows Blaschko's lines (*see also* 2.10). (From Clark A & Burn J (1991) *Med Genet* **28**: 330, *Courtesy of British Medical Association*)

Capillary microscopy

Although specialist equipment is expensive, an ophthalmoscope or dermatoscope can allow useful enhancement of capillary detail in nailfolds and other lesions; mineral oil should be applied to the skin first as it reduces reflection of light from the stratum corneum and thus improves the transparency of this layer (*see* Fig 19.41).

Hess test

Capillary fragility or platelet defects can be assessed semiquantitatively by the Hess test (tourniquet test). A sphygmomanometer cuff is applied to the upper arm at between systolic and diastolic pressure for 5 minutes, and the number of petechiae in a predetermined 5 cm diameter circle is counted after the pressure is released; more than five is considered abnormal (**Fig 4.20**). The integrity of the capillary wall depends on various factors, and an abnormal Hess test result may be the result of variety of problems including abnormalities of the vessel wall, thrombocytopenia and platelet dysfunction.

PALPATION

The importance of actually touching the skin during cutaneous examination must be emphasised. Skin texture and quality of scaling can be adequately assessed only by palpation, which is also essential for determining tenderness, consistency, surface changes and fixation of localised lesions. Abnormally warm or cold skin can be determined by palpation, and abnormalities of sweating can be detected by the observer as wet or dry skin with altered texture.

In addition to simply feeling the skin, specific manœuvres that can be useful are discussed below.

Linear pressure

Dermographic weals (*see* Fig 16.7) are elicited by scoring the skin using blunt pressure from a narrow but not sharp object, such as an orange stick or fingernail.

Shearing of clinically normal skin to form blisters can occur in intra-epidermal blistering disorders, notably pemphigus, and is known as Nikolsky's sign (*see* p. 236).

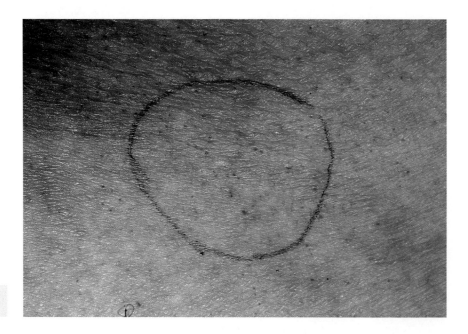

Figs 4.20 Hess test. Purpuric spots have appeared in a marked circle on the arm after application of a blood pressure cuff above venous pressure

Blunt pressure and point pressure

Fingertip pressure can be used to determine whether oedema can be pitted and also to assess capillary refill in circulatory disorders. Pressure produces blanching (*see also* diascopy above); capillary refill is normally visible as a rapid return of pinkness to blanched skin, but this is delayed in arterial disease.

Point pressure using a suspended weight can identify a specific type of physical urticaria known as delayed pressure urticaria. One version of this test uses a sling containing bricks or full wine bottles arranged so that the hanging weight compresses a marble on the flexor aspect of the horizontal forearm or on the extensor thigh with the patient sitting. The weight should be 2–10 kg and applied for 10–30 minutes. This type of urticaria appears about 8–12 hours after the stimulus and lasts for many hours.

Point pressure applied to some focal lesions may identify an underlying dermal defect through which the nodule can be partially compressed, e.g. neurofibromas, anetoderma (**Figs 4.21** and **4.22**). This has been likened to palpating a buttonhole. Pressure on the top of a blister may cause it to spread (*see* Figs 13.9 and 13.10).

Squeezing

Squeezing can be helpful in localisation of the level of a lesion. Because the dermis is fibrous, it can be picked up as a fold of skin and moved over subcutaneous nodules or deeper lesions within muscle or bone, unless these are fixed to the lower part of the dermis. Such manipulation may not be possible in areas where the skin is tight, such as the scalp, and in this case, deep nodules may seem to be attached to the skin. By contrast, squeezing a firm intradermal nodule, such as a dermatofibroma (**Fig 4.23**), may cause it to wrinkle or dimple at the skin surface.

Increased skin turgor also decreases the ability to squeeze a pinch of skin. A typical situation where this is applied as a diagnostic test is in lymphoedema of the foot. Normally, a pinch of skin can be obtained on the dorsum of the second toe, but this is impossible when there is established lymphoedema, as the skin becomes more rigid (Kaposi–Stemmer sign).

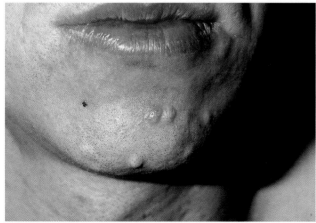

Fig 4.21

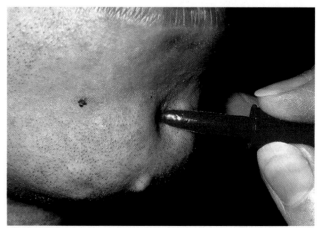

Fig 4.22

Figs 4.21, 4.22 Anetoderma. Lesions of anetoderma, in this case secondary to previous inflammation, are soft nodules of subcutaneous tissue (4.21), which protrude through a dermal defect identified by point pressure (4.22)

69

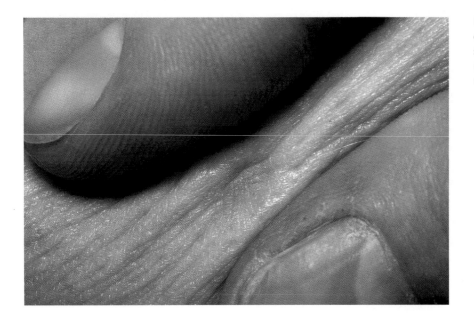

Fig 4.23 Squeezing a dermatofibroma. Squeezing the skin around a firm intradermal nodule, such as this dermatofibroma, may produce a dimple effect

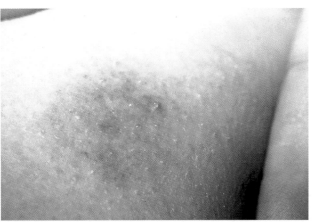

Fig 4.24

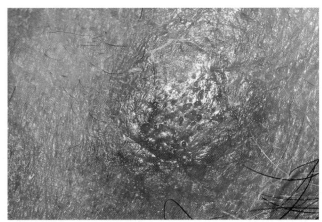

Fig 4.25

Figs 4.24, 4.25 Squeezing. In a disorder known as follicular mucinosis, squeezing the lesions may cause expression of visible mucin globules from the hair follicle orifice (4.24). **Squeezing acute eczema** (4.25). This may result in the expression of epidermal oedema fluid, which can be confused with mucin but is less viscid

Squeezing can sometimes cause extrusion of foreign material, such as splinters, or of abnormal endogenous material, such as cyst contents or mucin (**Figs 4.24** and **4.25**). By contrast, lateral stretching is used to produce blanching (*see* Diascopy, pp 62–63).

Stretching

Stretching the skin, typically using a thumb and index finger, produces blanching. It also allows improved visualisation of some firm deep nodules such as 'submarine' comedones in acne (**Figs 4.26** and **4.27**).

Rubbing

In cutaneous mast-cell disorders, typically urticaria pigmentosa (**Figs 4.28–4.30**, *see also* Fig 9.53), rubbing the lesions causes release of inflammatory mediators from mast cells, and the brown lesions become red with a surrounding flare known as Darier's sign. Rubbing a neuroblastoma releases vasoconstricting catecholamines and causes a pale halo around the red–blue nodule.

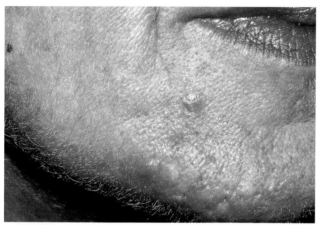

Fig 4.26

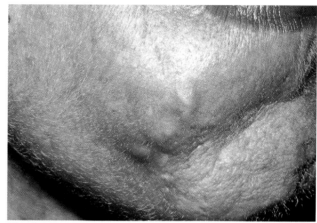

Fig 4.27

Figs 4.26, 4.27 'Submarine' comedones in acne. These may be difficult to see (4.26) until the skin is stretched (4.27). The easiest way to do this is for the patient to stretch the skin of the cheek by pressure from the tongue (From Cunliffe WJ *et al.* (2000) *Br J Dermatol* **142**: 1084–1091, *courtesy of Professor W Cunliffe*)

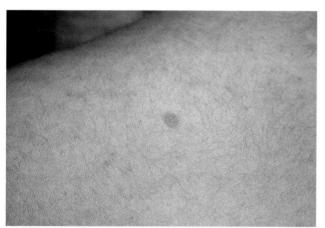

Fig 4.28

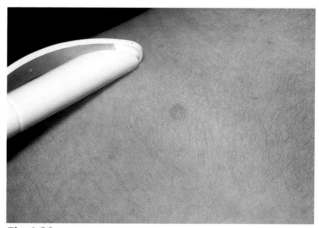

Fig 4.29

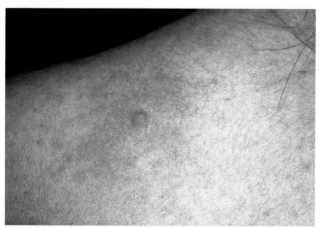

Fig 4.30

Figs 4.28–4.30 Darier's sign. When an urticaria pigmentosa lesion (4.28) is rubbed with a blunt object (4.29), it causes the release of histamine and other inflammatory mediators from mast cells; the effect is apparent within a few minutes (4.30) as oedema and erythema ('urtication') of the initially brown plaque (*see also* 9.53).

Scratching

Scratching the surface of a psoriatic plaque with a thumbnail gives the surface scale a noticeably silvery appearance (**Fig 4.31**), a technique known as grattage. Similarly, the fine scale of pityriasis versicolor can be accentuated by scratching over the surface of the lesions (*see* Figs 7.14, 7.15). Inadvertent minor scratches may produce linear purpura in amyloidosis (*see* Fig 17.24), cryoglobulinaemia and sometimes vasculitic disorders, such as Henoch–Schönlein purpura (*see* Fig 17.23).

Picking

Picking scale off the surface of a psoriatic lesion causes small bleeding points. This phenomenon, known as Auspitz's sign, is classically described in psoriasis but is not specific to this dermatosis. It is important to pick crust off ulcers or nodules to assess the features adequately (**Figs 4.32 and 4.33**).

Pricking

Impaired pin-prick sensation is an important feature of neuropathic ulcers and is a classic feature of leprosy. Development of lesions at the site of injection of serum or saline, after venesection or after other minor trauma, is known as pathergy and is characteristic of pyoderma gangrenosum and Behçet's disease.

Heat and cold

Localised heat and cold can be used to identify specific types of physical urticaria. Examples include the 'ice cube test' which is employed to recognise cold urticaria (*see* Fig 16.11), and warming the patient in a bath to show cholinergic urticaria (*see* Fig 16.10). This type of urticaria can also be provoked by exercise (**Figs 4.34 and 4.35**).

DIAGNOSTIC TIPS AND PITFALLS

- Feeling the skin and actively palpating the quality of scaling, texture of lesions, etc. is an integral part of cutaneous examination

- Scaling and crusting may obscure diagnostic features; physical removal of surface scabs may be of great value

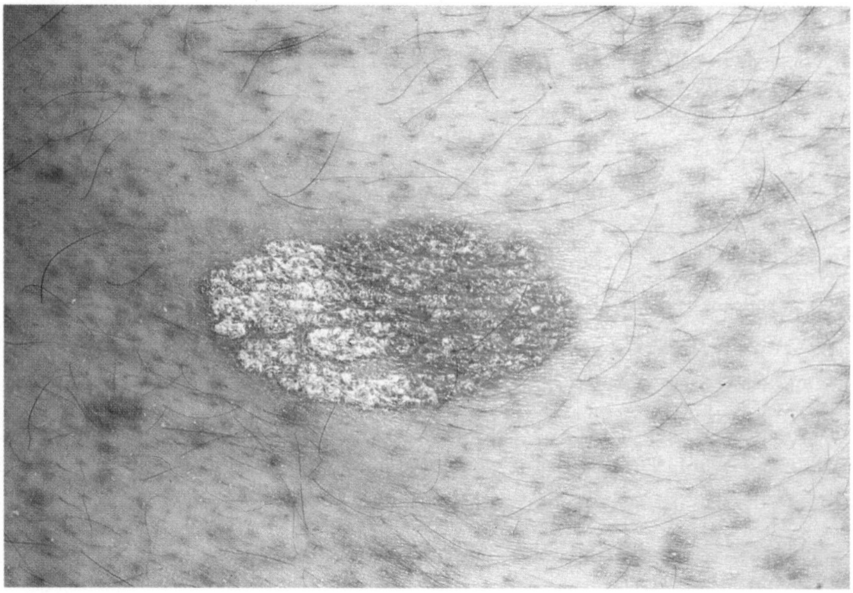

Fig 4.31 Typical silvery scale of psoriasis. Gentle scratching of half of this plaque of psoriasis shows the typical scale and the fact that this can be actively elicited

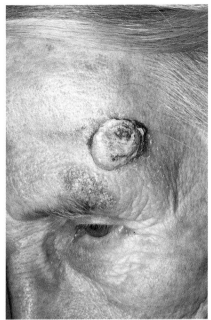

Fig 4.32

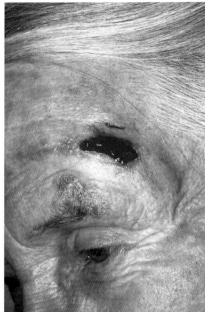

Fig 4.33

Fig 4.32, 4.33 Removal of crust.
Removing the crust from this
forehead lesion showed it to be oval
rather than rounded in shape.
Although this did not allow a
confident diagnosis in this case, it did
mean that excision could be
performed with primary closure of the
wound, which would not have been
easy for the larger rounded area
covered by the crust

SCALPELS AND SKIN SCRAPINGS

Paring the surface keratin from some lesions can be a helpful diagnostic manœuvre, especially in the differential diagnosis of warts and corns (**Figs 4.36** and **4.37**). The tiny black spots that constitute talon noir (*see* Fig 9.47) are due to old blood that has leaked from capillaries into the epidermis, and these can be pared off with a scalpel to provide reassurance about the nature of this disorder. Paring the surface of a nail may enable subungual haematomas to be visualised and may also allow samples to be taken to confirm the presence of blood, although this can be difficult to perform. Scoring the surface of the nail enables nail growth to be assessed; it can also confirm the movement of a subungual haematoma—the distance to the score mark or edge of the haematoma being measured from a fixed point, such as the distal part of the lunula.

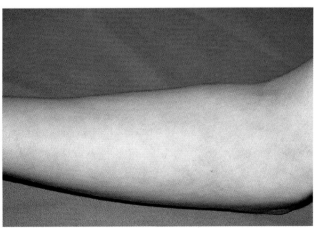

Fig 4.34

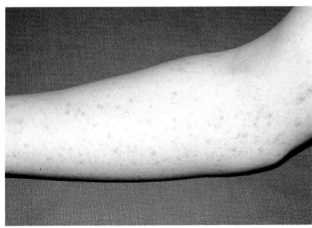

Fig 4.35

Figs 4.34, 4.35 Cholinergic urticaria. The normal skin of the arm in this patient (4.34) has developed numerous lesions shortly after a period of exercise (4.35)

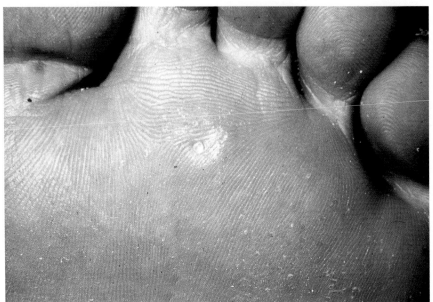

Fig 4.36

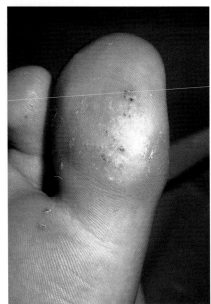

Fig 4.37

Figs 4.36, 4.37 Pared surface of a corn. This shows a central shiny area (4.36), compared with the small dark vessels of a pared wart (4.37)

Taking skin scrapings for mycological examination requires use of microscopy and is not strictly a clinical physical sign. However, the technique is one that can be used in the clinic without special tissue processing and is therefore illustrated (**Figs 4.38–4.42**). Scrapings are placed in 20% potassium hydroxide and warmed to soften the keratinous scales; spores and hyphae are visible without special stains, but ink enhances visualisation (**Fig 4.43**).

Another technique that requires microscopy and staining of specimens but no involved processing is the Tzanck smear test. This test is used as a rapid confirmation of herpesvirus infections. The base of a vesicle is gently scraped and the material placed on a glass slide, which is then stained with Giemsa or Wright's stain in the same way as a routine haematology blood film. Multinucleated giant cells confirm the diagnosis. However, compared with virology culture results, false positive results occur in about 5% of cases and false negative results in about 30%.

OTHER SENSES

Sense of smell can be important but is considered only briefly as it cannot be demonstrated in a textbook. Many smells are most apparent from the breath, e.g. ketones, or on clothing and are not discussed here. Several factors contribute to smell from the skin, including:

- The action of bacteria on sweat and sebum.
- Bacterial degradation of the stratum corneum, which has been softened by sweat (odour from feet, pitted keratolysis of the feet, intertrigo, disorders of keratinisation such as Darier's disease).
- Infections, especially anaerobic infection of leg ulcers or fungating tumours.
- Ingested foods, particularly onions and garlic.
- Endogenous metabolites, especially in amino acidurias. Some of these are very specific and recognisable, such as the fishy smell of trimethylamin-uria, although the smell is initially apparent in the urine rather than from the skin.
- Topical applications, including some medicaments.

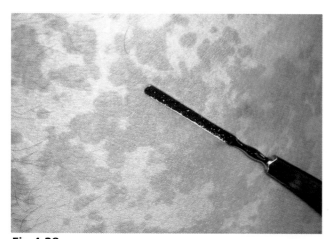
Fig 4.38

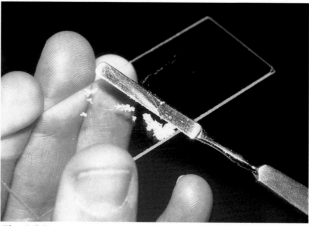
Fig 4.39

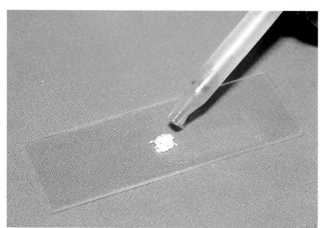
Fig 4.40

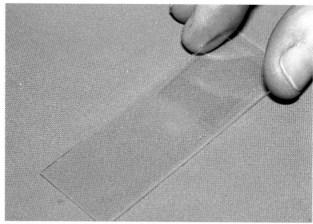
Fig 4.41

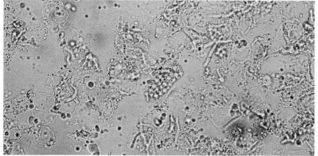
Fig 4.42

Figs 4.38–4.42 Mycological examination of skin scrapings in a patient with pityriasis versicolor. Scrapings are taken by gently scratching the skin surface (4.38), and scale is transferred to a microscope slide (4.39). Keratin is dissolved using 20% potassium hydroxide solution (4.40), a coverslip is applied to protect the microscope lens (4.41), and microscopy shows spores and hyphae of *Pityrosporum ovale* (4.42)

SPECIAL STRUCTURES

Hair

The following procedures can be useful in hair disorders:

- Wood's light examination for some fungi.
- Examination of scalp hairs (or eyebrows in some disorders) with a hand lens or a simple microscope may reveal abnormalities of the hair shaft, such as breaks or kinking (**Fig 4.44**).
- Hair is loose and easily pulled out in alopecia areata (*see* Fig 18.22) and in inflammatory ringworm infections (kerion).

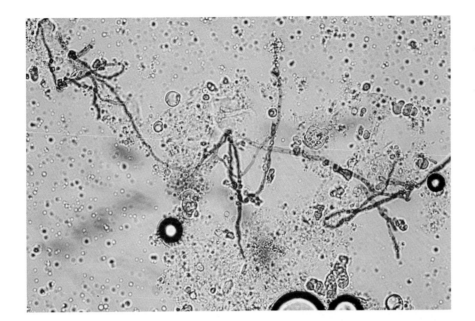

Fig 4.43 Visibility of spores and hyphae. This can be increased if they are stained with blue–black ink. In this case, *Trichophyton rubrum* hyphae have been stained with 'Quink' blue–black ink

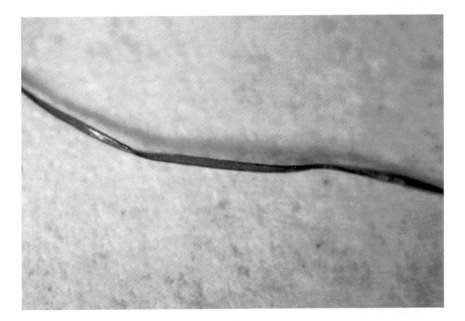

Fig 4.44 Examination of a 'corkscrew hair' in scurvy shows that the hair is irregularly kinked with flat, ribbon-like regions. Compare with the more common rolled hairs (*see* 6.4)

- Ingrowing beard hairs (pseudofolliculitis barbae, *see* Fig 14.10) can be identified by using a needle to lift up the ingrowing portion of the hair.
- A group of about 20 hairs can be pulled out to assess the proportion of actively growing hairs by counting anagen (growing) and telogen (resting) hair bulbs. This requires a degree of expertise and is generally performed only by experienced trichologists or dermatologists with a specific interest in hair disorders.

Teeth

Although rarely important in dermatological examination, teeth are accessible and should be routinely inspected in children with inherited skin disorders, as enamel deficiency is a feature of some types of epidermolysis bullosa, and abnormalities of dentition occur in several genodermatoses.

Eyes

Conjunctival or scleral vascular abnormalities are seen in disorders as diverse as rosacea and ataxia telangiectasia, whereas retinal vascular abnormalities are found in pseudoxanthoma elasticum, Fabry's disease (angiokeratoma corporis diffusum) and vasculitic disorders. Conjunctivitis occurs due to infections, and blistering disorders such as erythema multiforme (**Fig 4.45**) and cicatricial pemphigoid (**Fig 4.46**) may lead to conjunctival scarring.

Herpesvirus infections cause corneal ulceration.

Uveitis is found in sarcoidosis and Behçet's disease. Genetic disorders such as neurofibromatosis (Lisch nodules of iris) (*see* Fig 9.20) and tuberous sclerosis (retinal nodules) can have characteristic ocular signs.

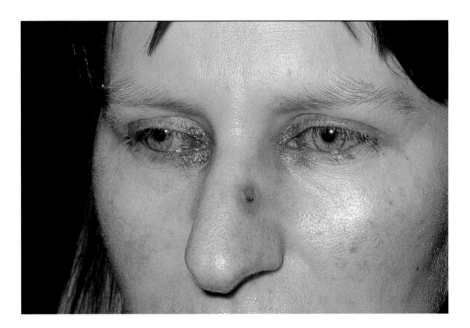

Fig 4.45 Severe conjunctivitis in a patient with Stevens–Johnson syndrome. Note that there is a lesion of erythema multiforme on the nose. Conjunctivitis can occur in cases of erythema multiforme without other mucous membrane involvement

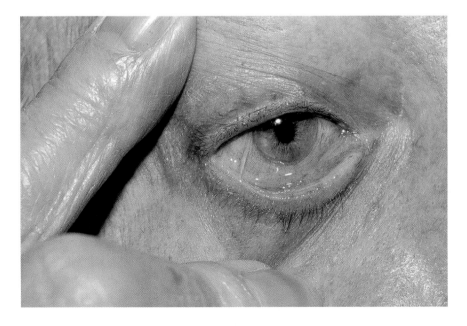

Fig 4.46 Cicatrical pemphigoid affecting the eye, causing scarring (symblepharon) and severe visual impairment. For this reason, the name 'benign mucous membrane pemphigoid' is something of a misnomer

5 Regional distribution

INTRODUCTION

The distribution of many dermatological disorders is determined by the presence of skin appendages (e.g. sebaceous glands, hair) or site variations in fat deposition of vascular supply. Similarly, external factors such as exposure to sunlight or contact with allergens or irritants may determine the body sites affected. Disorders associated with different anatomical sites are discussed in this chapter.

MIDLINE LESIONS

Midline lesions often arise owing to defects of embryological fusion and are of particular importance in children. Midline lesions of the face, scalp, nape of the neck and lower back are of particular concern as they can have deep connections to neural or meningeal structures. Lumbosacral hypertrichosis ('faun tail', **Fig 5.1**), naevi, vascular lesions or dimples may all occur in conjunction with spina bifida. Midline scalp nodules in babies or infants may represent encephalocoeles or meningocoeles. Such lesions may alter in size owing to crying or if the jugular vein is compressed (Furstenberg's sign).

SCALP

Hair disorders are considered in Chapter 18. Absence of scalp hair, especially male pattern baldness, exposes the scalp to sun damage so that actinic keratoses (*see* Fig 9.86), basal cell carcinoma (*see* Figs 9.73–9.77) and squamous cell carcinoma (*see* Fig 9.95) are common on the bald scalp. Presumably because of the high blood flow, the scalp is a relatively common site for cutaneous metastases (*see* Fig 9.78) from solid tumours (i.e. of the breast stomach, lung, uterus, large intestine, kidney, prostate ovary, liver, bone).

Rashes that usually, or sometimes exclusively, involve the scalp (**Table 5.1**) include psoriasis (**Fig 5.2**), seborrhoeic dermatitis (*see* Fig 18.53), dandruff and lichen simplex.

Fig 5.1 'Faun tail'

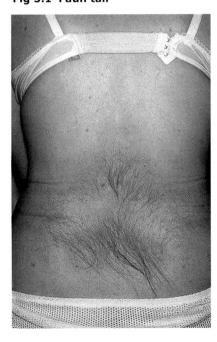

Table 5.1 Localised lesions and rashes that characteristically or commonly affect the scalp

Hair disorders	Alopecias, hair shaft abnormalities, infections and infestations (see chapter 18)
Rashes	Psoriasis (5.2, 8.14), seborrhoeic eczema (18.53), lichen simplex
Localised lesions	Epidermoid and pilar cysts, naevus sebaceous (syn. organoid naevus) (9.57) and hair follicle tumours, actinic keratoses (9.86), basal cell carcinoma, squamous cell carcinoma, cutaneous metastases (9.78)

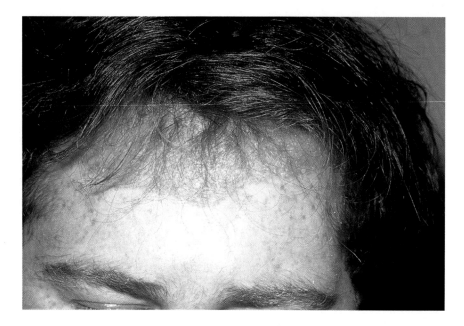

Fig 5.2 Scalp. Psoriasis often involves the scalp margin

Some localised disorders, such as epidermoid and pilar cysts, are common on the scalp. The term sebaceous cyst is a misnomer. These cysts are lined by a keratinising squamous epithelium. The foul-smelling contents are inspissated keratin.

Naevus sebaceous (organoid naevus) is a hamartoma containing sebaceous glands, which presents during childhood as a yellowish bald area. It is more common on the scalp than on other body sites. Various hair follicle neoplasms, such as cylindromas, also occur mainly on the scalp.

FACE

Consultations about facial rashes and lesions (**Table 5.2**) are common. The four most usual problems include eczema, acne, rosacea and discoid lupus erythematosus (*see* Fig 7.40). The presence of large numbers of sebaceous glands explains the distribution of acne (*see* Fig 14.6), rosacea (*see* Fig 2.44) and seborrhoeic dermatitis (*see* Fig 7.16) as these result from diseases of this skin appendage or its secretions. Ingrowing beard hairs cause pseudofolliculitis barbae (*see* Fig 14.10), and shaving may spread bacterial, viral wart (*see* Figs 9.54 and 8.26) and herpes simplex infections.

Exposure to sunlight can lead to chronic changes, for example elastosis (*see* Fig 6.17), lentigo (*see* Fig 9.21), actinic keratoses (*see* Figs 7.33 and 7.34) and tumours such as squamous cell carcinoma. Acute sun exposure results in burning and may aggravate rosacea, as well as causing several specific photodermatoses.

Many rashes affect the face, sometimes as part of a generalised distribution and sometimes as a specific site. They include atopic dermatitis, which

DIAGNOSTIC TIPS AND PITFALLS

- The four commonest causes of facial rashes are eczema (all types), acne, rosacea and discoid lupus erythematosus

- Atopic dermatitis affects the skin around the ears, eyelids and mouth

- Seborrhoeic dermatitis affects the scalp margin, ears, eyebrows and nasolabial folds

- Contact dermatitis may result from direct application (e.g. of cosmetics), rubbing the face with contaminated hands (e.g. rubber, metals and nail varnish) or by airborne exposure (e.g. perfumes, phosphorus sesquisulphide in red match heads)

- Psoriasis commonly affects the scalp margin (*see* **5.2**) and ears but can be found on any part of the face

- Rosacea produces redness, usually with papules and pustules, of the nose, cheeks, forehead and chin but typically spares the immediate perioral and periorbital skin

Table 5.2 Localised lesions and rashes that characteristically or commonly affect the face

Rashes

Any part of face	Eczema (seborrhoeic (7.27), atopic (15.24), allergic contact (15.40)) Photosensitivity (drugs (2.31), polymorphic light eruption, photosensitivity dermatitis) Acne (14.6) Discoid lupus erythematosus Psoriasis (5.2) Infections (herpes simplex, herpes zoster, impetigo (7.4)), Scleroderma (11.39) Angio-oedema (16.3)
Butterfly pattern	Rosacea (2.44) Systemic, some discoid, lupus erythematosus (8.21) Erysipelas (17.1) Lupus pernio (5.3)
Periorbital	Eczema (atopic, seborrhoeic blepharitis, contact allergy to nickel, eyedrops) Dermatomyositis ('heliotrope rash') (5.4, 5.5) Purpura due to the Valsalva manœuvre (periorbital petechiae) Amyloidosis (Panda sign of periorbital purpura) Neonatal lupus erythematosus ('owl facies')

Localised lesions

Naevi (9.25)
Seborrhoeic warts (9.79), solar lentigines (9.21)
Actinic keratoses (7.33)
Basal cell carcinoma (9.73), squamous cell carcinoma
Keratoacanthoma
Epidermoid cysts (9.56)
Appendage tumours—syringoma (eyelids)
Xanthelasma (eyelids) (3.36)

particularly affects the skin (*see* Fig 15.24) around the ears, eyelids and mouth, and seborrhoeic dermatitis, which affects the scalp margin, ears, eyebrows and nasolabial folds. Contact dermatitis is also common and may occur as a result of direct application of allergens (e.g. cosmetics), rubbing the face with contaminated hands (e.g. rubber, metals, nail varnish) or airborne exposure (e.g. perfumes, phosphorus sesquisulphide in red match heads).

Psoriasis commonly affects the scalp margin (*see* Fig 5.2) and ears but can be found on any part of the face.

Less common eruptions that characteristically affect the face include the chronic form of sarcoidosis, lupus pernio (**Fig 5.3**), and the rare acute (butterfly rash) form of lupus erythematosus (*see* Fig 17.5).

The eyelids consist of soft, thin skin that swells easily. Dermatomyositis causes oedema and a violaceous colour of the eyelids (**Figs 5.4 and 5.5**) known as the heliotrope rash (heliotropes are a plant species with purple flowers). Oedema at this site can also occur in eczema, angio-oedema, myxoedema, nephrotic syndrome, infectious mononucleosis, trichinosis (syn. trichiniasis, a parasitic worm infection) and superior vena cava obstruction.

Infections, such as impetigo (*see* Fig 7.4), often affect the face. The face is also a common site for erysipelas (*see* Fig 17.1) and herpes zoster.

Common discrete lesions on the face include naevi, which in time often evolve into flesh coloured, dome-shaped papules (*see* Figs 9.23–9.25) and seborrhoeic warts (*see* Fig 9.79). In black races, some normal variants, such as dermatosis papulosa nigra (*see* Fig 6.34), typically occur on the cheeks. Other localised facial lesions include milia (*see* Fig 6.48), xanthelasma (*see* Fig 3.36) and syringomata (*see* Fig 9.61).

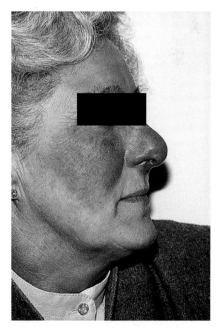

Fig 5.3 Face. Lupus pernio, a chronic form of sarcoidosis, characteristically affects the nose and cheek region and has a dusky purple colour. It is associated with other chronic features of the disease, such as those affecting the lungs and bone

81

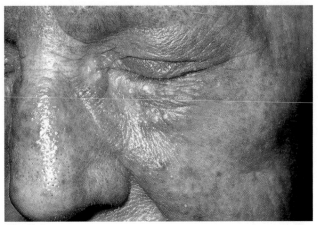

Fig 5.4

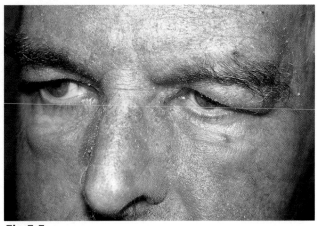

Fig 5.5

Fig 5.4, 5.5 Eyelids. These are a typical site in dermatomyositis, which causes the violaceous heliotrope rash seen here (5.4). Oedema may also be a prominent feature of dematomyositis (5.5)

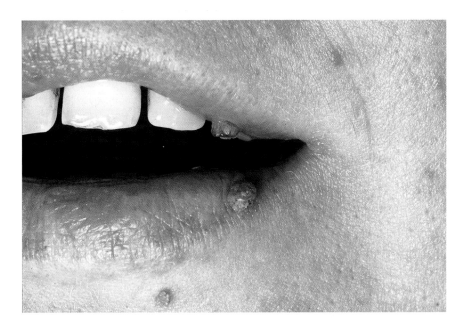

Fig 5.6 Lips. Viral warts are common on the lips. Two lesions on surfaces that are apposed are known as kissing lesions, particularly appropriate in this example (*see also* 9.85)

Lips

Infections such as viral warts (**Fig 5.6**) and cold sores due to herpes simplex virus, are common on the lips (**Table 5.3**).

Angular cheilitis occurring at the corners of the mouth (*see* Fig 1.10) may be the result of iron deficiency, local candidiasis or, more commonly, change in facial shape, especially in patients with worn dentures.

Eczema produces scaling, fissuring and oozing of the skin around the lips; the cause may be atopic dermatitis—an irritant effect of licking—or contact allergy to cosmetics (**Fig 5.7**) or toothpaste.

Swelling of the lips occurs as an episodic phenomenon in angio-oedema or a more fixed abnormality in granulomatous cheilitis (**Fig 5.8**) and Crohn's disease.

Erosions and blistering of the lips occur as a result of pemphigus vulgaris or with mucous membrane involvement in erythema multiforme (Stevens–Johnson syndrome) (*see* Fig 13.32).

Localised lesions on the lip include warts (*see* Fig 5.6), vascular abnormalities such as venous lake (*see* Fig 6.26) or hereditary haemorrhagic telangiectasia (**Fig 5.9**), lentigines and squamous cell carcinoma—which can be relatively subtle at this site.

Table 5.3 Localised lesions and rashes that characteristically or commonly affect the lips

Rashes	Eczema (atopic, 'lip-lick,' contact) Cheilitis (either angular (1.10), granulomatous, actinic, secondary to oral retinoid treatment, lip chewing) Infections (herpes simplex, impetigo, candidosis) Lichen planus (8.24), lupus erythematosus, Behçet's disease, CREST Bullous disorders (e.g. pemphigus vulgaris, Stevens—Johnson syndrome) Angio-oedema (16.4)
Localised lesions	Warts (5.6) Angiomas (hereditary haemorrhagic telangiectasia (5.9), pyogenic granuloma), venous lake (6.26) Lentigines (Peutz—Jeghers syndrome (9.15), Laugier–Hunziker syndrome, oral melanotic macules) Squamous cell carcinoma (9.95)

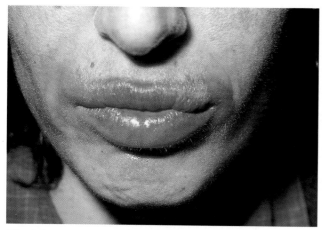

Fig 5.7 Contact allergic eczema. This patient was allergic to the strawberry flavouring in her 'organic' lip gel.

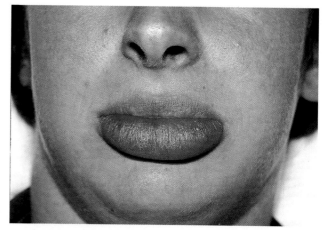

Fig 5.8 Orofacial granulomatosis. This causes swelling of the lips, cheek and tongue and often presents with swelling of the lower lip. Histology of the involved lip shows a granulomatous infiltrate. A small proportion of patients who present with these symptoms have Crohn's disease or sarcoidosis

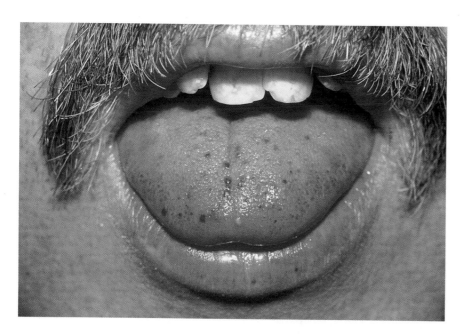

Fig 5.9 Lips. The small angiomatous lesions of hereditary haemorrhagic telangiectasia usually involve lips and tongue, as well as other skin and mucosal sites

Table 5.4 Causes of changes seen in the oral cavity

Site	Local	Systemic cause, or associated with a generalised skin disease
Tongue	Scrotal tongue Median rhomboid glossitis (5.12) Geographical tongue (5.10) Black hairy tongue (5.16) Leukoplakia (5.13) Carcinoma	Atrophic glossitis due to vitamin B12 deficiency Kawasaki disease (red tongue) Oral hairy leukoplakia in HIV infection (5.15) Hereditary haemorrhagic telangiectasia (5.9)
Gingiva	Gingivitis due to poor dental hygiene causing bleeding	Bleeding in leukaemia, HIV infections, clotting disorders, scurvy Immunobullous disease (pemphigus, mucous membrane pemphigoid, linear IgA disease) Gingival swelling caused by drugs (phenytoin, cyclosporin), Crohn's disease etc. 'Strawberry gingiva' of Wegener's granulomatosis Childhood dermatomyositis
Buccal and palatal mucosa	Candidiasis (5.11) Leukoplakia, carcinoma Lichenoid eruptions (buccal): lichen planus, lichenoid contact allergy (e.g. to dental amalgam (5.14) and frictional changes (along the bite line))	White patches caused by lichen planus, hairy leukoplakia in HIV infection (5.15)
Floor of mouth	Leukoplakia, carcinoma	
Any or all of the above	Lichen planus (may be intraoral only: mainly buccal (2.22), tongue, gingival) Mouth ulcers (5.17) (mainly buccal, gingival, tongue, see Table 12.6) Neoplasia Candidiasis (5.11)	Lichen planus (2.22) Mouth ulcers (mainly buccal, gingival, tongue; see Table 12.6) Hand, foot and mouth disease Kaposi's sarcoma in HIV infection

Oral cavity

Detailed discussion of purely intraoral diseases is beyond the scope of this text. Numerous skin disorders may have associated mucosal signs, and some are discussed here.

Lesions may occur in association with skin lesions or in isolation (**Table 5.4**). For example, palatal and buccal erosions are often present months before skin lesions develop in pemphigus vulgaris. Also, the buccal mucosa is abnormal in about 75% of patients with lichen planus (*see* Figs 2.22 and 8.22), even though it is usually asymptomatic and therefore easily missed. Palatal involvement is common in AIDS-related Kaposi's sarcoma.

Some oral diseases are specific to particular parts of the mouth (**Table 5.4**), such as geographical tongue (**Fig 5.10**) or median rhomboid glossitis (**Fig 5.12**), which is one presentation of candidiasis. By contrast, ulceration, erosion, the commoner pattern of oral candidiasis (**Fig 5.11**) and leukoplakia (**Fig 5.13**) can affect any part of the mouth, and the distribution is not usually helpful in differential diagnosis.

The range of responses of the oral mucosa is relatively limited, and several disorders may cause clinically similar lesions. For example, streaky white marks reminiscent of lichen planus (termed 'lichenoid') may occur owing to trauma, lupus erythematosus or contact allergic reactions (**Fig 5.14**). Occasionally, the appearance of an ulcer (e.g. minor aphthous ulcers, **Fig 5.17**) can be helpful in the diagnosis, but in general, the appearances of mouth ulcers in different diseases are similar in nature, varying only in extent. Persistent asymmetrical ulceration should always raise the question of intraoral neoplasia. Malignant ulcers in the mouth feel hard; the importance of palpation of such lesions is stressed.

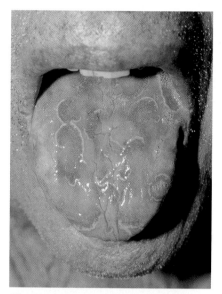

Fig 5.10 Geographical tongue (benign migratory glossitis). The annular pattern and atrophic areas change in a week. In most patients, the condition is painless

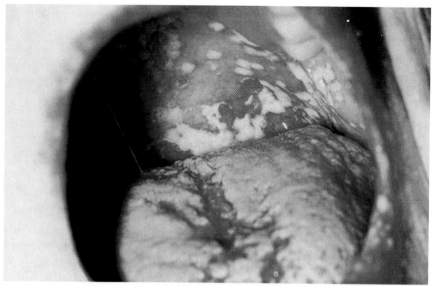

Fig 5.11 Oral candidiasis (thrush). These white or creamy lesions on the tongue and palate are called pseudomembranous candidiasis. The word thrush does not refer to any possible similarity between the thrush's plumage but to a Norse word for rotten wood. Oral candidiasis occurs in healthy neonates who have not yet developed immunity to the yeast, and other immune suppressed patients (those who have undergone organ transplantation and those who are HIV-positive particularly). Antibiotic and corticosteroid therapy also predispose to oral candidiasis

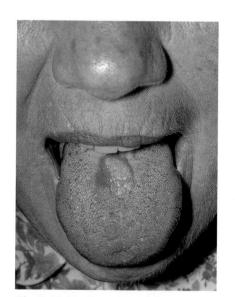

Fig 5.12 Median rhomboid glossitis. This is another variant of oral candidiasis and is more common in people who smoke, wear dentures or are immune compromised

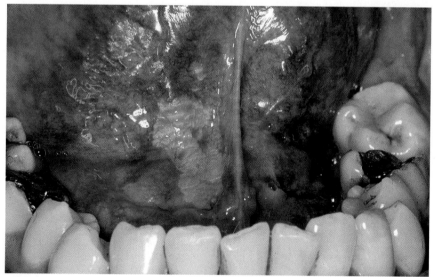

Fig 5.13 Leukoplakia under the tongue. Leukoplakias on the anterior floor of the mouth and the undersurface of the tongue have a particularly high risk of malignant change

Several systemic diseases have oral manifestations. Some of these are non-specific, such as oral ulceration in Behçet's disease. Crohn's disease may cause a variety of oral lesions, including a cobblestoned appearance of the mucosa, ulceration and persistent lip swelling (orofacial granulomatosis; see **Fig 5.8**). Others are useful clinical pointers, for example oral candidiasis (*see* Fig 5.11) is one of the earlier signs of AIDS. More recently described specific signs include the 'strawberry gingiva' of Wegener's granulomatosis.

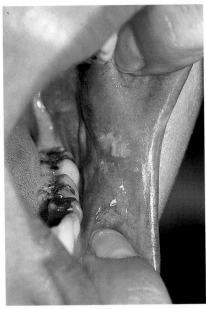

Fig 5.14 Lichenoid reaction to dental amalgam. Patients with old dental mercury containing amalgam can become allergic to the mercury and develop lichenoid reactions on the mucosa adjacent to the amalgam

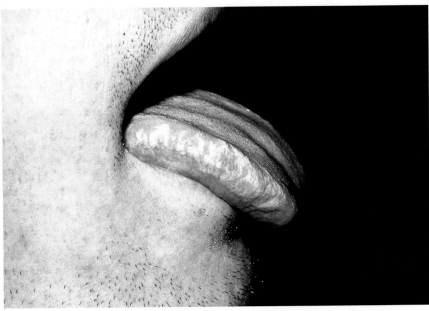

Fig 5.15 Oral hairy leukoplakia. This only occurs in people with a severe immune defect, especially those with HIV infection. The cause is probably due to opportunistic infection of tongue epithelium with the Epstein–Barr virus

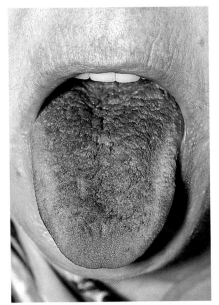

Fig 5.16 Black hairy tongue. This occurs in those with poor oral hygiene or dry mouth—sometimes due to the use of tricyclic antidepressants or broad-spectrum antibiotics. The long filiform papillae are stained by chromogenic micro-organisms, presumably similiar to the mould that grows on shower curtains

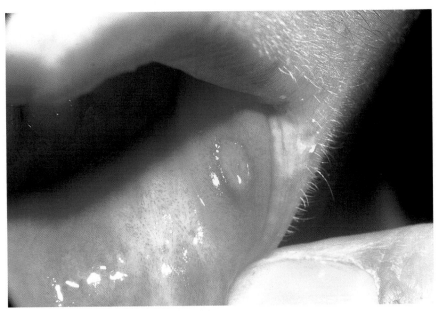

Fig 5.17 Aphthous ulcer. This shows the characteristics sharply defined circular painful mucosal ulcer usually less than 5 mm in diameter, with a bright red edge. The base of the lesion is covered in creamy coloured fibrin

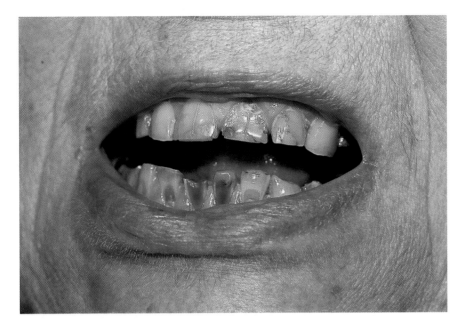

Fig 5.18 Dental changes in Sjögren's syndrome associated with progressive systemic sclerosis. Reductions in salivary flow due to the Sicca syndrome associated with systemic sclerosis have caused extensive dental caries in this patient

Dental abnormalities may be associated with skin disease (e.g. Gorlin's syndrome (*see* Fig 7.52) and anhidrotic ectodermal dysplasia) or may become abnormal as a result of the disease (**Fig 5.18**).

Ears

The ears are often involved in psoriasis and seborrhoeic dermatitis (both of which mainly affect the external auditory canal) (**Table 5.5**). Fissures at the junction of ear and scalp, especially at the earlobe, are a common finding in atopic eczema. Some rashes may localise to the ear for specific reasons, such as the very common finding of contact allergy to nickel in metal earrings. Ear piercing may also cause keloid scars (**Fig 5.19**). Localised, apparently 'eczematous' areas that do not correspond with pierced areas should always raise the suspicion of discoid lupus erythematosus (**Fig 5.20**), as should comedones in the concha in the absence of comedonal acne elsewhere on the face.

Disorders that are more specific to the ear include infections such as acute perichondritis and also an aggressive pseudomonas infection known as

Table 5.5 Localised lesions and rashes that characteristically or commonly affect the ears

Rashes	Psoriasis Eczema (atopic, seborrhoeic, contact (15.38; especially due to metals, in pierced ear lobes) Lupus erythematosus (5.20) Relapsing polychondritis (2.45) Infections (perichondritis, malignant otitis externa) Juvenile spring eruption
Localised lesions	Actinic keratosis Chondrodermatitis nodularis helicis (9.99) Malignancies: basal cell and squamous cell carcinoma, atypical fibroxanthoma Granuloma annulare Gout (tophi) (12.24) Keloids (5.19)

DIAGNOSTIC TIPS AND PITFALLS

- Scaling and itching of the external auditory meatus may be due to otitis externa, psoriasis or seborrhoeic dermatitis. Very rarely, patients are also allergic to applied remedies

- Fissures at the junction of ear and scalp, especially at the ear lobe, are a common finding in atopic eczema

- Ear-lobe crusting and scaling are usually due to contact allergy to nickel in metal earrings, but also remember discoid lupus erythematosus

- Lesions on the sides of the ear, typically the helix in men and the antihelix in women, are usually due to chondrodermatitis nodularis. This usually only occurs on the preferred sleeping side and results from compression of the ear during sleep

- Actinic keratoses and squamous cell carcinomas are caused by sun exposure and thus appear as a solitary crusted or scaling lesion on the top of the ear. Basal cell carcinomas more commonly affect the concha or behind the ears

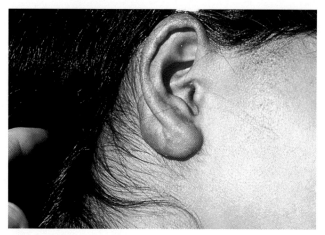

Fig 5.19 Ears. Ear piercing can cause a variety of problems. Localised allergic reactions to metals are the most common, but keloid scars (shown here) and lacerations of the ear lobe can also occur

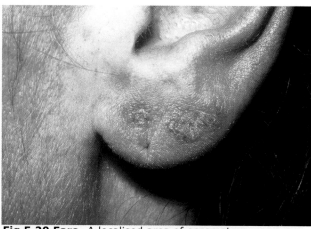

Fig 5.20 Ears. A localised area of eczematous appearance on the ear, not corresponding to a pierced hole, is suggestive of chronic discoid lupus erythematosus

malignant otitis externa, which occurs in diabetics. Relapsing polychondritis (*see* Fig 2.45) is an inflammatory multisystem disorder of collagen, which may present as a red, tender ear with characteristic sparing of the non-cartilaginous earlobe. Juvenile spring eruption is a photodermatosis, which characteristically affects the rim of the pinna, causing erythema and small, clear blisters.

Among localised lesions commonly found on the ears is chondrodermatitis nodularis helicis (*see* Fig 9.99), which typically occurs on the lateral aspect of the upper pole of the helix in men and the antihelix in women. Actinic keratoses (*see* Figs 9.86–9.88) also affect the upper pole of the helix, but on the superior, rather than the lateral, border. Squamous cell carcinomas (*see* Figs 9.95–9.97) tend to occur on the superior or posterior edge of the ear and basal cell carcinoma within the concha or behind the ears.

Less common nodules on the ears include those of granuloma annulare and gout; although uncommon, the ears are involved with disproportionate frequency.

Hands

The thicker stratum corneum on the palms and soles traps tissue fluid leaking from the inflamed skin in acute eczema. As a result, small blisters or vehicles develop, producing the appearance of pompholyx eczema (*see* Fig 1.7).

The hands may be involved as part of many widespread rashes (**Table 5.6**), including psoriasis and eczema, either of which may only affect the hands and/or feet. Eczema localised to the hands always raises the possibility of irritant or allergic contact dermatitis. Psoriasis at this site may seem typical of psoriasis elsewhere, be difficult to distinguish from eczema or present as a pustular variant (*see* Fig 14.2). Palmoplantar keratodermas (*see* Fig 7.1) may also need to be considered in the differential diagnosis of eczema or psoriasis.

Erythema multiforme often affects the hands, and typical target lesions on the palms suggest that the likely trigger is herpes simplex infection (*see* Fig 2.5). Dermatophyte fungal infection producing unilateral palmar rash (*see* Fig 7.18) can be easily missed unless both hands are examined. Fungal nail infections occur on the hands but are more common on the feet (*see* Fig 19.36). Other rashes that have a predilection for the hands include that of scabies infestation (finger web spaces and radial border of the palm; *see* Fig 15.12) and photosensitivity disorders (dorsum of the hands). Dermatomyositis classically causes thickened areas over the dorsum of the joints, known as Gottron's papules (**Fig 5.21**) or collodion patches, with

DIAGNOSTIC TIPS AND PITFALLS

- Endogenous eczema on the hands generally affects the palms, whereas exogenous (contact allergic or contract irritant) eczema affects the dorsal aspects

- Blisters are more common in palm and sole eczema because in acute eczema, the thicker stratum corneum at these sites traps tissue fluid leaking from the inflamed skin

- Unilateral nail dystrophy or rashes on the hands and feet must be considered to be fungal until proven otherwise. Always take scrapings from unilateral 'eczematous' hand rashes

- Recent onset itching associated with a rash on the hands is probably due to scabies. Check for burrows along the finger web spaces and radial border of the palm

- In infants or toddlers, scabies characteristically produces small pustules on the soles of the feet. This is rare in older patients

Table 5.6 Localised lesions and rashes that characteristically or commonly affect the hands

Rashes	Eczema (irritant and allergic contact dermatitis, atopic, dyshidrotic) (15.29–15.32)
	Psoriasis (7.2), palmoplantar pustulosis (14.2), Reiter's syndrome
	Dermatophyte infection (7.18)
	Palmoplantar keratodermas (7.1, 7.45)
	Scabies (15.12)
	Erythema multiforme (2.5)
	Photosensitivity (dorsum), porphyria cutanea tarda
	Dermatomyositis (dorsum) (18.9), scleroderma/CREST
	Vasculitis, telangiectasia (including hereditary haemorrhagic telangiectasia)
	Acrocyanosis, chilblains
	Acral chemotherapy reactions
	'Purpuric gloves and stockings' rash (parvovirus infection)
	Secondary syphilis
Localised lesions	Nail abnormalities and periungual lesions (see Chapter 19)
	Viral warts (9.83), orf, cowpox, Milker's nodule, herpetic whitlow
	Actinic keratoses (9.87), keratoacanthoma, squamous cell carcinoma
	Arsenical keratoses
	Pyogenic granuloma (9.65)
	Granuloma annulare
	Digital mucoid cyst (13.34)
	Accessory digits, acquired fibrokeratoma
	Picker's nodule, knuckle pads

sparing of the intervening skin. A streaky erythema (*see* Fig 17.9) can also occur (known as Gottron's sign). By contrast, the lesions of lupus erythematosus affect the skin on the dorsum of the finger but often spare the knuckles (**Fig 5.22**). Nailfold involvement occurs in both of these connective tissue disorders as well as in disorders in the scleroderma spectrum.

Viral warts are extremely common on the hands; granuloma annulare (*see* Fig 11.29) and pyogenic granuloma (*see* Fig 9.65) are less common, but the hands are a characteristic site. Lesions virtually specific to the hands include acquired fibrokeratomas (*see* Fig 9.101), accessory digits and digital mucoid cysts (*see* Fig 13.34), which occur on the dorsum of the terminal phalanx. Actinic keratoses (*see* Fig 9.87), keratoacanthoma (*see* Fig 9.93) and squamous cell carcinoma (*see* Fig 9.95) all affect the dorsum of the hands after chronic sun exposure.

DIAGNOSTIC TIPS AND PITFALLS

- Dermatomyositis classically causes thickened areas over the dorsum of the joints. By contrast, the lesions of lupus erythematosus affect the skin on the dorsum of the finger but often spare the knuckles

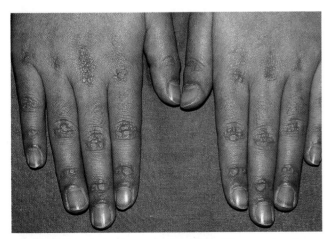

Fig 5.21 Hands in dermatomyositis. There are well-defined erythematosus papules coalescing on the knuckles and joints of this 12-year-old girl with juvenile dermatomyositis

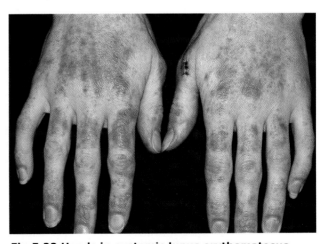

Fig 5.22 Hands in systemic lupus erythematosus. Here, the redness and scaling are localised to the skin between the joints rather than over the joints themselves, and the posterior nailfold changes are not as noticeable as with dermatomyositis

Table 5.7 Localised lesions and rashes that characteristically or commonly affect the feet

Rashes	Eczema (contact dermatitis, atopic, dyshidrotic; (15.33–15.35)) Juvenile plantar dermatosis (5.24, 7.46) Psoriasis, palmoplantar pustulosis (14.2), Reiter's syndrome Dermatophyte infection (athlete's foot), including nail infection (7.18) Palmoplantar keratodermas (7.45) Pitted keratolysis (5.23) Vasculitis (14.22, 17.35) Acrocyanosis, chilblains 'Purpuric gloves and stockings' rash (parvovirus infection) Secondary syphilis
Localised lesions	Nail abnormalities (see Chapter 19) Viral warts (verrucae) (4.37) Callosities and corns (4.36, 5.25) Granuloma annulare

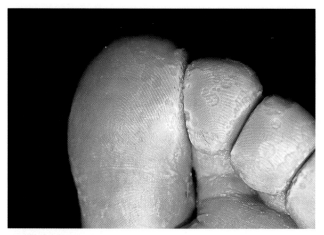

Fig 5.23 Pitted keratolysis. This is caused by an infection of the stratum corneum with a *Corynebacterium* species. The bacteria consumes stratum corneum leaving these areas of superficial pitting. Excessive sweating predisposes to pitted keratolysis, and the feet are usually foul-smelling

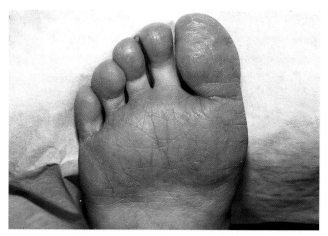

Fig 5.24 Feet. Juvenile plantar dermatosis of the soles is characterised by a red, 'glazed' appearance and fissures

Feet

The hands and feet (**Table 5.7**) often have the same patterns of eruption; disorders such as eczema, psoriasis, keratodermas (*see* Fig 7.1) and nail disorders affecting either or both. Dermatophyte infections are much more common on the feet than on the hands, especially affecting the nail plate and lateral toe web (*see* Fig 7.17). Eruptions that seem to be specific to plantar skin include pitted keratolysis due to corynebacterial infection (**Fig 5.23**) and a disorder known as juvenile plantar dermatosis (**Fig 5.24**), which is seen in children. Scabies often affects the feet in infants (*see* Fig 15.15), characteristically producing small pustules, but is rare in older patients. The effects of gravitational pressure on the structure of capillary and venule walls cause vasculitic lesions to commonly localise to the lower leg (*see* Fig 17.35). Widespread eczema and exanthemata also have a purpuric element on the lower leg, but this is not present on the trunk and upper arms. Localised lesions, such as warts, corns and callosities (**Fig 5.25**), are all common; the distinction between warts and corns is discussed in Chapter 4. Granuloma annulare on the dorsum of the feet (*see* Fig 11.29) is often mistaken for a fungal infection, but this can be excluded clinically by the absence of surface scaling.

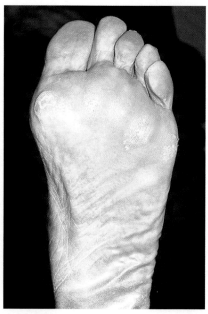

Fig 5.25 Feet. Callosities are common on both the sole (heels and metatarsal heads) and the dorsum of the foot (especially in women)

Limbs

Several forms of eczema commonly affect the limbs and generally have a more readily recognisable pattern on limbs than on the trunk. Discoid eczema commonly appears on the legs. The knee and elbow flexure distribution of atopic eczema (*see* Fig 15.2) and the involvement of the shins in asteatotic eczema (*see* Fig 15.4) and lichen simplex are characteristic. Keratosis pilaris (*see* Fig 7.36) causes follicular keratinisation and occurs mainly on the lateral aspect of the upper arms and thighs.

Vascular disorders, including arterial and venous diseases (*see* Chapter 17), are often apparent in the limbs rather than on the trunk. Venous disease may be accompanied by eczema, lymphoedema and episodes of cellulitis. Bacteria causing cellulitis may also gain entry via small fissures caused by tinea pedis. Lymphoedema can develop from a congenital or inherited abnormality or as a result of scarring or malignant obstruction of lymphatics.

Other disorders where limb involvement is typical are listed in **Table 5.8**. Lower limbs are exposed to sunlight in women who usually wear skirts. This results in photosensitivity disorders and chronic actinic damage resulting in the lower leg being the common site for Bowen's disease (intra-epidermal carcinoma; *see* Fig 8.17) in women. Other hazards of exposure are cold, which causes chilblains (*see* Fig 17.41) on the toes and over fat-insulated areas such as the upper outer thigh. Insect bite reactions, such as the nodules and blisters of papular urticaria (*see* Fig 13.1), occur on the lower leg, and cat flea bites occur around the ankles. Dermatofibromas (*see* Fig 9.50) commonly occur on limbs, possibly because they arise at old sites of insect bites.

FLEXURES

Flexural involvement in psoriasis (**Table 5.9**, *see* Fig 8.15) is common but unusual in eczema, and should arouse suspicion of a contact dermatitis—for example, to deodorants, hygiene wipes, clothing or, around the neck, airborne dust. Friction, moisture, heat, secondary infection and irritants, including soaps, urine or faeces all play a part in the development of intertrigo, nappy rash and pruritus ani. Irritant napkin eruptions in children (**Fig 5.26** and **5.27**) are becoming less common with disposable nappies, but other conditions may present at this site (**Fig 5.28** and **5.29**).

Infections commonly occur in flexures. Dermatophyte infections may spread from an infected toe web (*see* Fig 15.20), and candidiasis, erythrasma (**Fig 5.30**) and trichomycosis axillaris (*see* Fig 18.51) all occur. The axillae and perineum are common sites of staphylococcal carriage.

Table 5.8 Localised lesions and rashes that characteristically or commonly affect the limbs

Rashes	Eczema (atopic 16.1), asteatotic (16.4), lichen simplex (8.5), discoid (2.1, 8.3), venous (8.2) Photosensitivity (arms) (7.20) Keratosis pilaris (7.36) Psoriasis (8.13) Lichen planus (8.22) Dermatitis herpetiformis (14.20) Necrobiosis lipoidica (11.10) Vasculitis, panniculitis, erythema nodosum, chilblains (17.41) Papular urticaria (14.1) Vascular disorders (arterial, venous, lymphatic) (17.43–17.46) Streptococcal cellulitis (mainly legs) Fixed drug eruption
Localised lesions	Dermatofibroma (9.50) Bowen's disease (mainly in women) (8.17)

Table 5.9 Localised lesions and rashes that characteristically or commonly affect the flexures

Rashes	Psoriasis (8.15) Contact dermatitis, seborrhoeic dermatitis Intertrigo, nappy rash Infections (candida (5.26), staphylococci, dermatophytes, erythrasma (5.30), trichomycosis axillaris (18.51) Hidradenitis suppurativa Acanthosis nigricans (3.17) Hailey–Hailey disease Pemphigus vegetans Histiocytosis X (Langerhans' cell histiocytosis) Metabolic: acrodermatitis enteropathica and zinc deficiency (5.28, 5.29), necrolytic migratory erythema (due to glucagonoma) Cutaneous lesions of Crohn's disease
Localised lesions	Fibroepithelial polyps (skin tags) (5.31) Freckles in neurofibromatosis (Crowe's sign) (9.19) Fox—Fordyce disease (6.3) Pseudoxanthoma elasticum

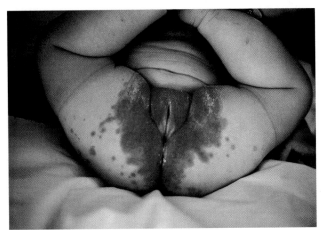

Fig 5.26

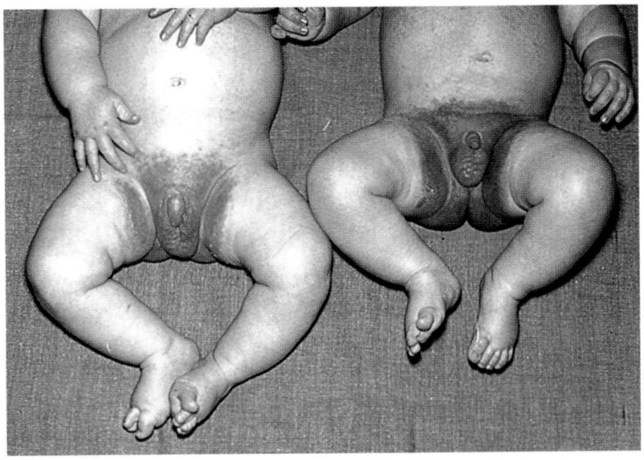

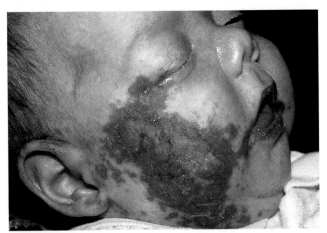

Fig 5.27

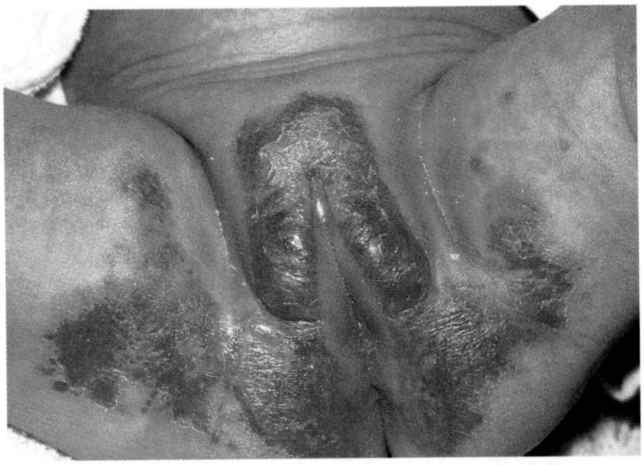

Fig 5.28

Fig 5.29

Fig 5.26–5.29 Napkin area. Examples of nappy rashes. Candidiasis (5.26) has a characteristic scarlet-red appearance with a glazed surface, satellite spots and sometimes pustules. In 5.27, an irritant eruption due to urine and faeces is shown. The creases are typically spared, and satellite lesions are not a feature. Zinc deficiency, in this case due to prematurity, is a rare cause of nappy rash (5.28). Facial rash in the same child is shown in 5.29. The rash of acrodermatitis enteropathica (an inherited defect of zinc metabolism) is identical. The child's nails are shown in 19.48

The localisation of apocrine glands explains the axillary and perineal distribution of hidradenitis suppurativa. The reason why these sites are affected by acanthosis nigricans (*see* Fig 3.17) is less well understood.

Fibroepithelial polyps (skin tags) are common in axillae (**Fig 5.31**) and around the neck. Less common, but a characteristic physical sign, is the presence of axillary freckling in neurofibromatosis (Crowe's sign, *see* Fig 9.19).

Umbilical

Several eruptions that occur at other flexural sites may affect the umbilicus, such as lesions due to scabies. Some umbilical lesions occur owing to embryological factors, e.g. persistent vitellointestinal duct, paraumbilical hernia. Sister Mary Joseph's nodule, a metastasis of bowel carcinoma to the umbilicus, and Crohn's disease affecting the umbilicus, may also affect this site for similar lesions. Mucous membrane pemphigoid may affect the umbilicus (sometimes in isolation), and purpura due to *Strongyloides* causes a periumbilical 'thumb-print' pattern.

GENITALIA

Several dermatoses may affect the genital skin as part of a generalised eruption, whereas others are confined to this site (**Table 5.10**). Several infections of the genitalia, such as genital herpes, genital warts or a primary syphilitic chancre, are sexually transmitted. Molluscum contagiosum (*see* Fig 9.3) often involves the perineum and genitalia in young children but not as a result of sexual spread in this age group. Pubic lice and scabies infestations may affect the genitalia, the latter causing nodular lesions (*see* Fig 15.17). Non-infective genital ulcers may also occur, for example in Behçet's disease.

Psoriasis, Reiter's syndrome (**Fig 5.32**), lichen planus, lichen sclerosus (*see* Fig 17.30) and lichen simplex of the scrotum or labia majora may be confined to genitalia but are usually also present at other sites. Lichenification of genital skin is often treated by a wide range of medicaments, and contact allergic dermatitis may result from this. The glans penis is a characteristic but unexplained site of fixed drug eruptions, leading to persistent pigmentation (**Fig 5.33**). The

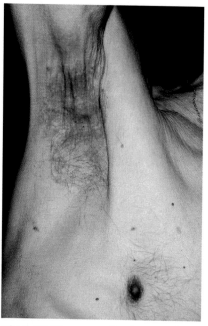

Fig 5.30 Flexures. Erythrasma produces a brownish coloured and often very chronic eruption in axillae and groins

Table 5.10 Localised lesions and rashes that characteristically or commonly affect the genitalia

Rashes	Sexually transmitted infections and infestations, including genital warts
	Scabies nodules
	Candidosis
	Psoriasis, Reiter's syndrome (5.32)
	Lichen planus
	Lichen sclerosus (8.29) (balanitis xerotica obliterans in males)
	Lichen simplex (penis, scrotum, vulva)
	Contact dermatitis
	Fixed drug eruption (5.33)
	Behçet's disease (ulcers)
	Fabry's disease
	Fournier's gangrene
Localised lesions	Angiokeratoma of Fordyce (5.35)
	Normal variants (see Chapter 5.34)
	Zoon's balanitis (5.34)
	Scrotal cysts, leiomyoma
	Bowen's disease-erythroplasia of Queyrat
	Squamous cell carcinoma

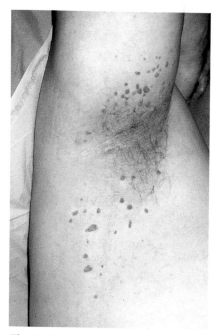

Fig 5.31 Flexures. Fibroepithelial polyps are one of the causes of lesions commonly known as skin tags; they often occur around the neck and in flexural sites and are soft, pedunculated, flesh coloured or slightly pigmented lesions

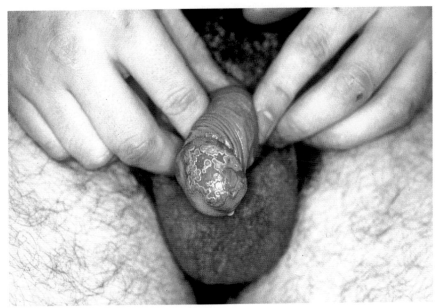

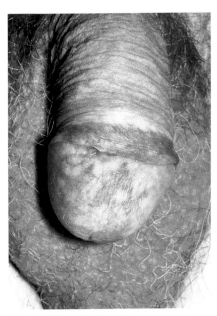

Fig 5.32 Genitalia. Circinate balanitis in Reiter's syndrome associated with urethritis. The discoid patches have coalesced to form a so-called circinate balanitis, which surrounds the entire glans penis. Note also the purulent urethral discharge (*photo courtesy of Dr Belinda Stanley*)

Fig 5.33 Genitalia. The glans penis is a relatively common site for fixed drug eruption and may become noticeably pigmented

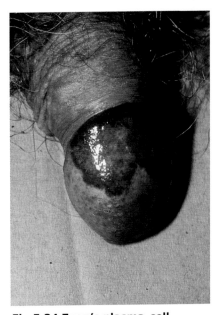

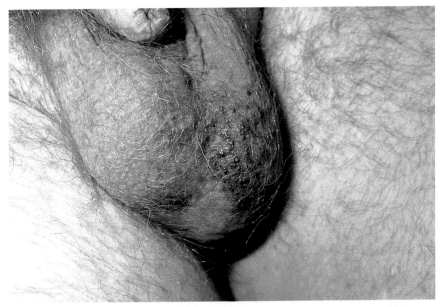

Fig 5.34 Zoon's plasma-cell balanitis. Zoon's balanitis is a condition of unknown aetiology, which causes erythema, sometimes with weeping or erosions of the glans penis and mucosal surface of the foreskin

Fig 5.35 Angiokeratoma of Fordyce. Typical small purple angiomas of the scrotum. These are clinically identical to angiokeratomas of Anderson–Fabry disease, but patients with Anderson–Fabry disease also have lesions around the pelvic girdle region and have a systemic disease with neurological, cardiac and renal involvement

inflammatory non-infective condition of Zoon's plasma cell balanitis (**Fig 5.34**) characteristically affects the glans penis and the corresponding undersurface of the prepuce; plasma cell vulvitis is the equivalent process in women.

Among non-infective localised lesions that have a predilection for genitalia are grouped angiokeratomas on the scrotum, known as angiokeratoma of Fordyce (**Fig 5.35**), and some normal variants such as sebaceous glands on the shaft (*see* Fig 6.42) and pearly penile papules around the corona of the penis

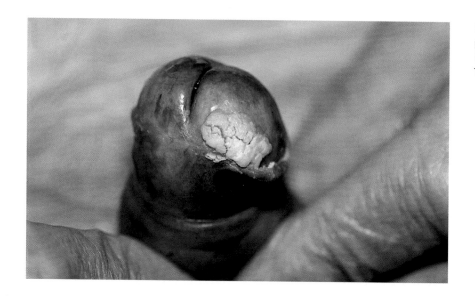

Fig 5.36 Bowen's disease of the penis. This patch of hypertrophic Bowen's disease had to be excised. There was no evidence of invasion

(*see* Fig 6.41). Rare causes of angiokeratoma, such as Fabry's disease (an X-linked disorder), also often involve the genitalia in males. Tumours of the genitalia include benign scrotal cysts and leiomyomas (a smooth muscle tumour); the most common malignant tumour is Bowen's disease (**Fig 5.36**), which may lead to squamous cell carcinoma.

USEFUL SITE COMBINATIONS

Although many of the eruptions discussed in this chapter can affect several different body sites, they may nevertheless involve only one specific area. For example, psoriasis may be generalised but can also affect the hands, flexures, scalp or genitalia alone. Such eruptions have therefore been considered under several headings. Some rashes, however, most commonly affect multiple sites at the same time and may therefore have a characteristic distribution pattern (Table 5.11).

Table 5.11 Examples of rashes and localised disorders that show characteristic combinations of body sites involved

	Scalp	Face	Chest	Back	Palms	Soles	Dorsum of hand	Forearm	Extensor elbow	Flexor knee	Extensor knee	Genital
Atopic eczema	+	+						Flexor elbow		+		
Psoriasis	+			Sacrum					+		+	
Lichen planus		Mouth						Wrist				+
Seborrhoeic eczema	+	+	+	+								
Acne		+	+	+								
Tinea	+					+						+
Scabies					+	+	+	Wrist	+			+
Warts		+			+	+	+					+
Photosensitivity		+	Neck				+	Dorsal forearm				
Dermatomyositis		+	+				+					
Dermatitis herpetiformis	+			Sacrum					+		+	

95

Normal variants and common anomalies

SWEAT GLAND AND HAIR VARIANTS

The skin appendages include eccrine and apocrine sweat glands, the sebaceous glands and hair and nails.

Sweat glands

The density of eccrine sweat glands varies with site and ranges from 120/cm^2 on the thigh to 620/cm^2 on the soles of the feet. The sweat ducts empty directly on to the skin surface and are not visible under resting conditions. However, they can be identified on the finger pulps with the aid of a hand lens as tiny pits on the print pattern ridges, some of which contain a minute, shiny droplet of sweat. Sweat production can be shown using the

DIAGNOSTIC TIPS AND PITFALLS

- Many normal variants may be erroneously diagnosed as pathological, creating concern for the patient

97

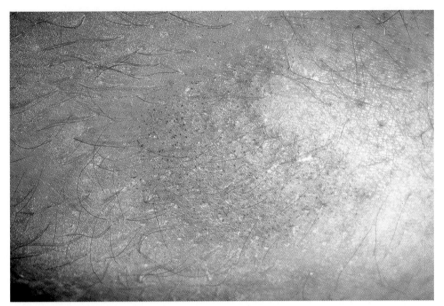

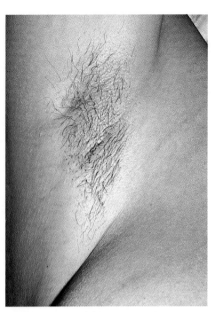

Fig 6.1 Hair follicle and sweat duct density in normal skin. Sweating has been provoked by poldine iontophoresis and sweat production identified by the ferric chloride–tannic acid reaction. Note that the sweat duct density is considerably greater than the hair follicle density (*photo courtesy of Dr Celia Moss*)

Fig 6.2 Hyperhidrosis in the axilla. Excessive axillary sweating is due to eccrine gland secretion and causes salt deposition and discoloration of clothing. In axillary hyperhidrosis, axillary odour is usually not a problem because the odoriferous apocrine sweat gland secretions are flushed away by the large volume of eccrine gland secretion

starch–iodine test (*see* Figs 4.18 and 4.19) or ferric chloride–tannic technique (**Fig 6.1**). Sweating is increased on the palms and axillae in situations of anxiety and excitement. Noticeable hyperhidrosis (**Fig 6.2**) occurs in some individuals under resting conditions (this is the reason for applying antiperspirants before sleeping), although sweating triggered by emotional stimuli is reduced nocturnally. Symptoms can become so disabling that ablation of nervous stimulation (by sympathectomy or injection of botulinum toxin) or even axillary vault excision may be required. Blockage of eccrine sweat ducts results in miliaria (**Fig 6.10**, *see also* Fig 14.16).

Apocrine glands grow to their full size at adolescence and are found in the axillae, nipples, perineum and genitalia. Apocrine sweat empties into the hair follicle, not directly on to the skin, unlike eccrine sweat. Only very small amounts of oily apocrine sweat are produced each day. Excessive axillary sweating is eccrine rather then apocrine in origin. Apocrine sweat may be coloured but is odourless at first; it becomes smelly owing to bacterial degradation of sweat constituents. Blockage of apocrine sweat ducts results in chronic itchy papules localised to the apocrine gland-bearing areas; this is known as Fox–Fordyce disease (**Fig 6.3**).

Hair follicles and sebaceous glands

In healthy subjects, the number of hair follicles remains constant throughout life, so that a newborn infant has a greater hair density—approximately $1100/cm^2$—compared with an adult—about $600/cm^2$. The hair shaft diameter is, however, smaller in the child and steadily increases to a maximum at around 10 years of age. Follicular orifices can be seen on the body as small, regularly placed pits, most of which contain fine hairs. On the scalp, terminal hairs are bunched together, and as many as four or five may emerge from the same point, although they are derived from separate follicles (*see* Fig 18.3). Abdominal hairs in obese men sometimes form a neat coil, because they grow without penetrating the stratum corneum (**Fig 6.4**). These should not be confused with the corkscrew hairs of vitamin C deficiency (*see* Fig 4.44) in which there is also follicular hyperkeratosis and a purpuric component.

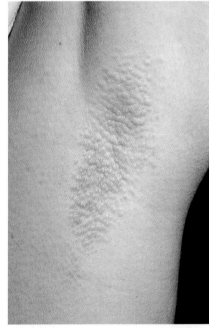

Fig 6.3 Fox–Fordyce disease. The skin-coloured axillary papules are due to apocrine duct obstruction and are associated with loss of hairs

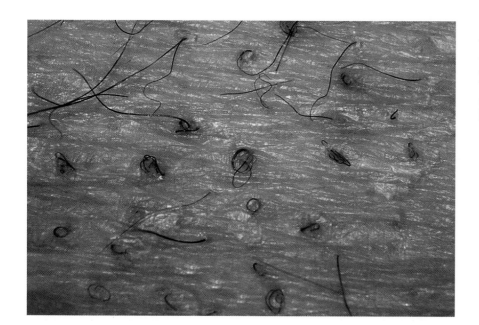

Fig 6.4 Rolled hairs. These form on the sites where clothing is tight, e.g. anterior abdominal wall, back and extensor surfaces in obese hairy men. The hair rolls up under the stratum corneum and can be uncoiled if the horny layer is broken with a needle

Each hair has an associated sebaceous gland, which produces an oily secretion; this causes the greasy feel to skin, best appreciated on the forehead, nose and hair. At most sites the sebaceous gland secretions empty via the sebaceous duct into the follicular canal. The size of the sebaceous gland does not correspond to the hair size, as witnessed by the huge sebaceous glands but tiny vellus hairs on the nose. At several sites, sebaceous glands empty directly on to the skin, including the nipples, genitalia and upper lip, where they may be considered abnormal by an inexperienced observer (**Fig 6.42**). Ectopic sebaceous glands are sometimes seen on the buccal mucosa, lips (where they are termed Fordyce spots; **Fig 6.44**) and genitalia.

Sebaceous gland secretions are under androgenic hormonal control. In children, sebaceous glands are tiny, and virtually no sebum is secreted until puberty, when the secretions produce greasy skin and hair and lead to the development of acne. Newborn infants may have large sebaceous glands due to the stimulatory effect of maternal hormones that have crossed the placenta (**Fig 6.9**).

NEWBORN SKIN

Erythema neonatorum (neonatal toxic erythema)

Erythema neonatorum occurs in approximately 50% of all full-term infants, but most cases are not seen by dermatologists. Starting during the second to the fourth day of life, blotchy macular erythema develops, principally on the trunk (**Figs 6.5 and 6.6**). The red areas may be a few to many hundreds but fade within a day. Very occasional weals or papules may appear, sometimes with an overlying pustule, in which case they need to be distinguished from infections or miliaria (*see* Fig 6.10, *see also* Fig 14.16).

Post-mature baby

Infants born after 42 weeks are considered post-mature. They have no lanugo hair, little vernix, long nails, short hair and white, cracked, skin that peels easily (**Figs 6.7 and 6.8**).

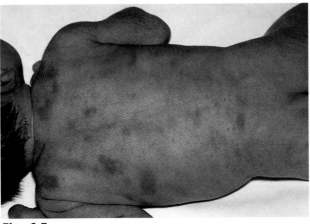

Figs 6.5

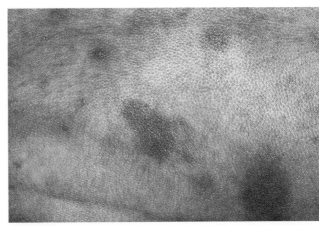

Figs 6.6

Figs 6.5, 6.6 Erythema neonatorum. This baby developed a characteristic erythematous macular eruption 24 hours after birth. Approximately 50% of newborn infants develop similar but less severe appearances in the first 4 days of life. It is rarely present at birth and spontaneously resolves after 2–3 days. Papular and pustular changes have also been described. 6.6 shows a close-up view of 6.5

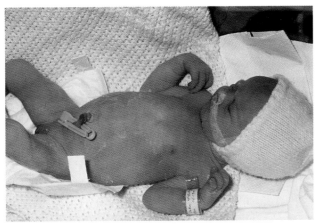

Figs 6.7

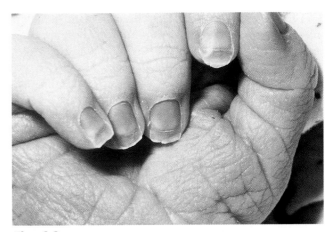

Figs 6.8

Figs 6.7, 6.8 Post-mature babies. Post-mature infants (6.7) have white parchment-like or desquamating skin. The nails are commonly long; this infant (6.8) was born 14 days post-term (6.7 *courtesy of Dr Andrew Cant*)

Sebaceous gland hypertrophy

Under the influence of maternal or placental hormones, sebaceous glands hypertrophy and appear as multiple pinpoint, yellow papules, best seen on the nose and cheeks (**Fig 6.9**). These changes fade within approximately 2 months. Other phenomena resulting from the same stimulus include breast swelling and secretion of milk (witches' milk), pigmentation of the linea alba and swelling of female and male genitalia.

Milia (milk spots)

Milia are pearly white, about the size of a pin-head, and are seen on the cheeks, chin and nasolabial folds in 40% of normal babies in the first 4 weeks of life. Histologically, these are keratin-filled cysts derived from the hair follicle. There is often difficulty in distinguishing pustular miliaria from milia on babies' faces, which has caused much confusion and contradiction in the definitions of these common conditions. Milia do not have an inflamed base, whereas pustular miliaria usually arise on an erythematous base; miliaria are generally more widespread. It is probable that the two conditions co-exist in many cases.

Miliaria

Sweat duct blockage causes different physical signs depending on the level of the block. Superficial blockage produces tiny, clear blisters that look like beads of sweat (*see* Fig 13.11) and that rupture when pressed. Deeper blockage tends to occur with greater humidity and results in very small, intensely itchy, red papules.

At birth, sweat ducts are not fully formed, so that duct blockage occurs readily. Almost all neonates develop transient crops of miliaria, usually provoked by being kept wrapped up in a warm room. In children, the blisters may be cloudy or even pustular (*see* Fig 14.16) even when not infected (**Fig 6.10**). Staphylococcal infection readily occurs in miliaria, and this must be excluded in babies with pustular miliaria.

Stork marks (salmon patches)

Stork marks are present at birth in approximately 50% of infants as pink, flat areas of telangiectasia on the nape of the neck, glabella or mid-forehead and the eyelids (**Fig 6.11**). They fade quickly on the eyelids, but are slower to clear from the glabella. Fifty per cent of 1 year olds and 40% of school children still have salmon patches on the nape of the neck (**Fig 6.12**).

Mongolian spots

Mongolian spots are poorly circumscribed, solitary or multiple areas of slate-brown or blue–brown discoloration on the sacral area. They are seen in over 90% of Asian and black babies, about 50% of Hispanic babies and 5–10% of white babies. The individual lesions range in size from a few millimetres to 10 cm. They may be very extensive and mistaken for bruises but usually fade in early childhood (**Fig 6.13**); even in Japanese people, less than 5% are still

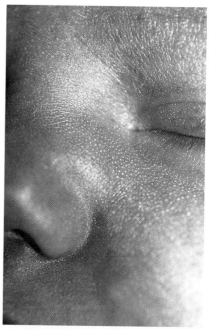

Fig 6.9 Sebaceous gland hypertrophy in a newborn infant. Tiny pinpoint yellow papules visible on the tip of the nose and cheeks are present in virtually all children less than 3 months old. These tiny yellow papules are normal sebaceous glands hypertrophied due to the effect of maternal oestrogens; they can be easily distinguished from milia and miliaria (*see* 6.10)

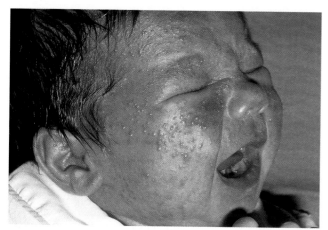

Fig 6.10 Pustular miliaria. There are tiny yellow papules, with surrounding erythema on the cheeks and nose. Miliaria or sweat-retention pustules may be visible at other body sites. In contrast to milia, there is surrounding erythema

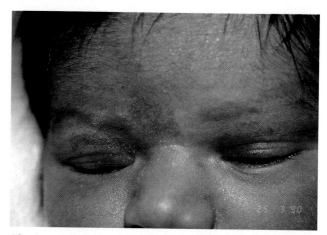

Fig 6.11 Glabella stork mark. As well as the nape of the neck, other areas of the face, including mid-forehead and eyelids, may be involved. Lesions on the eyelids fade rapidly, but those on the glabella may last for several months; very few persist into early childhood (*photo courtesy of Dr DWA Milligan*)

detectable by adolescence. They are considered to be due to functional dermal melanocytes that are still migrating from the neural crest to the basal layer of the epidermis.

AGED SKIN

Actinic (senile) purpura

Actinic (senile) purpura presents as areas of purpura, sometimes greater than 20 mm in diameter, which occur suddenly on the dorsum of the hands and forearms (**Fig 6.14**). Fresh lesions often have an irregular shape, but individual lesions fade and may merge with fresher areas over time. They develop as a result of intradermal bleeding after minor trauma. Dermal vessels are inadequately supported by dermal collagen and shear easily due to a combination of senile atrophy and actinically induced collagen damage. This condition may be compounded by the additive effects of topical or oral steroid use. In such cases, the patient's skin is characteristically transparent (**Fig 6.15**), allowing clear visualisation of underlying extensor tendons and larger veins; there is also a greater likelihood of associated generalised osteoporosis.

Actinic (senile) comedones

Actinic comedones are seen on and around the eyelid, cheeks and nose in association with thickening, wrinkling and yellowing of the skin (**Fig 6.16**).

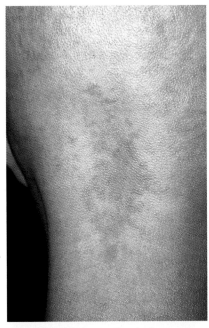

Fig 6.12 Stork mark on the neck. This is a variety of naevus flameus, sometimes called a salmon patch. These are present in up to 70% of neonates. Approximately 40% of school children have neck salmon patches. This one in an adult became visible when the patient developed alopecia totalis

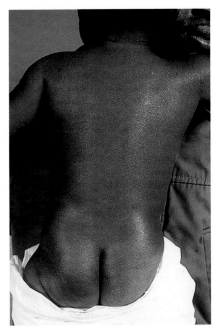

Fig 6.13 Mongolian spots. These may range from a few millimetres to several centimetres in diameter, and the colour varies from slate-brown to blue. They are present almost always on black babies, but in approximately 10% of white babies only (*photo courtesy of Dr Andrew Illchyshyn*)

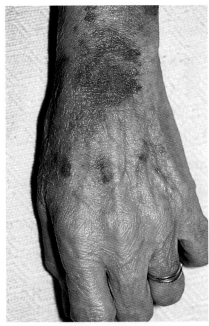

Fig 6.14 Actinic (senile) purpura. Dermal vessels are poorly supported by actinically damaged and atrophic collagen. Minor trauma leads to rupture of the vessels. Purpura is easily shown by applying a sheer force to a skinfold, using the forefinger and thumb. The purpura is very slowly reabsorbed compared with deeper bruise purpura

This condition is also known as nodular elastoidosis or Favre–Racouchot syndrome. The blackheads are formed from dilated pilosebaceous openings, without sebaceous gland hyperplasia, and they contain a mixture of altered keratin, a sebum-like substance, and melanin, which produces the black colour of the comedone.

Solar elastosis

Solar elastosis presents as yellowish plaques, made up of almost coalescent individual yellow papules. It is best seen on the forehead (**Fig 6.17**), nose and cheeks, with relative sparing of the deep skin creases of the face. The yellowing is due to changes in dermal collagen and elastin, caused by sun-induced damage. Cutis rhomboidalis is another variant, with thickened, yellowish areas of involved skin divided by uninvolved deep skin creases (**Fig 6.18**). The changes are restricted to the sun-exposed areas of the neck and thus stop abruptly below the collar line.

Stellate scars

Stellate scars are seen, in association with other signs of collagen atrophy, on the sun-exposed forearm and dorsum of the hand. The condition is believed to be due to minor trauma, although in most patients, no such history is forthcoming (**Fig 6.19**).

Sebaceous hyperplasia

Sebaceous hyperplasia is a common condition, presenting as yellowish, solitary or multiple papules, approximately 2–5 mm in diameter, with a central depression occurring on the face (**Fig 6.20**). They characteristically have an umbilicated centre, as the enlarged sebaceous glands are tethered to a central pilosebaceous follicle; oily material may be expressed from the umbilicated centre. If solitary, these papules may be confused with basal cell carcinoma, although small papular basal cell carcinomas are less yellow in colour, they are dome-shaped rather than umbilicated when small, and oily material cannot be squeezed out of them.

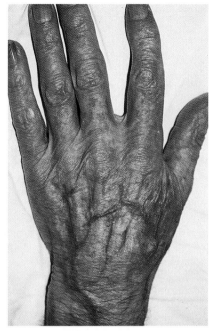

Fig 6.15 Atrophic/transparent skin. Tendons and veins can be easily seen through the transparent skin. There is commonly associated senile purpura. Patients with atrophic or transparent skin often have generalised osteoporosis

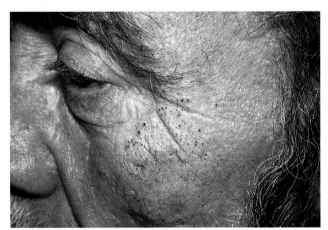

Fig 6.16 Actinic (senile) comedones. These blackheads or comedones are formed from dilated pilosebaceous openings without any sebaceous gland hyperplasia

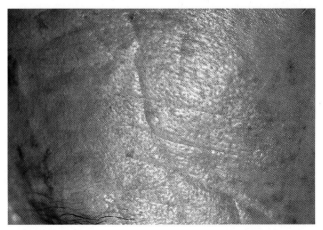

Fig 6.17 Solar elastosis. Diffuse, reticulate or striated, yellowish-coloured infiltration of the skin on the lateral side of the forehead and sparing of the central forehead. This condition is due to actinically induced collagen damage and an increase in elastin-like fibres within the dermis

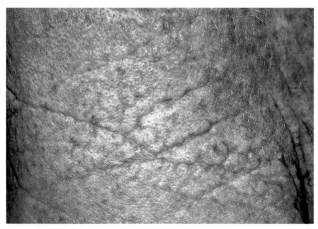

Fig 6.18 Cutis rhomboidalis. Thickened, yellowish skin appears on the back of the neck, divided into rhomboid shapes by deep skin creases. There is a sharp cut-off point at the level of the collar. This condition generally occurs in people repeatedly exposed to the sun, usually owing to an outdoor occupation

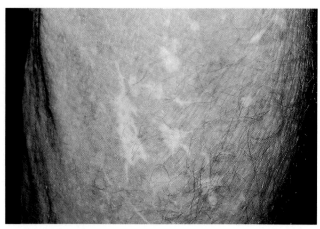

Fig 6.19 Stellate scars. These are star-shaped or linear, best seen on the forearms, and arise after minor injuries. They are commonly associated with actinic purpura

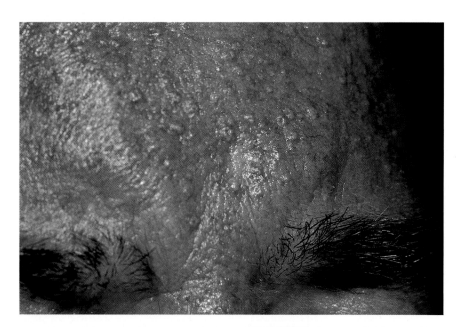

Fig 6.20 Sebaceous hyperplasia. Multiple yellowish papules with a central depression on the forehead, from which oily material can sometimes be expressed by gentle pressure. Solitary lesions may be difficult to distinguish from basal cell carcinoma

COMMON VASCULAR ANOMALIES

Physiological vascular mottling

Physiological vascular mottling presents as purplish, reticulate, vascular markings, which are common on the limbs of normal individuals, usually in cold conditions. In children, this condition is called cutis marmorata (marbled skin, **Fig 6.21**), and it is present, to some extent, in virtually all babies, usually on the arms and legs in cold conditions.

Idiopathic livedo reticularis and livedo mottling are terms used to describe a similar appearance seen especially in older children and women (**Fig 6.21**), many of whom seem to have a predilection for chilblains, acrocyanosis or erythrocyanosis. Mottling of this type never completely disappears in adults on warming, but it does fade considerably.

The position of the mottling is fixed and is believed to be related to the normal vascular supply to the skin. The white areas represent high skin blood

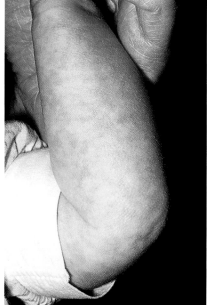

Fig 6.21 Cutis marmorata—physiological. Generalised purplish mottling of the skin at any site, but usually the arms and legs in children. It is more commonly seen in the cold and disappears on warming

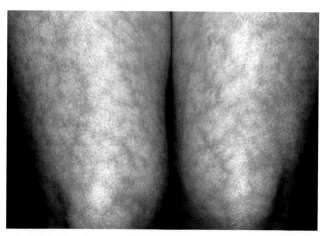

Fig 6.22 Livedo reticularis. This is a uniformly distributed, purplish mottling usually seen on the legs of women and children in cold weather. It is essentially the same as the cutis marmorata mottling present in normal children, except that in adults the changes do not completely disappear on rewarming. Patches of livedo mottling separated by normal skin, sometimes referred to as broken livedo, are abnormal (*see* 17.16)

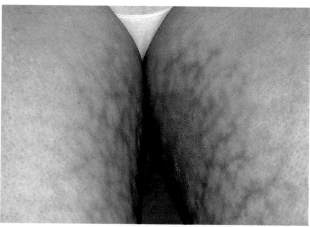

Fig 6.23 Erythema ab igne. Haemosiderin staining of the normal physiological, reticulate, vascular markings on the skin occurs after recurrent heat damage, such as a hot-water bottle (as in this case) or sitting next to a fire

flow from a deep, central feeding vessel, and the purple, net-like patterns correspond to areas of relatively sluggish blood flow at the boundaries of adjacent areas of arterial blood supply.

Disease may localise within this region of sluggish flow in vascular mottling. Erythema ab igne (**Fig 6.23**) is caused by haemosiderin staining and epidermal dysplasia, which occurs in the boundary areas of sluggish blood flow owing to reduced heat dissipation; in hyperviscosity states, such as cryoglobulinaemia, purpuric change may produce a reticulate purpura (*see* Fig 17.28). Reticulate mottling is a feature of cutis marmorata telangiectasia congenita (*see* Fig 17.15) and Rothmund–Thompson syndrome (*see* Fig 17.7).

Localised reticulate vascular patterns with apparently normal intervening skin may indicate a collagen vascular disorder such as polyarteritis nodosa (*see* Fig 17.16).

Flush pattern

Physiological flushing (*see* Fig 17.4) on the face, and particularly the upper chest and neck, is due to transient vasodilation of superficial dermal plexus vessels. It may be provoked by emotion, alcohol or heat.

Campbell de Morgan spots (cherry angiomas)

Campbell de Morgan spots usually present as dark red or pink angiomas, 2–5 mm in diameter, predominantly on the trunk (**Fig 6.24**). They occur more commonly with advancing age and histologically are angiokeratomas with dilated capillaries underlying a hyperkeratotic epidermis. Multiple tiny, cherry angiomas can sometimes be confused with a vasculitis or capillaropathy (**Fig 6.25**).

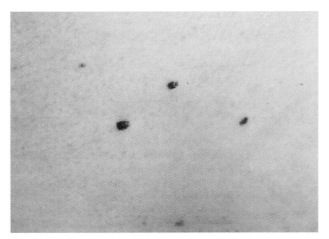

Fig 6.24 Campbell de Morgan spots. These are bright red angiomas, usually on the trunk. They are benign and are not associated with any systemic disease

Fig 6.25 Multiple minute Campbell de Morgan spots. There are multiple tiny, purple Campbell de Morgan spots, which may sometimes be confused with purpura or vasculitis (*see also* 17.15)

Venous lake

Venous lakes present as purple or blue, slightly raised, soft lesions, which are common on the lips (**Fig 6.26**) but are also often seen on the face and ears of elderly people (*see* Fig 9.67). Histologically, these are dilated veins.

Thread veins

Thread veins are common on women's legs (**Fig 6.27**). These normal vessels are not associated with abnormal deep veins, but are dilated normal horizontal venous plexus vessels. If they are a cosmetic embarrassment they can be destroyed by injection of sclerosants.

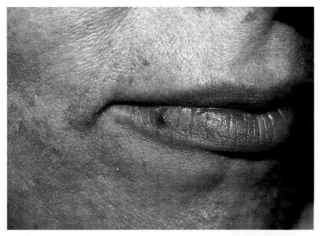

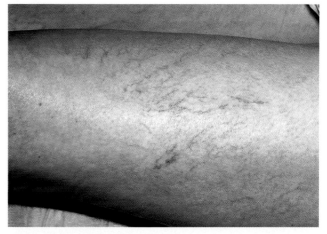

Fig 6.26 Venous lake of the lip. These are purplish, slightly elevated papules usually seen on the lower lip, and they are more common in women. They are dilated veins and may be up to 1 cm in diameter. They are simply destroyed by electrodesiccation or cryotherapy.

Fig 6.27 Thread veins. These purplish red, venous blood vessels are larger than telangiectatic capillaries or post-capillary venules. Vessels of this size can be injected with sclerosing solutions

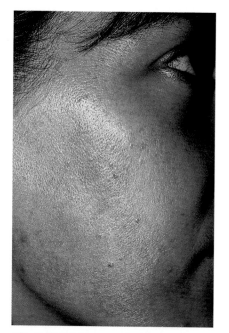

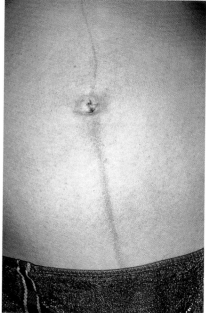

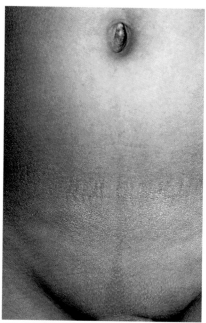

Fig 6.28 Chloasma (melasma).
Hyperpigmentation of the forehead, cheeks and temples in pregnancy and in women taking oral contraceptives is common. Pigmentation becomes more pronounced in sun exposure and takes several years to disappear. Melasma also occurs in men of Middle Eastern or Asian origin

Figs 6.29

Figs 6.30

Fig 6.29 6.30 Linea nigra. Temporary linear pigmentation between the xiphisternum and public region occurs during pregnancy (6.29). Linear pigment between the umbilicus and public region seems to be a normal variant in Asian children (6.30) and some adults

PIGMENTATION

Pigment changes in pregnancy

Oestrogens stimulate melanin production, producing chloasma (melasma), a symmetrical pigmentation of the brow, cheeks and temples in pregnancy (**Fig 6.28**). It also occurs in 10–20% of women taking oral contraceptives and usually in men of Middle Eastern or Asian origin. The pigmentation takes several years to fade and is made more obvious by sun exposure.

Linea nigra, a line of discrete hyperpigmentation between the public hair and the umbilicus, also occurs in most pregnant women (**Fig 6.29**) and seems to be a normal variant in some Asian children (**Fig 6.30**) and adults. Common naevi temporarily darken in pregnancy.

Racial pigment variants

Palmar pigmentation

In black people, the palmar skin creases are normally pigmented, whereas this only occurs in disease states in white people (**Fig 6.31**). Hyperpigmented macules also occur on the palms and soles in about 50% of black-skinned people.

Pigmentary demarcation lines

Pigmentary demarcation lines refer to sharply distinct and contrasting areas of normal and hypopigmented skin and have also been termed Voigt's lines

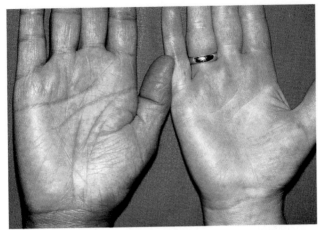

Fig 6.31 Palmar creases. Black skin compared with white skin: palmar skin crease pigmentation is normal in black-skinned people, but is present in people with white skin only in pathological states, such as Addison's disease (*see* 3.4)

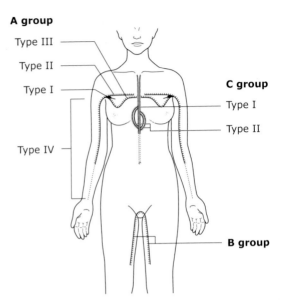

Fig 6.32 Pigmentary demarcation lines. Linear zones of hypopigmented skin adjacent to normal pigmented skin are a common occurrence. Similar patterns are seen in Afro-Carribean and Japanese people. The commonest are groups A and C (from Selmanowitz VJ & Krivo JM (1975) *Br J Dermatol.* **93:** 371, *courtesy of Blackwell Scientific Publications*)

and Futcher's lines. These lines are seen in black and Japanese people as a series of different patterns, some of which run true in particular families (**Fig 6.32**). The most common variant described in Afro-Carribean Americans is the midline vertical hypopigmentation line, which overlies the sternum in approximately 70% of Afro-Carribean children. This becomes less visible with increasing age; approximately 30% of adults are affected. The other relatively common type is the transition from darker dorsal to paler ventral skin on the anterior aspect of the upper arm, which has suggested the theory that the demarcation may have a photoprotective role.

Beaded juxtaclavicular lines

Beaded juxtaclavicular lines, which occur on the upper anterior trunk, are hyperplastic pilosebaceous follicles; they are relatively common, but more usual and more easily visible in black skin (**Fig 6.33**).

Nail pigmentation

Almost 90% of Afro-Caribbeans have pigmented bands on the nails. Several nails are commonly affected (*see* Fig 19.6).

Dermatosis papulosa nigra

Dermatosis papulosa nigra describes small, darkly pigmented, pedunculated and warty papules appearing on the face of Afro-Carribeans (**Fig 6.34**). They are very common and probably represent hyperpigmented seborrhoeic warts, although they are present at a younger age than seborrhoeic warts in white people.

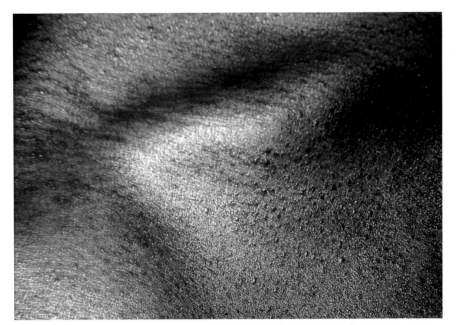

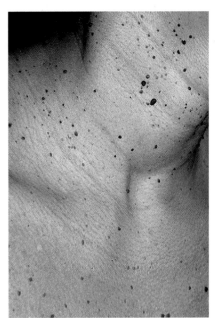

Fig 6.33 Beaded juxtaclavicular lines. These clustered papules on the upper anterior chest are a normal feature of both black and white skins, although they are easier to see in black skin, particularly over the clavicle where they appear to be linearly arranged. They may be confused with a disorder termed recurrent infundibulofolliculitis but are non-inflammatory and asymptomatic; although also described as an abnormal hamartoma under the name of hamartoma moniliformis, they are actually hairless pilosebaceous follicles and seem to be a normal finding in all individuals

Fig 6.34 Dermatosis papulosa nigra. Presenting as small, pigmented, warty lesions, these are very common in Afro-Carribean people. They appear to be deeply pigmented seborrhoeic warts, although they develop in a younger age group than seborrhoeic warts do in people with white skin. Note also the beaded juxtaclavicular lines (as shown in a different patient in 6.33)

SCARS AND POST-INFLAMMATORY CHANGES

Striae

Striae, or stretch marks, are common in adolescence due to the growth spurt. They occur on the back as horizontal, parallel lines, which are sometimes referred to as whiplash striae (**Fig 6.33**). Indeed, they have been confused with child abuse. They also occur on the thigh, buttocks and arms. In pregnancy, striae appear on the breasts and abdomen as they enlarge. Striae are common on the upper arms, chest and thighs of body builders and other people putting on weight rapidly. Topical, oral and endogenous corticosteroids (the latter in Cushing's syndrome) all cause collagen damage and accentuation of these otherwise physiological changes. However, patients with physiological striae on the lower back can be readily distinguished from those with Cushing's syndrome owing to their rapid increase in height rather than an increase in fat.

Scars

Several types of scarring may occur in acne, including ice-pick scars (**Fig 6.36**), flat scars on the face, white papular lesions, which occur particularly on the chest (**Fig 6.37**) and back and, less commonly, keloid scars (usually on the shoulders and upper trunk). Bridged comedones (**Fig 6.38**) are common in older men who have had severe acne, particularly on the back or perineal region, and form part of the follicular occlusion triad with hidradenitis suppurativa and dissecting cellulitis of the scalp.

109

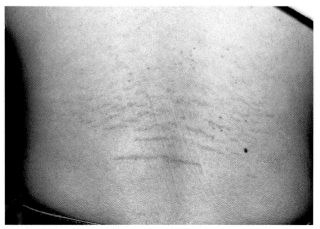

Fig 6.35 Whiplash striae. Stretch marks are common in the adolescent growth spurt. On the back they appear as horizontal parallel lines, where they are fancifully referred to as whiplash striae

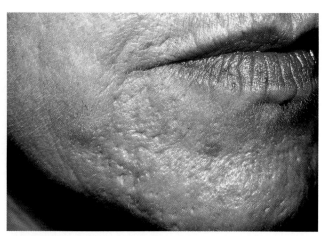

Fig 6.36 Ice-pick scarring due to acne. Deep or ice-pick scars can be excised with a punch biopsy. These are too deep for removal by dermabrasion

Fig 6.37 Papular lesions on the chest due to acne. Multiple flesh-coloured papules are present. Some lesions may show characteristic changes of anetoderma (*see* 4.21)

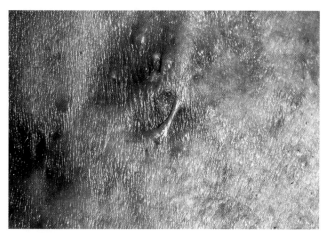

Fig 6.38 Bridged or fistulated comedones after acne. These occur, mainly on the back, in an aggressive form of acne known as acne conglobata. Other lesions in patients with this pattern of acne have multiple pores containing melanin-pigmented black comedones

Chicken-pox scars are usually depressed with a small crateriform edge to produce a 'punched out' appearance (**Fig 6.39**). Molluscum contagiosum initially heals with small scar-like lesions, which fade with time. In black skin, scars may become hypopigmented or hyperpigmented (**Fig 6.40**).

NORMAL VARIANTS AT SPECIFIC SITES

Genitalia

Pearly penile papules

Pearly penile papules are smooth, dome-shaped lesions. They are found around the penile corona, appearing after puberty and being entirely normal (**Fig 6.41**). Histologically, they are angiokeratomas.

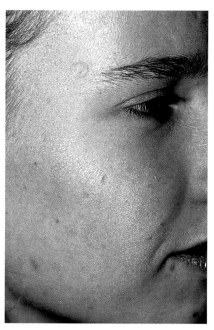

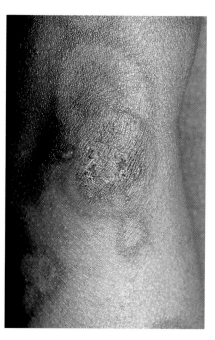

Fig 6.39 Chicken-pox scars.
These are characteristically crateriform scars that seem to occur after secondary infection of chicken-pox lesions

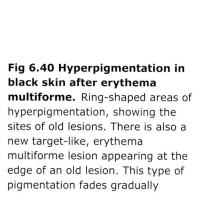

Fig 6.40 Hyperpigmentation in black skin after erythema multiforme. Ring-shaped areas of hyperpigmentation, showing the sites of old lesions. There is also a new target-like, erythema multiforme lesion appearing at the edge of an old lesion. This type of pigmentation fades gradually

Sebaceous glands on the genitalia

Sebaceous glands on the genitalia are tiny yellow papules, visible at the base of hairs on genital skin. They are also seen on the shaft of the penis (**Fig 6.42**), foreskin and frenulum without an associated hair. They may be a cause of anxiety in adolescent men and are occasionally confused with viral warts. Reassurance alone is required.

Axillae

Disorders related to the apocrine sweat apparatus are discussed on p98.

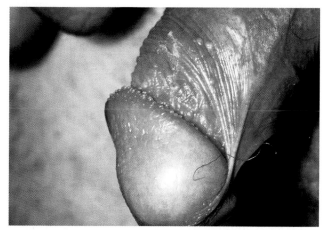

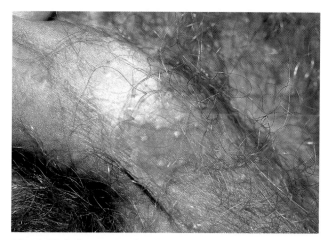

Fig 6.41 Pearly penile papules. These pink, shiny papules, which are symmetrically arranged around the base of the glans penis, are perfectly normal

Fig 6.42 Sebaceous glands on base of penile shaft. Sebaceous glands at this site may be large compared with the associated hair. They appear as geometrically arranged, yellowish papules and are best seen on the base of the penile shaft or scrotum. These are entirely normal, but sometimes cause alarm when they first appear in adolescence

111

Axillary tags

Axillary tags are small, flesh-coloured, pedunculated tags that are common in either sex around the neck (**Fig 6.43**) and in flexural areas such as the axillae and groin and beneath the breasts in women. Larger, pigmented tags also occur. Histologically, these are fibroepithelial polyps. Larger lesions may be confused with neurofibromas or pedunculated naevi.

Trichomycosis axillaris

Trichomycosis axillaris presents as yellowish concretions on axillary skin due to a build-up of the bacterium *Corynebacterium tenuis* (*see* Fig 18.51). The matted hairs are best removed by shaving, and then the condition can be prevented from reappearance by regular washing.

Head and neck

Fordyce spots—ectopic sebaceous glands of the lips and oral mucosa

Fordyce spots are multiple small, yellowish-white papules visible on the lips or buccal mucosa. They represent residual sebaceous glands at these hairless skin sites (**Fig 6.44**). The papules should not be confused with Wickham's striae due to lichen planus or with white plaques of candida.

Pre-auricular sinus

Pre-auricular sinus is usually a minor defect just visible as a tiny pit on the ascending portion of the helix (**Fig 6.45**). Larger sinuses, sometimes becoming granulomatous, are usually situated just in front of the ear. A pre-auricular sinus may become secondarily infected and cause recurrent facial cellulitis.

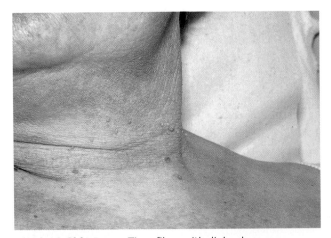

Fig 6.43 Skin tags. Tiny, fibroepithelial polyps are commonly seen around the axillae and neck, particularly in obese people. They are not warts

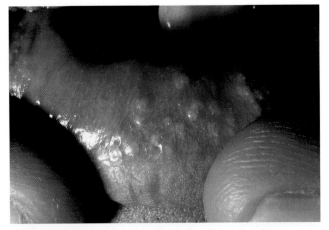

Fig 6.44 Sebaceous glands of the lips—Fordyce spots. Ectopic sebaceous glands without associated hair follicles can sometimes be seen as yellowish papules on the buccal mucosa and lips. These may be confused with lichen planus or candidiasis but are distinguished by being asymptomatic, yellow, uniform in size and without confluent, linear or reticulate patterning. Compare this with Wickham's striae of the lips (8.44)

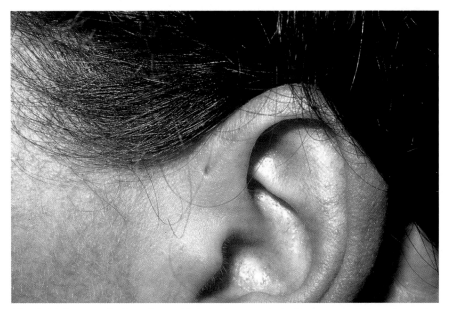

Fig 6.45 Pre-auricular sinus. This is characteristically seen as a tiny pit on the ascending portion of the helix. Larger sinuses are usually situated in front of the ear. The latter may become secondarily infected and have multiple irregular sinus tracts

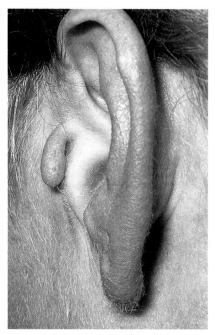

Fig 6.46 Accessory auricle. There is a fleshy papule just anterior to the ear. This may sometimes contain a cartilaginous core

Accessory auricle

Accessory auricles appear, sometimes bilaterally, just in front of the tragus or anterior to the sternomastoid muscle as a soft (**Fig 6.46**) or cartilaginous nodule.

Ear lobe crease

The presence of an ear lobe crease (**Fig 6.47**) is associated with an increased prevalence of major coronary artery disease and a cardiovascular cause of death. It is not related to obesity.

Milia

Milia are tiny white papules of epidermal-lined keratin that arise from a sweat duct epithelium. Originating in the dermis, they slowly migrate upwards through the skin. They are common on the cheeks and around the eyes of adults (**Fig 6.48**) and newborn babies.

Legs and feet

Dimpled fat (cellulite)

On thighs and buttocks, particularly in women, deposition of excessive subcutaneous fat is uneven because the fibrous septae joining the skin to the deep fascia limit smooth swelling of the subcutaneous tissue. This creates an irregular, dimpled surface, which has been called cellulite (**Figs 6.49** and **6.50**). A similar appearance can be seen on the bottoms of plump, healthy babies.

Piezogenic (pressure-induced) pedal papules

Piezogenic pedal papules are small, fatty lumps, usually asymptomatic, which occur on the medial side of the foot on standing (**Fig 6.51**). They are due to

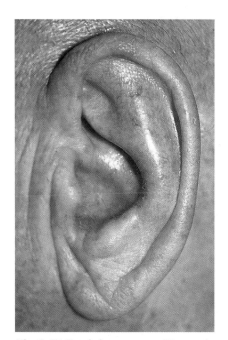

Fig 6.47 Ear lobe crease. Diagonal ear lobe creases are present in 30% of adults; they run diagonally back at approximately 45 degrees from the external meatus to the edge of the ear lobe. Their presence correlates with coronary artery disease

113

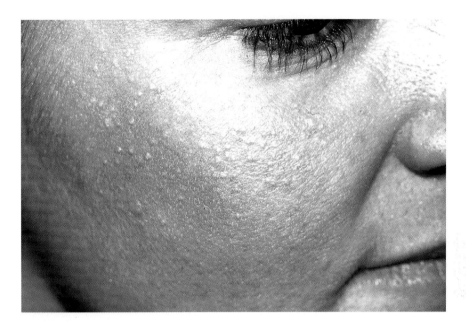

Fig 6.48 Milia. These small, yellowish papules are commonly seen on the cheeks of healthy individuals. They are not closed comedones, but are small, epithelial line cysts that can be removed only after piercing the overlying skin with a sharp needle. They are derived from sweat duct epithelium, and if left alone they slowly migrate through the dermis and epidermis until shed

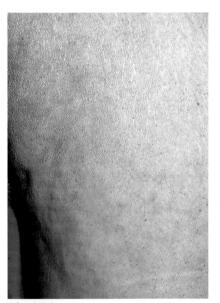

Fig 6.49

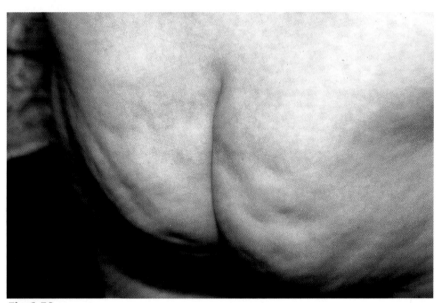

Fig 6.50

Fig 6.49, 6.50 Cellulite. Dimpling of the fat on the thighs and buttocks is very common, particularly in women (6.49). It also occurs on the buttocks in chubby children, as shown here in this 1-year-old boy (6.50)

fatty herniations into the dermis. Although present in 75% of the population, they become painful or more pronounced in some people for obscure reasons. Similar papules are seen at the palmar aspect of the wrist in 85% of normal individuals.

Muscle herniations of the leg

Muscle herniations are soft swellings visible on the lateral aspect of the shins on standing (**Fig 6.52**). Palpation normally reveals a small defect in the underlying deep fascia, usually the entry point of a vessel or nerve through the tibialis anterior muscle, through which muscle herniates. Such herniations are more common in muscular individuals.

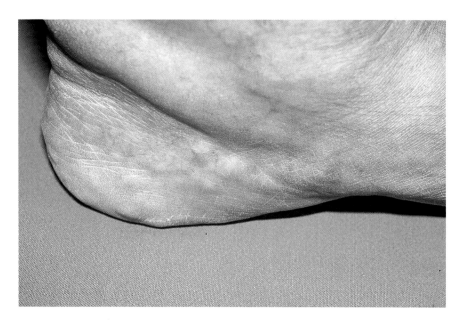

Fig 6.51 Piezogenic pedal papules. These small, fatty herniations are commonly seen on the side of the heel (best seen with the patient standing) and also occur at the wrist. They are present in virtually everyone. Occasionally they become painful

Hands

Palm crease pits

Small pits can be identified in the palm creases of approximately 20% of normal individuals (*see* Fig 7.49). They are more common in black people and are not a consequence of manual labour. Palmar pits seen in Darier's disease (*see* Figs 7.50 and 7.51) and basal cell naevus syndrome (*see* Fig 7.52 and Table 7.4) are not limited to palm crease lines.

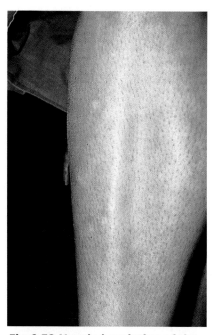

Fig 6.52 Muscle herniation of the leg. This is caused by herniation of muscle through the deep fascia where it is perforated by communicating veins. It presents as nodules on the anterior lateral aspect of the lower leg. The nodules are soft and compressible and can be accentuated by sitting with the legs crossed and pressing the calf hard on the opposite knee

7 Scale, crust and thickened skin

DEFINITIONS

Keratoderma

Keratoderma is a pattern of increased thickness of keratin, which produces an exaggeration of the normal features, with a relatively smooth surface (**Fig 7.1**) but none of the loose flakes seen in a scaling disorder and without the craggy roughness of hyperkeratosis.

Scales

Scales are thin, dry plates of desquamated epithelial cells, formed as a result of either increased or abnormal keratinisation (**Fig 7.2**).

Hyperkeratosis

Hyperkeratosis is thickening of the keratin layer and thus is similar in mechanism to scaling. The difference is that in hyperkeratosis, the keratin is adherent rather than loose and thus creates a craggy rough surface (**Fig 7.3**), mounds or horns rather than the plate-like morphology of scales.

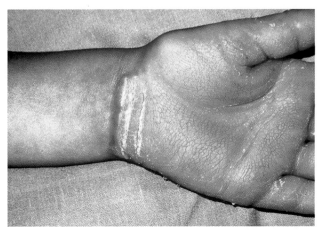

Fig 7.1 Diffuse palmar keratoderma or tylosis. There are several varieties of diffuse keratoderma. Most are inherited and have no systemic significance, although one type, described in just three families, is strongly associated with carcinoma of the oesophagus. Acquired palmoplantar keratoderma has been associated with carcinoma of the bronchus and adenocarcinoma of the stomach

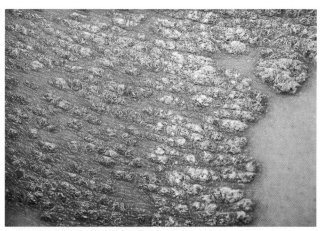

Fig 7.2 Psoriatic scale and rubbing. The right side of the plaque has been rubbed with a wooden spatula. This results in the appearance of white scale on the plaque surface, as more light is reflected from the multiple air–keratin interfaces produced

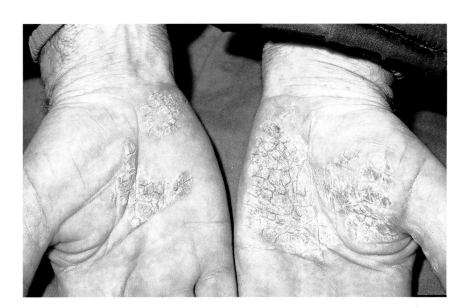

Fig 7.3 Hyperkeratotic palmar eczema. This chronic condition usually affects both palms and is thought by some to be the result of repeated trauma; it is more common in men and is not due to contact allergies

Crusts

Crusts or, more colloquially, scabs are formed from dried blood (brownish-red colour), serum (yellow) or purulent (yellowish-green) exudate, as in impetigo (**Fig 7.4**). A crust may be thick or thin, friable or adherent.

KERATODERMA

Differences between hyperkeratotic plaques and keratoderma

Confluent psoriasis (*see* Fig 8.16) or eczema (**Fig 7.3**) results in sheets of flaking, which may become hugely hyperkeratotic, with a hard, craggy rough surface. Within such plaques, there are often deep fissures caused by splitting of the thick skin during flexion and extension.

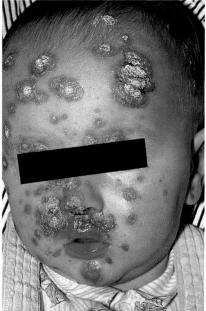

Fig 7.4 Impetigo crusts. This child has extensive crusted lesions on his forehead and oozy lesions around his nose

In keratoderma, the horny layer of the epidermis is formed normally, but is not shed at the correct rate. Thus, the horny layer becomes thicker, producing a waxy layer of thick, yellow keratin (*see* Fig 7.1) similar in colour to that seen in a simple corn. The thickened skin in keratoderma is not scaly and cannot be picked off, in contrast to the hyperkeratotic disorders such as psoriasis and hyperkeratotic eczema. In the latter disorders, epidermal cells are produced in excess, and because they are not properly formed, they scale or flake-off easily, particularly when rubbed or scratched.

Palm and sole keratoderma

Most types of keratoderma affect the palms and soles, and occasionally, the knees, elbows and heels are also involved. The keratoderma may result in confluent involvement of the whole palm and sole or focal islands of keratoderma (**Fig 7.45**). In contrast to hyperkeratosis, the overlying keratin at these sites is usually relatively flexible and does not scale or fissure. Contrast this with the shiny and fissured scale of juvenile forefoot dermatosis (**Fig 7.46**, *see also* Fig 5.24) and the hyperkeratosis of chronic eczema (**Fig 7.3**). In psoriasis of the hands, linear hyperkeratotic psoriatic lesions may appear on the sides of the fingers (**Fig 7.47**), over the joints and on the palms.

TYPES OF SCALE

Psoriasiform

Psoriatic scale is made from imperfectly formed, poorly adherent, parakeratotic epithelial cells, identified histologically by the retained nuclear remnants. Gentle rubbing disrupts the loose layers of parakeratotic cells, producing multiple air–keratin interfaces, which reflect rather than transmit light. Hence, as the scaly plaque is rubbed, the surface stratum corneum loses its transparency and turns white (*see* Fig 7.2). Continued rubbing results in the appearance of pinpoint bleeding, as the thin, suprapapillary epidermis is removed, and the dermal vessels are breached. This appearance is sometimes referred to as Auspitz's sign. It is not specific to psoriasis, being seen also in Darier's disease, seborrhoeic warts and actinic keratoses.

Ichthyotic scale

Diffuse ichthyotic scaling resembles fish scale, although unlike fish skin, the scales do not overlap, and the plates of dry skin are separated by cracked edges. There are a variety of inherited types of ichthyosis (**Table 7.1 and Figs 7.5–7.12**), the commonest being ichthyosis vulgaris (*see* Figs 7.5 and 7.6), which is associated with atopic eczema. Acquired ichthyosis occurs in malnutrition, starvation and lymphoma and is indistinguishable from ichthyosis vulgaris. Patients with ichthyosis vulgaris often also have exaggerated skin creases (*see* Fig 7.6). Ichthyosis is seen in its most severe form in babies born with a variant of non-bullous ichthyosiform erythroderma. These children are encased in rigid hyperkeratotic scale, which splits, producing an appearance not unlike a harlequin's costume. These babies invariably died, hence the term harlequin fetus (**Fig 7.10**). Since the mid-1980s, some have survived with the use of oral retinoids, and the term harlequin ichthyosis has been coined.

Some ichthyoses, such as erythrokeratoderma variabilis and ichthyosis linearis circumflexa (the skin eruption of Netherton's syndrome), consist of changing annular and polycyclic lesions (**Fig 7.12**) rather than diffuse ichthyosis. The affected sites still have the same fine flakes of scaling on the inside of the extending margin. In ichthyosis linearis circumflexa, this appearance is described as 'double-edged.'

Table 7.1 Types of ichthyosis

Type	Inheritance	Clinical features
Ichthyosis vulgaris (7.5)	Autosomal dominant	Small white shiny plaques, with sparing of the flexures
Non-bullous ichthyosiform erythroderma (7.7)	Autosomal recessive	Generalised redness and fine scaling of the entire skin surface
Bullous ichthyosiform erythroderma	Autosomal dominant	At birth, generalised erythema, scaling and blister formation at frictional trauma sites. In adult life, verrucous hyperkeratosis at flexures and peculiar digitate keratoses ('porcupine man')
Lamellar ichthyosis (7.8)	Autosomal recessive	Large thick dark brown scales associated with ectropion. Affected children present as collodion babies at birth (7.9)
Steroid sulphatase deficiency (7.11)	X-linked (males only)	Large darker brown scales and ichthyosis vulgaris. Flexural involvement occurs, but some sparing is always present, usually of antecubital and popliteal fossae (1.11)

Fine (pityriasiform) scale

Fine scale is seen in the xerosis or dry skin of atopic eczema (**Fig 7.13**), pityriasis rosea, pityriasis versicolor (**Fig 7.14** and **7.15**), seborrhoeic eczema (**Fig 7.16** and **2.9**) and fungal infections (**Fig 7.17**).

In endogenous eczema and psoriasis, the rash is usually symmetrical, in contrast to a fungal infection (**Fig 7.18**). Incorrect diagnosis leading to the use of topical steroid therapy for a dermatophyte infection may initially mask some of these features by reducing the local inflammatory response (*see* 15.19).

In fungal infections due to dermatophytes ('ringworm' fungi) or to *Pityrosporum ovale* (the yeast that causes pityriasis versicolor, now more strictly termed *Malassezia globosa*), gentle scraping of the skin using a blunt scalpel produces a small heap of feathery, delicate scale. Examination of this scale under a microscope, using potassium hydroxide to dissolve the keratin, reveals the presence of hyphae (*see* Fig 4.42). In pityriasis versicolor infections, the abnormal scaling resolves with treatment, but the affected skin often remains depigmented until further sun exposure. Occasionally, pigment loss is permanent. Persistent scaling implies that treatment has been inadequate.

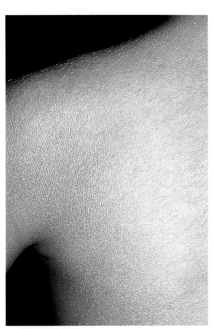

Fig 7.5 Ichthyosis vulgaris. Fine white scale on the back of a Chinese child with extensive ichthyosis vulgaris

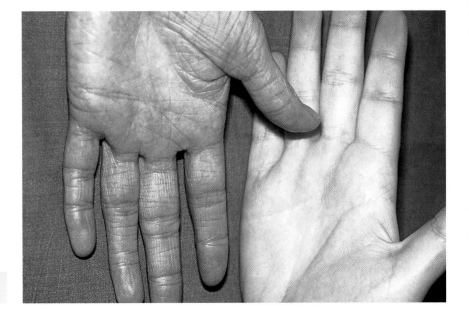

Fig 7.6 Exaggerated skin crease in ichthyosis vulgaris compared with a normal palm. Both are palms of females in their mid-thirties. The palm on the left belongs to a patient with ichthyosis vulgaris and atopic eczema. Skin crease lines are greater in number, wider and a darker pink than those of the normal palm

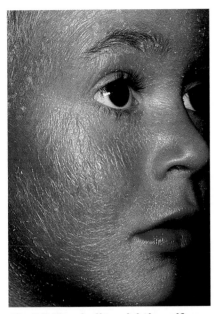

Fig 7.7 Non-bullous ichthyosiform erythroderma. This child has generalised red skin with fine scaling. He was a severely affected collodion baby but now has relatively mild, non-bullous ichthyosiform erythroderma requiring topical treatment only

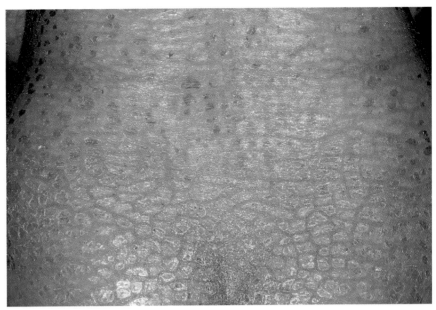

Fig 7.8 Lamella ichthyosis. The scales are large dark plates; all sites are affected, including the flexures. At birth, affected children may be collodion babies (*see* 7.6)

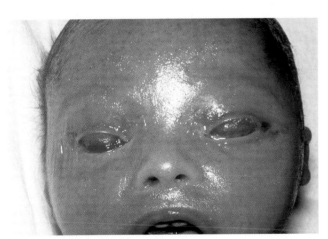

Fig 7.9 Collodion baby. Children with this condition are born with this shiny cellophane-like covering of skin, which splits. The tight scale constricts, producing an ectropion and interfering with feeding. The skin is shed within a few weeks, and the child goes on to manifest either lamella ichthyosis, X-linked ichthyosis, non-bullous ichthyosiform erythroderma or, occasionally, normal skin (*photo courtesy of Dr D W A Milligan*)

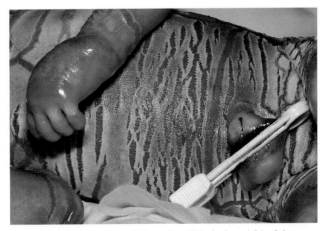

Fig 7.10 Harlequin ichthyosis. This baby girl is 8 hours old. She is encased in a thick scale. Note the oedematous hands covered in a mucoid membrane. The scale forms *in utero* from the abnormal keratin and does not stretch to allow the child to grow. The child then becomes encased in a rigid scale, which splits as the baby grows (as shown here), or the child's face produces grotesque eversion of the eyelids and lips so that only the mucosal surfaces are visible. Here, the scale has been kept moist by careful nursing in a high-humidity incubator; in a drier atmosphere, the scale would dry out and form what has been described as a 'coat of armour'

The fine scaling seen in atopic xerosis is considered by some to be a mild form of ichthyosis vulgaris. Others, including ourselves, use the term ichthyosis vulgaris to describe light-reflecting, fish-like scales adhering to the skin and sparing the flexures. We consider xerosis and ichthyosis vulgaris to

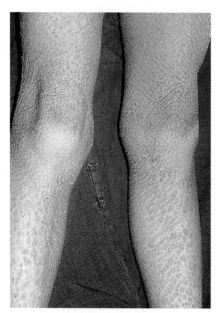

Fig 7.11 Steroid sulphatase deficiency. There are large dirty-brown scales over the entire body. Although flexures are involved, there is usually some sparing around the antecubital and popliteal fossae (*see* 1.11)

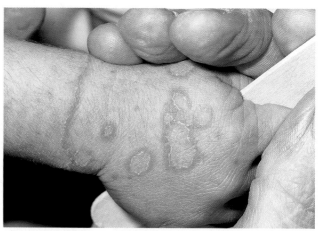

Fig 7.12 Erythrokeratoderma variabilis. This uncommon inherited disorder of keratinisation presents with slowly migrating or changing annular or polycyclic lesions with fine ichthyotic scaling at the margin

Fig 7.13 Atopic xerosis. Fine scaling on the limbs of a 9-year-old boy with atopic eczema. The scale may be seen better if the skin is rubbed gently with the finger nail. It is easier to appreciate the 'dryness' or fine scaling and slight roughness of the skin by touch than it is by sight

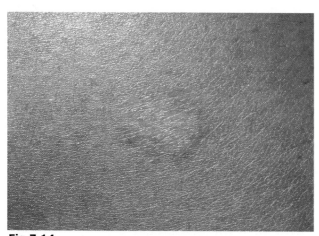

Fig 7.14

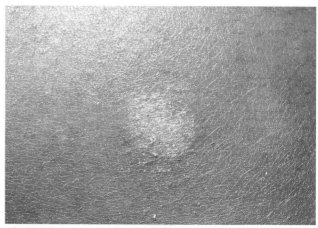

Fig 7.15

Fig 7.14, 7.15 Pityriasis versicolor scaling. Fine scale on the pigmented lesion (7.15) can be shown by scraping the surface with a blunt scalpel (7.14). The causative yeast can be identified on microscopic examination of potassium hydroxide preparation (see 4.42)

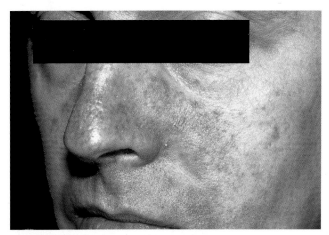

Fig 7.16 Seborrhoeic eczema of the face. Fine, rather greasy scaling on the cheeks, nasolabial folds, eyebrows, ear canals and scalp is common in seborrhoeic eczema. The same patient is shown in 2.9. Thicker scaling also occurs (*see* 7.27). Scalp changes are shown in 18.53

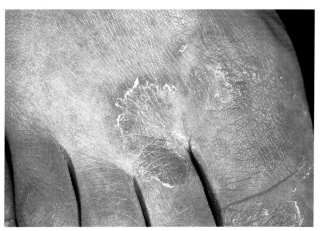

Fig 7.17 Scaling annular edge in tinea pedis. In active fungal infections, there is an advancing edge with an inward-pointing scale. The scaly border of fungal infections commonly reaches the extreme red border, unlike the inward-pointing scaly border of pityriasis rosea (*see* 7.22), which starts a few millimetres from the red edge. Skin scrapings from tinea pedis will show fungal hyphae (*see* 4.43)

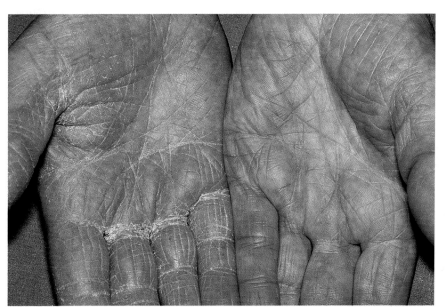

Fig 7.18 Fungal infection of palms. *Trichophyton rubrum* infections on the palms and soles produce widespread, fine, white scaling that may be easily overlooked. Asymmetrical involvement is an important clue; the right hand is affected. Note the deeper pink colour and white scale visible in the skin creases on the thenar eminence

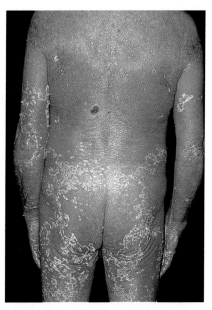

Fig 7.19 Erythrodermic psoriasis. There is generalised fine scaling in this man with erythrodermic psoriasis. It is impossible to diagnose the cause of confluent erythroderma from the skin changes alone; previous history, medications and results of skin biopsy may all be important

be separate entities for the following reasons; atopic xerosis affects all sites, whereas ichthyosis spares the flexures; fine scale occurs in xerosis compared with the larger scales seen in ichthyosis; and, functionally, atopic xerosis behaves like low-grade eczema.

Generalised scale or exfoliative dermatitis

Virtually complete skin involvement with redness and fine scaling is referred to as erythroderma or exfoliative dermatitis (**Fig 7.19**). There are several

123

causes of erythroderma (*see* Table 2.4), but in the fully developed case, these may be clinically indistinguishable.

Annular scaling

Annular lesions may have well formed large flakes of 'psoriasiform' scaling (e.g. psoriasis, secondary syphilis) or smaller flakes of fine scaling (e.g. tinea corporis, lupus erythematosus (**Fig 7.20**) and eczema).

A collarette or thin rim of inward-pointing scale is also seen in disorders such as pityriasis rosea (**Figs 7.21** and **7.22**), drug eruptions (**Fig 7.23**), viral exanthemata and porokeratosis (**Figs 7.24–7.25**). Lesions of erythema annulare centrifugum may have a 'trailing edge' of scale, as the annular lesions gradually expand (*see* Fig 2.3).

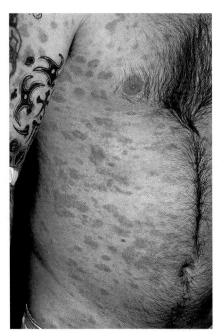

Fig 7.21 Pityriasis rosea. Fir-tree distribution of pityriasis rosea on the trunk. Lesions are oval, with their long axis sloping out and downwards from the midline

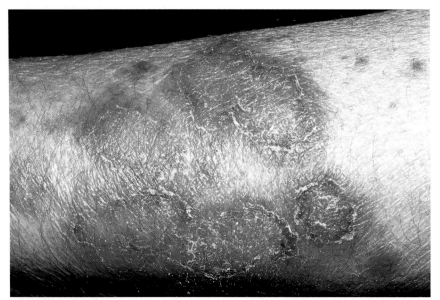

Fig 7.20 Subacute lupus erythematosus. Annular scaling lesions and photosensitivity are the two characteristics of subacute lupus erythematosus

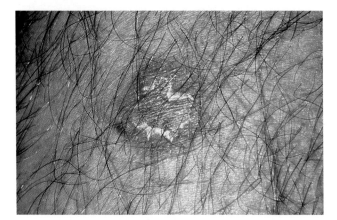

Fig 7.22 Pityriasis rosea—herald patch. The herald patch is larger than the eruptive lesions, but otherwise identical in morphology. The word pityriasis refers to the bran-like or feathery, delicate, fine, fluffy nature of the scale. In pityriasis rosea, the unattached margin of scale points towards the centre of the lesion and starts several millimetres inside the outer margin of the red papule—unlike in a fungal infection, where scaling is present at the outermost margin of the red area

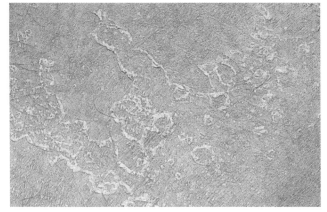

Fig 7.23 Collarettes of scaling in a resolving drug eruption. A similar pattern occurs after sunburn

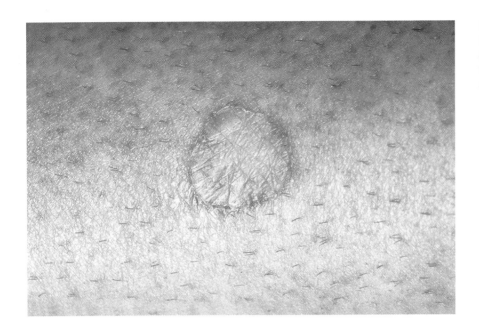

Fig 7.24 Porokeratosis. Individual lesions of porokeratosis are similar in all variants. They are annular lesions with a rim of inward-pointing scale and an atrophic centre

Pityriasis rosea

Pityriasis rosea principally affects people aged 10–35 years. A single, scaly, oval, herald patch appears, usually on the trunk or proximal limbs. Approximately 7–14 days later, multiple scaly lesions appear on the trunk and proximal limbs (**Fig 7.21**). These are usually oval patches 1–2 cm in diameter and covered with a fine scale, which rapidly begins to peel centrally, leaving a collarette of fine scale attached at the rim, with the free edge pointing towards the centre of the patch (**Fig 7.22**). Scaling does not extend to the edge of the lesion, which has a red, slightly raised margin. On the trunk, the lesions characteristically follow the skinfold lines (**Fig 7.21**), and the overall pattern has been likened to a fir-tree shape. Pityriasis rosea-like eruptions occur in some types of drug reactions, including those to gold, captopril, metronidazole and barbiturates. Similar lesions can be seen in eczema and psoriasis, and secondary syphilis should always be considered in the differential diagnosis.

Post-inflammatory scale

In the late stages of drug eruptions, viral infections (*see* Fig 10.2) and simple sunburn, it is common to see scaling or peeling at the margins of resolving lesions. There is often an appearance of annular peeling within the affected region, forming 'collarettes' (**Fig 7.23**). Similar small collarettes of scaling are seen on the palms in the resolving phase of a pompholyx or dyshidrotic eczema.

Porokeratotic scale

Individual lesions of porokeratosis (**Fig 7.24**) are oval or round, 5–15 mm in diameter, with a ridge of horny scale that points upwards and inwards towards the centre of the lesion. The skin in the centre of the lesion is atrophic, and there may be a central follicular keratosis in early lesions. The commonest form, in which individual lesions are small, is disseminated superficial actinic porokeratosis. This relatively common condition is seen on the lower legs (**Fig 7.25**) and other sun-exposed sites, usually in women, and must be distinguished from actinic keratoses. A more severe variant, known as porokeratosis of Mibelli, occurs on the trunk, face and genitalia. On the limbs, lesions may be reticulate or grouped in a linear fashion (**Fig 7.26**).

DIAGNOSTIC TIPS AND PITFALLS

- In patients with pigment loss due to pityriasis versicolor, the presence of scaling indicates persistent infection

- Psoriatic plaque scale turns white on rubbing because of the creation of multiple light-reflecting keratin—air layers

- Crust indicates the presence of exudate; scale indicates a disorder of keratin production or damage to a normally formed stratum corneum

- The differential diagnosis of pityriasis rosea includes drug reactions (gold, captopril, metronidazole and barbiturates), eczema, psoriasis and secondary syphilis

- Malignant transformation of actinic keratosis to squamous cell carcinomas occurs in less than 1% of cases

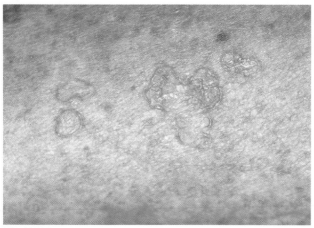

Fig 7.25

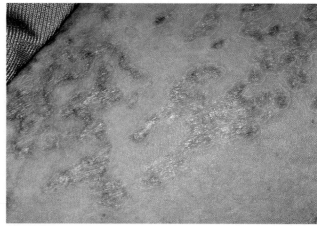

Fig 7.26

Fig 7.25, 7.26 Porokeratosis. There are two common types of porokeratosis: disseminated superficial actinic porokeratosis, in which the lesions are discrete and scattered and usually seen on the legs in women (7.27); and the more severe porokeratosis of Mibelli, in which lesions merge together to form a reticulate pattern (7.28). Note the slightly wrinkled appearance of the atrophic skin centrally within each lesion

Peeling and glazed desquamation

In some dermatoses, sheets of keratin may be shed. This can happen in several acute transient eruptions, such as sunburn or drug eruptions; in these conditions, small collarettes of scaling are often prominent.

Desquamation of the palms and soles may occur in the form of sheets of keratin, owing to the thickness and self-adherent nature of the horny layer. This may also occur after an acute dermatosis or systemic illness or may be caused by drugs such as systemic retinoids. It typically leaves a rather red shiny or 'glazed' appearance of the underlying skin—similar to that seen in juvenile plantar dermatosis (*see* Fig 7.46).

Sheets of desquamation with a shiny or glazed appearance also occur in kwashiorkor, in which the appearance of the skin has been termed the 'enamel paint sign'.

Greasy adherent yellow–brown scale

Greasy adherent yellow–brown scale is present in seborrhoeic eczema and Darier's disease.

Seborrhoeic eczema

In seborrhoeic eczema the scaling tends to occur on the central face (**Fig 7.27**), central chest or interscapular area and around the ears. This is probably due to the high density of sebaceous glands at these sites; seborrhoeic eczema is caused by a *Pityrosporum ovale* infection or overgrowth, and this yeast feeds on the secretions of the sebaceous gland.

Darier's disease (keratosis follicularis)

Darier's disease is an autosomal dominant skin disorder that produces lesions on the trunk, neck, face, palms (**Figs 7.50 and 7.51**), mouth, hands and nails (*see* Fig 19.25). Multiple papules become grouped into sheets of oozy, sometimes foul-smelling plaques, especially on the central chest, under the breasts (**Fig 7.28**), around the ears and on the flexures. The individual lesions are

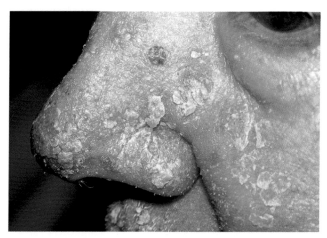

Fig 7.27 Crusted seborrhoeic eczema. Thick, yellow crusted scales are present on the face of this elderly man with seborrhoeic eczema. Inadequate washing is probably a contributory factor

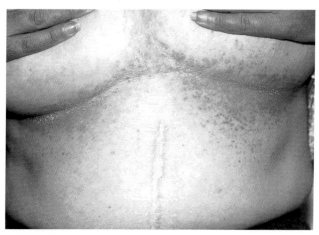

Fig 7.28 Darier's disease of the chest. There are symmetrical confluent brown papules under the breasts in this woman with Darier's disease. Her nails are shown in 19.25

warty papules, 1–3 mm in diameter (**Fig 7.29**), which in places may appear distributed in a follicular pattern because of the close-set, geometric arrangement. However, the papules are closely packed, having a higher than normal follicular density; they may arise at sites that do not contain follicular epithelium (e.g. the mouth, palms), and histologically, they do not arise from follicular epidermis, although keratotic plugs may, by chance, fill follicles. On the back of the hands, flat, warty papules resembling plane warts are visible (**Fig 7.30**), whereas on the palms, small pits can be seen (*see* Fig 7.50 and 7.51).

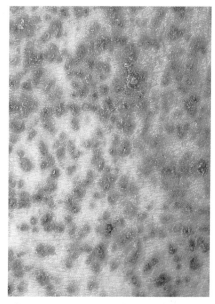

Fig 7.29 Close-up view of Darier's papules. These conical brown papules are covered by a dirty-brown hyperkeratotic crusted scale. When this is removed, a tiny oozy pit remains. Papules on the body, the acrokeratosis verruciformis lesions, and palm pits all share the same histological features of suprabasal clefts and acantholysis

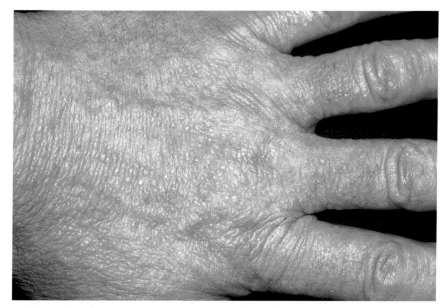

Fig 7.30 Acrokeratosis verruciformis in Darier's disease. On the dorsum of the hands, multiple or sometimes solitary small warty papules can be seen. These acrokeratosis verruciformis lesions may be confused with plane warts. Acrokeratosis verruciformis and nail changes (*see* 19.25) are the first features to appear in affected children

Initial reports suggested that many people with this condition were mentally retarded, but it is now clear that most affected individuals are of normal intelligence.

HYPERKERATOSIS

Focal lesions

Warty scaling is a common feature of some solitary lesions such as seborrhoeic warts (*see* Fig 9.79–9.82). It is also seen in association with chronic oedema (**Fig 7.31**, *see also* Fig 17.46).

Discrete areas of hyperkeratotic scaling, especially on the lower legs, are a common presenting feature. These may be due to generalised skin disease such as psoriasis or eczema, but there is also a variety of non-follicular keratoses that produce similar changes with multiple small keratotic lesions.

Some of the common causes of multiple, discrete, scaly papules have been discussed earlier in this chapter and are listed in **Table 7.2**.

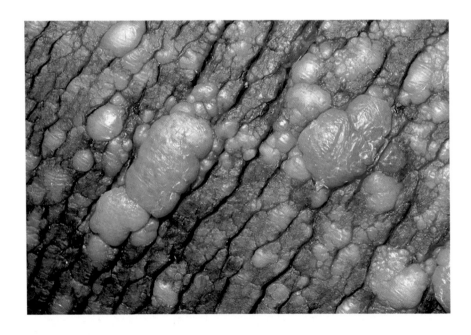

Fig 7.31 Warty change in chronic oedema. Deep clefts and slightly warty nodules are a feature of longstanding lymphoedema (*see also* 17.46)

Table 7.2 Common causes of multiple discrete scaly or hyperkeratotic papules

Psoriasis (8.11)

Eczema (2.1)

Disseminated superficial actinic porokeratosis (7.25)

Flegel's disease (hyperkeratosis lenticularis perstans)

Kyrle's disease (7.32)

Actinic keratoses (7.33, 7.34)

Arsenical keratoses (7.48)

Seborrhoeic warts (9.79)

Stucco keratoses (7.35)

Flegel's disease and Kyrle's disease

Flegel's disease and Kyrle's disease are discussed together because they are difficult to distinguish clinically and are possibly variants of the same condition. In its classic form, Flegel's disease appears on the trunk and limbs as small, warty papules with overlying psoriasiform scale. In Kyrle's disease (**Fig 7.32**), similar grouped follicular papules, with a central keratotic plug that may reach 20 mm in diameter, are seen.

Actinic keratoses

Actinic keratoses are patches of dyskeratosis or abnormal keratinocyte maturation caused by excessive sun exposure and are common on exposed sites in people with white skin. Initially, they appear as small areas of telangiectasia with a very fine overlying scale (**Fig 7.33**). These areas progress to patches of ill-defined scaling (**Fig 7.34**), which may be pigmented. Scaling may be thickened or only just apparent but is characteristically hard and spiky in texture,

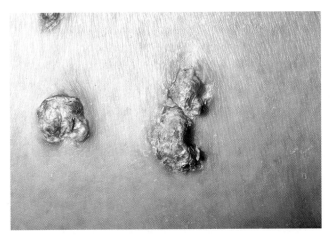

Fig 7.32 Kyrle's disease. This disorder of keratinisation is characterised by hard keratotic nodules, which are partially buried within the skin and leave a deep crater when removed

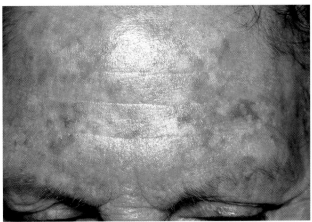

Fig 7.33 Actinic keratosis—telangiectatic type. Multiple small oval and round scaly telangiectatic areas of actinic keratoses are present on this patient's forehead

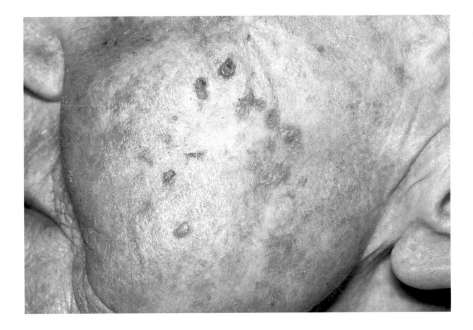

Fig 7.34 Actinic keratosis—scaly type. There are multiple warty keratoses on the cheek of this elderly woman who had never had a holiday abroad. Note also the general yellowing of her skin (*see also* 9.86–9.88)

129

to the extent that the palpable abnormality is more striking than the visual appearance of the lesions. Malignant transformation to squamous cell carcinomas probably occurs in less than 0.1% of cases; in addition, the tumours created have a low rate of metastasis in comparison with squamous cell carcinomas arising on skin not damaged by sun exposure or in a patch of Bowen's disease.

Stucco keratoses

Stucco keratoses are tiny, whitish, warty papules seen on the lower limb of elderly patients (**Fig 7.35**). They are very similar to small seborrhoeic warts except that they do not pigment.

Follicular lesions

Follicular hyperkeratosis

Hyperkeratosis localised to follicular orifices (**Table 7.3**) is commonly seen in keratosis pilaris (**Fig 7.36**) and pityriasis rubra pilaris (**Fig 7.37**). Careful inspection of plaques of lichen sclerosis et atrophicus (**Fig 7.39**) and discoid lupus erythematosus (**Fig 7.40** and **7.41**) may reveal multiple follicular, keratotic plugs in the affected areas. Digitate keratoses (**Fig 7.42**) are often not follicular in origin but may be confused with follicular keratoses as they have a similar distribution density on the skin surface.

Table 7.3 Recognised causes of follicular keratoses
Discoid lupus erythematosus (7.40)
Psoriasis (8.9–8.13)
Lichen planus (8.22)
Keratosis pilaris (7.36)
Pityriasis rubra pilaris (7.37)
Lichen sclerosis et atrophicus (7.39)
AIDS-related pityriasis rubra pilaris (7.38)

DIAGNOSTIC TIPS AND PITFALLS

- Digitate keratoses may be acquired or familial; they are multiple small finger-like projections, which resemble follicular keratoses but may not be follicular in origin and are thus potentially more densely packed

- The tin-tack sign is produced by the presence of keratin moulds of follicular orifices—it occurs in discoid lupus erythematosus, pemphigus erythematosus, seborrhoeic eczema, some drug eruptions and radiation-damaged skin

- Keratoderma produces yellow, flexible, thickening of the stratum corneum of the palms and soles. By contrast, in hyperkeratosis, the thickened keratin is craggy, white and fissured

- A crust on a solitary lesion obscures most of the physical signs. The crust must therefore be removed before attempting to make a diagnosis

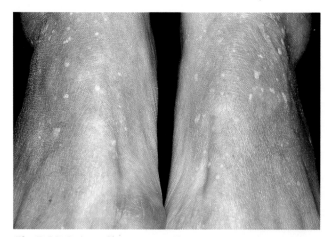

Fig 7.35 Stucco keratoses. These are tiny white warty papules, seen here on the dorsum of the foot and ankle. They are considered to be a variant of seborrhoeic warts

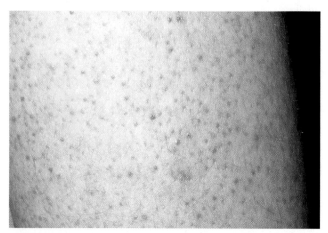

Fig 7.36 Keratosis pilaris. A form of follicular hyperkeratosis, which is most common on the outer thigh and outer upper arm. Individual lesions are small spikes of hyperkeratosis, with mild inflammation in some cases

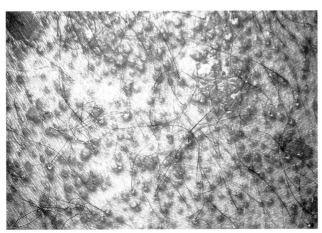

Fig 7.37 Pityriasis rubra pilaris. Follicular papules have a broader inflammatory component than keratosis pilaris. Five types are generally recognised, based on age group and location (*see also* 2.43)

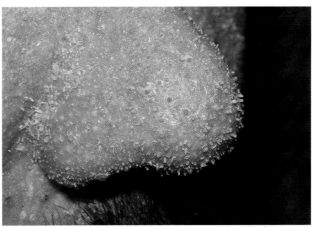

Fig 7.38 Follicular keratosis on the nose in HIV infection. This severe variant of pityriasis rubra pilaris has been described in AIDS patients who also have pronounced pustular acne

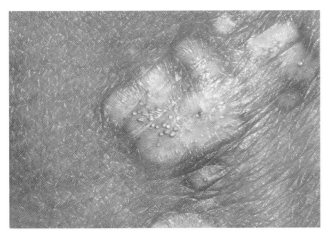

Fig 7.39 Lichen sclerosus et atrophicus follicular keratoses. There are little follicular plugs in this ivory-coloured plaque of lichen sclerosus et atrophicus. Compare this with the classic lichen sclerosus et atrophicus extragenital lesions shown in 8.29

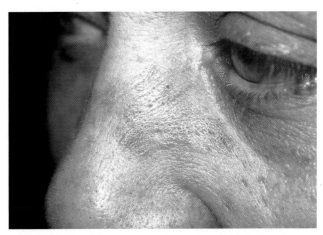

Fig 7.40 Discoid lupus erythematosus showing follicular plugs. Follicular plugging in plaques of discoid lupus erythematosus can be seen on the side of this woman's nose

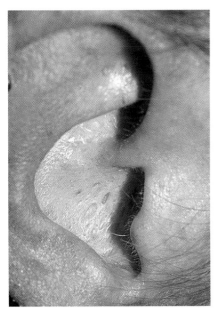

Fig 7.41 Follicular plugging of the concha in discoid lupus erythematosus. Large follicular plugs are seen in approximately a third of patients with this condition

Fig 7.42 Digitate keratoses. These small spikes of keratin are finger-shaped and probably occur in several disorders. They may be provoked by radiotherapy, and in some instances, they appear as a transient phenomenon

Perforating dermatoses

The perforating dermatoses are diseases in which damaged or abnormal dermal material such as red cells, micro-organisms or altered connective tissue is extruded through the epidermis as a secondary phenomenon (for example, damaged collagen in perforating granuloma annulare). This process is also termed transepidermal elimination.

In some perforating disorders, such as elastosis perforans serpiginosa, perforating folliculitis and Kyrle's disease (*see* Fig 7.32), transepidermal elimination is considered to be the primary disorder. Interestingly, a similar range of perforating dermatoses (reactive perforating collagenosis) are often seen in patients with chronic renal failure and diabetes. The extruded material is not keratin but is often extruded into the upper portion of a follicle and forms a hard plug; where the extrusion occurs through interfollicular epidermis, the epidermis is often thickened and has a central pit through which the extruded material passes. Thus, all these conditions share the ability to produce lesions, which, even if not necessarily follicular or keratotic, resemble multiple follicular keratoses.

Tin-tack sign

Removal of adherent scale sometimes reveals adherent keratin plugs attached to the undersurface of the scale that are reminiscent of carpet tacks; these are keratin moulds of follicular orifices (**Fig 7.43**). The tin-tack sign is present in discoid lupus erythematosus, pemphigus erythematosus (**Fig 7.44**), seborrhoeic eczema, some drug eruptions and radiation-damaged skin.

Palmar lesions

Palmar pits and keratoses

In healthy individuals, palmar crease pits (*see* pp 134–5) and keratoses may be present. Palmar keratoses and pits can also occur as a result of arsenic ingestion (**Fig 7.48**), Darier's disease (*see* Figs 7.50 and 7.51), basal cell naevus syndrome (**Fig 7.52**) and some types of keratoderma (**Fig 7.53**); they may be an incidental finding in other more widespread skin diseases (**Table 7.4**).

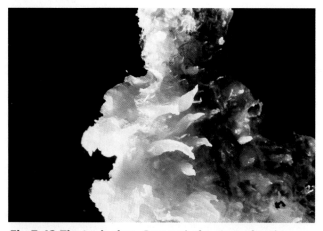

Fig 7.43 Tin-tack sign. Removal of a piece of scale reveals these casts of keratin stuck to the undersurface of the scale

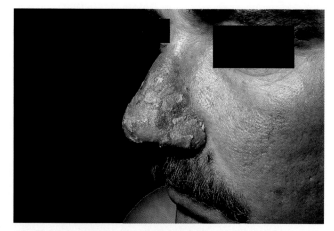

Fig 7.44 Pemphigus erythematosus of the nose. Crusted lesions appear on the face, scalp, chest and back. Compare this to the yellowish crusted lesions occasionally seen in seborrhoeic eczema (*see* 7.27)

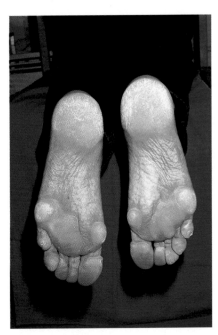

Fig 7.45 Focal palmoplantar keratoderma. Thickened areas of yellow keratin have formed on the pressure points of this patient's feet. Focal keratodermas can be readily distinguished from the diffuse variants, where the thickened keratin covers the sole. Several clinical patterns of keratoderma have been described; many in just a few families. Study of the genetics has provided information on keratin gene mutations

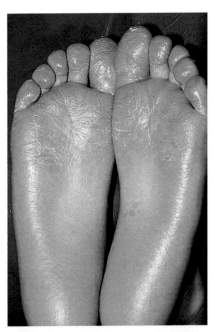

Fig 7.46 Juvenile plantar forefoot dermatosis. Symmetrical scaling of the forefoot. Painful fissures develop on the scaly areas

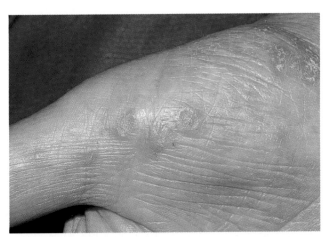

Fig 7.47 Senear–Caro ridge. Non-pustular psoriasis of the hands causes lesions over the extensor surfaces of the finger joints, palms and finger tips. Characteristic linear, saucerised plaques of psoriasis may develop along the lateral aspects of the index fingers and palms—sometimes referred to as the Senear–Caro ridge

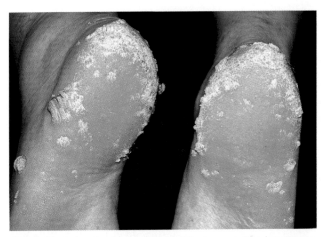

Fig 7.48 Arsenical keratoses. These corn-like keratoses arise on the palms and soles years after arsenic ingestion. Much smaller keratoses also occur. Squamous cell carcinomas may develop in the keratoses, but most skin cancers arise on sun-exposed skin. Patients show a high prevalence of internal malignancy of the lung, breast, pancreas, stomach, etc.

Arsenical keratoses

Long-term arsenic ingestion due to either a contaminated water supply or earlier therapeutic use in psoriasis and other skin diseases can result in discrete corn-like keratoses on the palm and soles (*see* Fig 7.48). Squamous cell carcinomas may arise in these lesions, and patients also show a higher prevalence of solid visceral tumours.

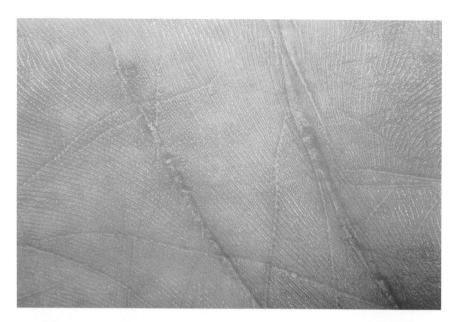

Fig 7.49 Punctate palmar pitting of palmar creases. Small keratotic papules in the palm and finger crease lines. These are more common in Afro-Caribbean people but also occur in white people. When present, they are of no pathological significance

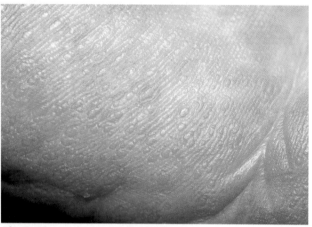

Fig 7.50

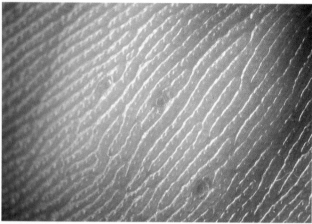

Fig 7.51

Fig 7.50, 7.51 Darier's palms. Palmar pits are characteristic of Darier's disease. In some patients, they can be seen to merge with acrokeratosis verruciformis lesions and are multiple (7.50). In others, just a few pits are visible (7.51). Histologically, they are identical to the papular lesions found elsewhere, thus showing that papules in Darier's disease are not derived from follicular structures (*photo courtesy of Dr Colin Munro*)

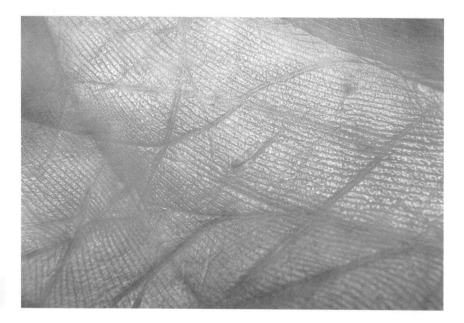

Fig 7.52 Palms—basal cell naevus syndrome. Patients with this autosomal dominant condition have multiple basal cell carcinomas and characteristic skeletal abnormalities. Affected children have a high prevalence of medulloblastoma. Sixty-five per cent of affected adults have visible pits. The pits are fewer and less easy to see than those of Darier's disease. Histologically, they are the result of premature loss of the dense palmar keratin occurring over an area of abnormal basaloid epidermal cells. Exceptionally, basal cell carcinomas may arise in the pits

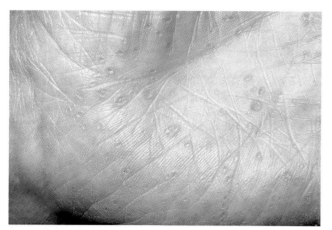

Fig 7.53 Punctate palmar keratoderma. This disorder may be familial and affects palms and soles. Typical lesions are slightly yellow, translucent umbilicated hyperkeratotic papules

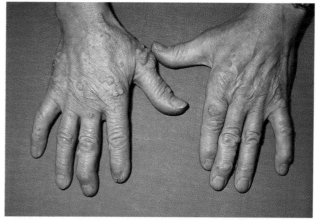

Fig 7.54 Multiple hand warts. Warts usually occur on the dorsum of the hands. They are uncommon in elderly people, unless immune suppressed, and their appearance in an adult should raise the possibility of immune deficiency due to HIV infection, chronic lymphatic leukaemia or Hodgkin's disease

Table 7.4 Discrete palmar keratosis and pits

Arsenical keratoses	Hyperkeratotic papules appear on the palms and soles as small, corn-like keratoses many years after arsenic ingestion (7.48)
Palmar crease pits	Small pits start as hyperkeratotic papules and evolve into small conical pits. They are found only on the palm and in digital creases (7.49)
Darier's disease	Punctate keratoses or palmar pits occur in patients and apparently unaffected relatives. The pits are pathognomonic of Darier's disease (7.50, 7.51)
Basal cell naevus syndrome	Palmar pits are 2–3 mm in diameter, up to 1 mm deep and have a perpendicular edge. Punctate hyperkeratosis is also seen in some patients. Histologically, the pits are the result of premature desquamation of the horny layer of the epidermis. Exceptionally, basal cell carcinomas arise on the palms and soles in these patients (7.52)
Punctate keratoderma	Familial and non-familial forms have been described. Papules 2–3 mm in diameter on the palmar surface sometimes become confluent. Other types of keratoderma produce generalised increased yellowish thickening of the palms and soles (7.1)
Others	Lichen planus, common warts (7.54), psoriasis (7.47) and corns all commonly produce keratotic changes on the palms, but rarely present diagnostic problems with the changes at other sites

CRUST

Multiple lesions

In exudative rashes such as subacute eczema (**Fig 7.55**) and excoriated eruption (*see* Chapter 16) and in blistering diseases (*see* Chapter 13), extensive crusted lesions may occur as the exudate dries on the skin surface. In the blistering diseases pemphigus foliaceous and pemphigus erythematosus (*see* Fig 7.44), crusted lesions, particularly on the nose and scalp, may be the presenting feature. The epidermal split in these conditions is high in the epidermis, so the blister roof is fragile and easily burst by minimal trauma; crusted lesions are therefore more common than intact blisters.

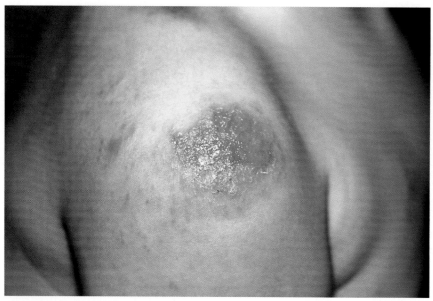

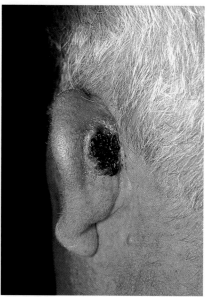

Fig 7.55 Subacute eczema with crusting. Crusts are beginning to appear on the margin of this oozy eczematous plaque

Fig 7.56

Solitary lesions

Individual lesions may produce crusts due to dried blood (e.g. bleeding pyogenic granuloma), serum (e.g. thermal burn) or purulent exudate caused by infection (e.g. impetigo, *see* Fig 7.4). In localised crusted lesions, it is essential to remove the crust before attempting to make a diagnosis because most of the physical signs will be obscured by this (**Figs 7.56** and **7.57**, *see also* Figs 4.32 and 4.33). In some tumours, such as Bowen's disease and squamous cell carcinomas (**Figs 7.56** and **7.57**), crusting due to exudation, secondary infection and hyperkeratotic scaling contributes to the crusted surface. These are discussed further in Chapter 9.

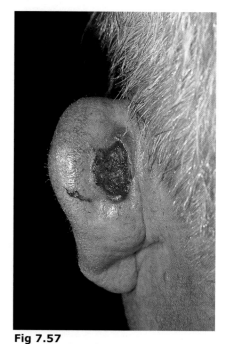

Fig 7.57

Figs 7.56, 7.57 Crusted squamous cell carcinoma. There is a blood-stained crust overlying the tumour and obscuring the examination. Removal of the crust, after first softening it by soaking, reveals the underlying tumour

8 Plaques

INTRODUCTION

A plaque (plate) is an area, usually greater than approximately 20 mm in diameter, of slightly elevated skin with colour and/or textural change. A similar change in a smaller area would be referred to as a flat-topped papule. Multiple papules and nodules can coalesce to form plaques. The term plaque is also used for similar-sized areas of flat skin with palpable textural change.

SCALING, HYPERKERATOTIC AND CRUSTED PLAQUES, USUALLY MULTIPLE

Overview

It is difficult to produce a consistently useful classification of plaques, as features overlap. For example, plaques of psoriasis are usually multiple but may be solitary; additionally, psoriatic plaques are usually characterised by having large silvery scales but may be hyperkeratotic, have a smooth shiny surface (especially in the flexures) or have a weeping eczematous morphology when inflamed. These features may vary from time to time or may even be present simultaneously at different body sites in a single individual. Similarly, seborrhoeic dermatitis may have psoriatic or eczematous features. Nevertheless, the predominant morphology of a plaque or plaques is an important part of describing these lesions and in reaching a diagnosis. Some of the skin diseases that present most commonly as multiple scaly plaques are listed in **Table 8.1**.

Eczematous plaques

The morphology of eczematous plaques is one of the most difficult clinical features to describe in dermatology. Eczematous plaques are usually not very sharply demarcated (**Figs 8.1** and **8.2**), but in some cases, such as discoid eczema (**Fig 8.3**) or acute contact dermatitis, the borders of the plaques may be quite sharp. The erythema and other inflammatory features are most

Table 8.1 Skin diseases commonly associated with multiple scaly plaques

Psoriasis (8.9)

Eczema, including seborrhoeic, atopic, lichen simplex (8.4)

Pityriasis rosea (7.21) and viral exanthemata (*see* Chapter 10)

Lichen planus (8.22)

Pityriasis rubra pilaris

Parapsoriasis (8.8)

Mycosis fungoides (8.6, 8.7)

Discoid lupus erythematosus (8.21)

Fungal infections (7.18)

Secondary syphilis

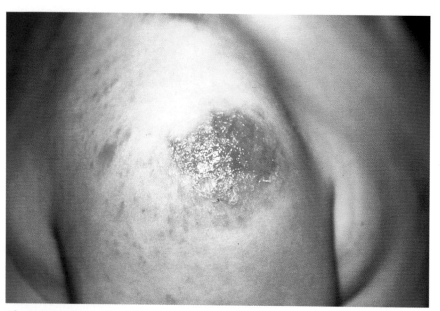

Fig 8.1 Oozing subacute eczema. In infants with atopic eczema, the rash is usually localised to the face, with diffuse or patchy involvement of the trunk (*see also* 15.22). In some children, this can be quite discoid in pattern but still with relatively poorly defined borders

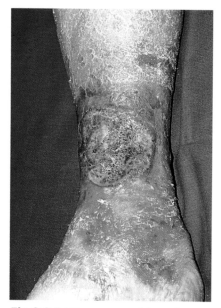

Fig 8.2 Eczema around leg ulcer. There is extensive eczema around this venous leg ulcer. Patch tests showed a positive reaction to thiuram mix, a rubber ingredient, although the patient was not using an elasticated support stocking or bandage containing rubber

intense centrally and fade at the edges, where there may be an appearance of breaking up into smaller lesions. At the acute end of the spectrum of eczematous morphology, the presence of weeping and oozy skin with associated crusting is characteristic (**Fig 8.3**). Mild eczema may just have a poorly demarcated redness with fine dry scaling. In more chronic eczema, there are features of lichenification (**Figs 8.4** and **8.5**). In between these extremes, subacute eczema consists of slightly oozy, red, smooth and shiny skin, an appearance that commonly occurs around chronic leg ulcers (**Fig 8.2**).

Lichenified plaques

Lichenification (**Figs 8.4** and **8.5**) results from repeated scratching and rubbing. It may be localised to areas such as the shins or nape of the neck (lichen simplex) or may be more widespread with several affected areas, notably in atopic individuals. The skin becomes palpably thickened, with a rough dry

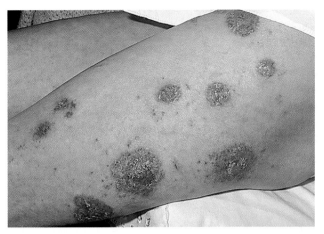

Fig 8.3 Discoid eczema. Multiple red scaly lesions on the arms and legs are typical

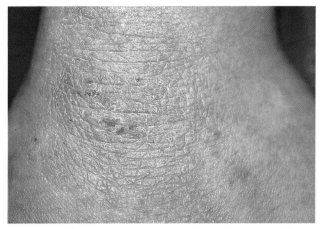

Fig 8.4 Lichenified eczematous plaque. A patch of lichenified skin with increased skin markings on the dorsum of the hand is evident in this girl with atopic eczema

Table 8.2 Stages of mycosis fungoides

1. Eczematous
2. Plaques
3. Papules
4. Nodules
5. Ulcerated lesions

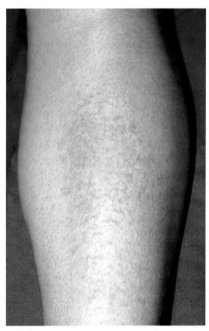

Fig 8.5 Cobblestoned lichenification. This man has chronic idiopathic eczema. On his left leg are areas of confluent papules, producing a cobblestoned appearance

appearance, and the normally barely visible skin crease lines become obvious (**Fig 8.4**). Fissures may appear within lichenified plaques of eczema (*see* Figs 12.2 and 12.4). On the trunk, shins or dorsum of the hand, lichenification may assume a cobblestoned appearance, produced by the confluence of multiple papules (**Fig 8.5**, *see also* Fig 11.28).

Mycosis fungoides and parapsoriasis

Mycosis fungoides and parapsoriasis are conveniently discussed here as both are most commonly confused with eczema, although the plaques in either disorder are generally more sharply defined than typical eczematous plaques. In some instances, psoriasis may also be considered in the differential diagnosis, although neither mycosis fungoides nor parapsoriasis typically has a psoriasiform type of scaling.

Mycosis fungoides is a cutaneous T-cell lymphoma of the skin, which passes through a number of stages (**Table 8.2**) over several years. At the plaque stage (**Fig 8.6**), large, irregular, just palpable, reddish-brown patches of skin develop, distributed asymmetrically on the body. As the disease progresses, these plaques become thickened or infiltrated. In established mycosis fungoides, a characteristic feature is the presence of lesions of different colours, superimposed on red- or brown-coloured background lesions (**Fig 8.7**). Lesions with an annular or arciform morphology are common. Some body sites, especially the buttocks, may show features of poikiloderma with atrophy, telangiectasia and pigmentation (*see* Figs 1.16 and 11.6). Further progression leads to the development of nodules, and finally ulcerated tumours (*see* Fig 12.29) in a very small proportion of cases.

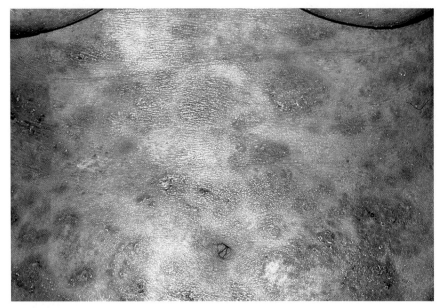

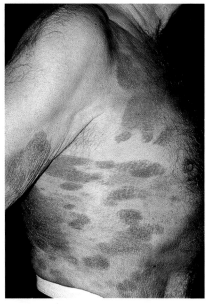

Fig 8.6 Mycosis fungoides—plaque stage. Multiple red and pigmented infiltrated plaques can be seen on this woman's trunk

Fig 8.7 Mycosis fungoides. Superimposed lesions of different colours in mycosis fungoides

In the early stages, it may be impossible to clinically identify those patients who will go on to develop nodules (*see* Fig 12.29) and ultimately die from lymphoma from those whose rash remains a barely troublesome patch of slightly wrinkled skin. At this early, pre-mycotic stage or eczematous phase of mycosis fungoides, the term parapsoriasis is used (**Fig 8.8**). This is perhaps one of the few instances where the descriptive skills of early dermatologists were poor, as (apart from rather sharp demarcation) the surface morphology of lesions of parapsoriasis more resembles that of eczema than of psoriasis. Features that suggest a benign course of parapsoriasis include small, uniformly shaped and sometimes digitate or finger-like plaques (*see* Fig 2.14) with a slight yellowish tinge, symmetrically distributed, particularly around the trunk, and clearing temporarily after sun exposure. Features suggesting a greater possibility of progression to mycosis fungoides include large, irregular and oddly shaped plaques, palpable plaques and the presence of poikiloderma (*see* Figs 1.16 and 11.6).

DIAGNOSTIC TIPS AND PITFALLS

- A particularly useful diagnostic clue for mycosis fungoides is the presence of plaques of different colours, which may appear superimposed on top of each other

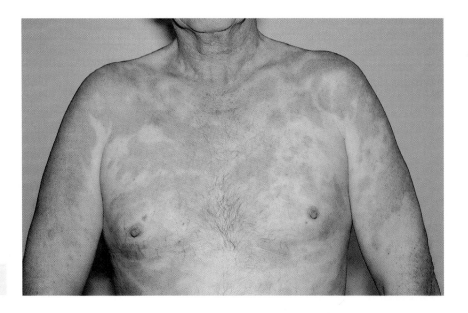

Fig 8.8 Large plaque parapsoriasis. Lesions are well demarcated but do not have psoriasiform scaling, or the marginal accentuation that can occur in psoriasis (compare with 8.9)

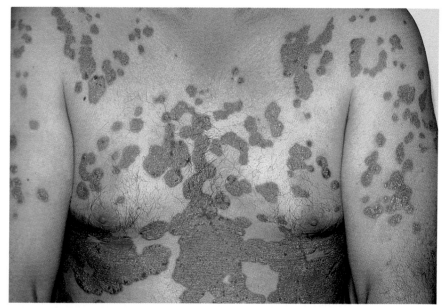

Fig 8.9 Chronic plaque psoriasis. Extensive scaly red plaques here have become confluent on the chest and abdomen

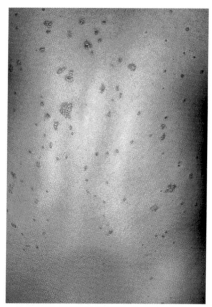

Fig 8.10 Small plaque psoriasis. The plaques on this woman's back, although small, are larger and more variable in size than those seen in guttate psoriasis

Psoriasiform plaques

Plaques of this pattern have a sharply demarcated border, generally uniform erythema (unless hidden by scaling), and are usually not moist or weeping (Fig 8.9).

Psoriasis

Psoriasis is characterised by well-defined, scaly plaques that are typically localised to the elbows (*see* Fig 1.4) and knees in patients with the chronic plaque pattern, although they may affect any site. Other recognised patterns include small plaque (**Fig 8.10**), guttate (**Fig 8.11**), annular (**Fig 8.12**), hyperkeratotic (**Fig 8.13**) and pustular (*see* Figs 14.7 and 14.20) psoriasis. Small plaque psoriasis should be distinguished from guttate (drop-like) psoriasis; the latter is triggered by a streptococcal infection in approximately 60% of cases and will usually resolve spontaneously. Small plaque psoriasis shares the same unpredictable prognosis as other non-pustular variants. Psoriasis also commonly involves the scalp (**Fig 8.14**), flexures (**Fig 8.15**) and fingernails (*see* Figs 19.21 and 19.50).

The scaling component in psoriasis is typically silvery in colour (**Fig 8.16**), especially when scratched (*see* Fig 4.31), and consists of rather large flakes. However, the degree of scaling varies between individuals and is influenced by body site (often absent at moist flexural sites, *see* Fig 8.15), topical applications and the degree of associated inflammation.

SCALY, HYPERKERATOTIC AND CRUSTED PLAQUES, USUALLY SOLITARY OR FEW

Bowen's disease

Bowen's disease is an intra-epidermal neoplasm, which presents as red, scaly plaques, usually on the lower legs of women. In contrast to psoriasis, in Bowen's disease, there is crusting rather than hyperkeratosis, and the margin

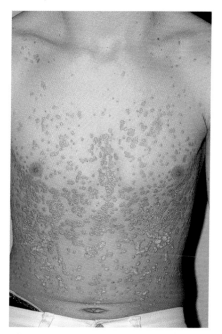

Fig 8.11 Guttate psoriasis. This is characterised by multiple small or drop-like spots of psoriasis. The rash often occurs after streptococcal infection and clears spontaneously after 6–8 weeks. Lesions are usually 2–3 mm in diameter and thus considerably smaller than those seen in small plaque psoriasis

141

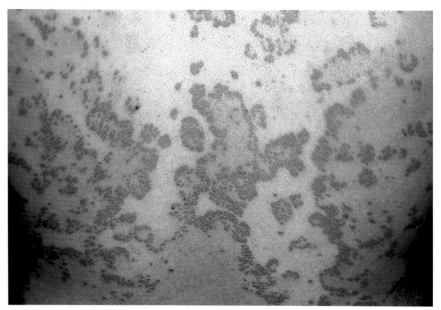

Fig 8.12 Chronic plaque psoriasis—annular pattern. With methotrexate therapy, plaques of psoriasis have started to clear from the centre, leaving a rim of psoriasis (same patient as in 8.9, 3 years later)

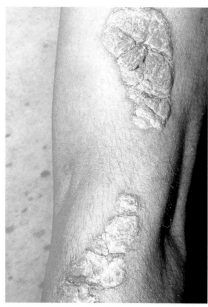

Fig 8.13 Hyperkeratotic psoriasis. Thick, hyperkeratotic plaques of psoriasis have developed on this man's arm

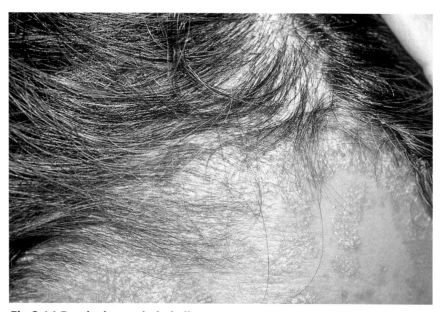

Fig 8.14 Psoriasis—scalp hair-line appearance. Psoriasis of the scalp commonly spreads to the forehead and ears

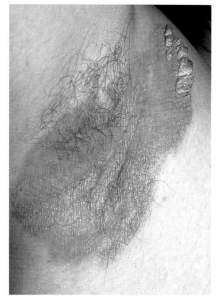

Fig 8.15 Psoriasis—flexural. Axillary psoriasis is less hyperkeratotic than plaques at other sites (same patient as in 8.13)

is irregular with little tongues of plaque extending into the surrounding skin (**Fig 8.17**). However, in patients with several small lesions, it may be impossible to distinguish psoriasis from Bowen's disease purely by clinical inspection.

Paget's disease

Paget's disease may affect the breast or pubic and perineal regions.

Paget's disease of the breast presents as a solitary plaque of oozy, crusted skin around the nipple and is due to local cutaneous spread from an

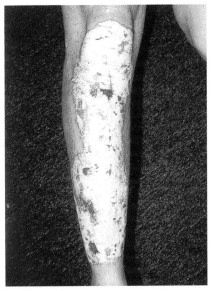

Fig 8.16 Plaques of psoriasis. This plaque shows silvery coloured thick scaling with some areas of excoriation. This is important therapeutically as penetration of topical agents will be poor unless a keratolytic agent is incorporated in the regimen

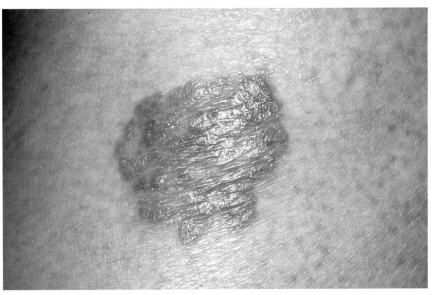

Fig 8.17 Bowen's disease of the shin. Plaques of Bowen's disease are usually solitary or few in number and most common on the lower legs in women. The features are a reddish-brown colour, scaling and crusting, and a sharply defined border that is more irregular than a plaque of psoriasis

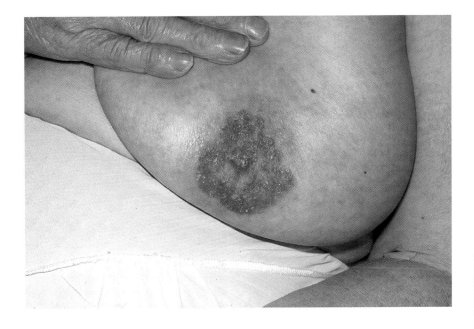

Fig 8.18 Paget's disease of the breast. This eczematous appearance involves the whole of the areola and is spreading on to the skin of the breast. Paget's disease should be suspected in any unilateral eruption affecting the areolar skin

intraductal carcinoma of the breast (**Fig 8.18**). By contrast, eczema of the nipple is usually, but not always, bilateral and is not uncommon in atopic eczema (**Fig 8.19**). Psoriasis, also generally bilateral, can affect the nipples and areola during breast feeding.

Extramammary Paget's disease generally presents as an asymmetrical, itchy, crusted, oozing or croded area around the vulva, anus (**Fig 8.20**), penis, scrotum or groin. It should be suspected if an eruption of eczematous appearance is unilateral in flexural regions of the perineum. Approximately 15% of patients have an associated carcinoma of an adjacent structure, such as the cervix, rectum or urinary tract. The prognosis is worse in this group. In the

DIAGNOSTIC TIPS AND PITFALLS

- There are occasions when it can be impossible to distinguish clinically between psoriasis and Bowen's disease. The most common pattern to cause this diagnostic dilemma is in elderly patients with a small number of well-defined erythematous scaly plaques on the legs

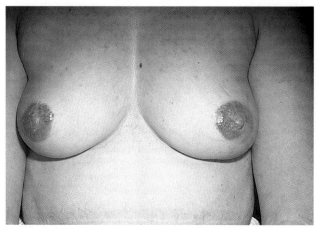

Fig 8.19 Eczema affecting the nipples and areolae.
By contrast to Paget's disease (*see* 8.18), eczema affecting
this region is typically bilateral, although not necessarily
symmetrical. In this example, the changes are rather more
inflammatory and more sharply conforming to the areolar
margin than is typical in Paget's disease, but less well-
circumscribed lesions may occur in atopic patients

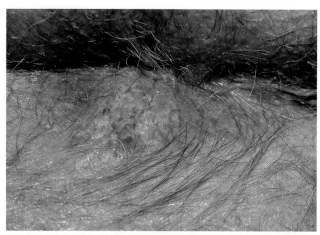

Fig 8.20 Extramammary Paget's disease. There is a
unilateral plaque of red, papillomatous skin with a white,
oozy surface on the perianal skin

remaining 85% of patients, tumour cells arise within the epidermis of the
adjacent skin, probably from apocrine duct cells or pluripotent germinative
cells.

Discoid lupus erythematosus

In discoid lupus erythematosus plaques usually occur on sun-exposed sites
(**Fig 8.21**). They are sharply demarcated and exhibit a combination of
changes, including redness, scaling, atrophy (*see* Fig 11.1), follicular
plugging (*see* Fig 7.40), telangiectasia and, usually in older lesions, hypopigmentation—sometimes with perilesional hyperpigmentation. Similar
changes are seen in the scalp, where follicular damage produces scarring
alopecia (*see* Fig 18.27).

COALESCENT PAPULES/COBBLESTONED PLAQUES

Several conditions may cause localised plaques with a cobblestoned appearance due to multiple closely grouped papules (**Table 8.3**). Numerous dermal
degenerative and deposition disorders (mucinoses, amyloidosis, etc.) cause
this pattern.

Lichen planus

The violaceous papules of lichen planus (**Fig 8.22**) may coalesce to form
plaques that have a cobblestoned surface and irregular edge, often with individual papules visible at the margins (**Fig 8.23**). Thick plaques also occur,
especially on the shin, in a variant known as hypertrophic lichen planus
(**Fig 8.24**). Lichen planus may also affect the buccal mucosa (*see* Fig 2.22) and
tongue, vulva and penis. Wickham's striae (*see* Fig 2.22) are seen in the buccal mucosa with a lacy, white pattern but are also visible on the skin as tiny,
fine, lacy lines running across the top of the papule (*see* Fig 4.16).

   Lichen planus is characterised by the appearance of lesions within areas of
skin damage (**Fig 8.22**), known as Koebner's phenomenon (*see* pp 20–21).

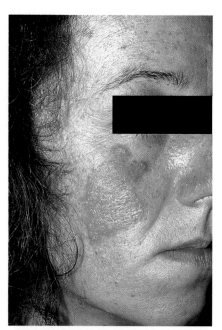

**Fig 8.21 Discoid lupus
erythematosus.** This woman has a
large, red, scaly plaque with a
hyperpigmented border on her cheek.
There are similar plaques on her
forehead

Table 8.3 Causes of plaques with a cobblestoned surface

Inflammatory	Lichen planus (8.23, 8.24) Lichenification (8.5) Papuloerythroderma (2.42) Granuloma annulare
Deposition	Lichen amyloidosis (8.25) Lichen myxedematosus
Degenerative	Colloid milium Solar elastosis (16.17) Diabetic finger pebbles (11.24)
Others	Multiple plane warts (8.26, 9.54)

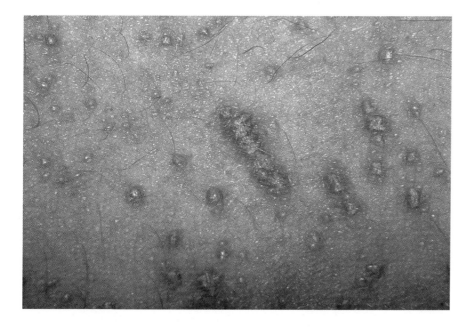

Fig 8.22 Lichen planus. A close view of papules on the arm shows several linear lesions, which appeared when lichen planus formed in the scratched skin—an example of Koebner's phenomenon

A variety of other skin diseases can localise to, or arise at, sites of skin damage (*see* Table 2.2).

A lichenoid eruption, normally due to a drug, resembles lichen planus but does not share all of the latter's characteristics. Clinical differences include atypical distribution, absent mucous membrane changes and features such as scaling and eczematous change, which are not encountered in typical lichen planus. Histologically, eosinophils are more prominent in drug-induced lichenoid reactions and are not seen in lichen planus.

Granuloma annulare

Granuloma annulare may present as annular, palpable, beaded lesions (*see* Fig 11.29), subcutaneous nodules (*see* Fig 9.1), generalised, multiple, tiny dermal papules, perforating papules or flat, red–brown plaques. The last group merge clinically and histologically with necrobiosis lipoidica (*see* Figs 11.10 and 12.37).

FLAT SMOOTH PLAQUES

In morphoea (**Fig 8.27**), lichen sclerosus (**Figs 8.28** and **8.29**) and necrobiosis lipoidica (*see* Figs 11.10 and 12.37), the predominantly dermal inflammatory process and subsequent fibrous tissue changes result in areas of skin with

DIAGNOSTIC TIPS AND PITFALLS

- Strictly, unilateral eczema of the nipple and areola should be assumed to be Paget's disease until histologically proven otherwise. Atopic eczema at this site is much more common but is bilateral (even if asymmetrical in degree)

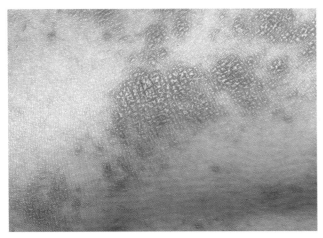

Fig 8.23 Coalescence of papules in lichen planus. This produces an irregular cobblestoned plaque

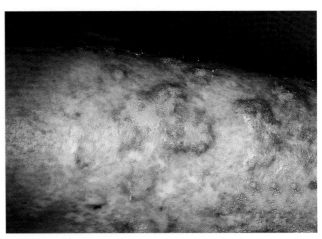

Fig 8.24 Hypertrophic lichen planus on the leg. This variant is often chronic and may cause considerable pigmentary disturbance, as in this case

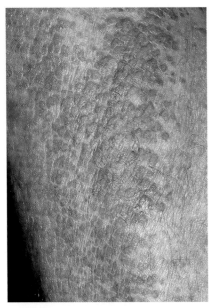

Fig 8.25 Lichen amyloidosis. Cobblestoned lesions on the legs, which probably represent a form of lichenification but histologically show amyloid deposition

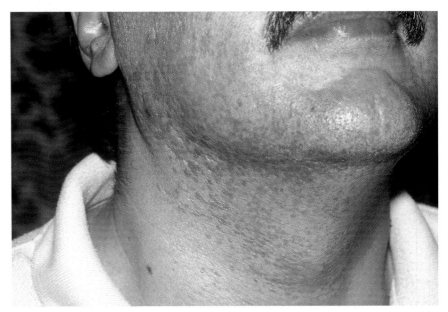

Fig 8.26 Plane warts. Multiple plain warts can occur on the face in men who practise wet shaving, as this encourages dissemination of the virus. Multiple tiny, warty papules become confluent, producing a tan-coloured plaque. Pigmentation in warts is much greater in patients with black skin

altered colour and texture. Chronic sarcoidosis of the skin may produce diffuse, brown–red, sometimes nodular, plaques on the trunk and limbs.

Morphoea

In morphoea, areas of shiny white skin with a purple/red border occur (Fig 8.27). On palpation, the skin feels stiff and may be attached to deeper structures, including bone. The margins of the early lesions may be elevated, compared with the surrounding skin. Later, the surface of the plaque is often depressed, compared with the surrounding normal skin, and in the atrophoderma variant of morphoea, it may be pigmented (*see* Fig 11.15).

Lichen sclerosus

Lichen sclerosus produces small, porcelain white areas, which become confluent (**Fig 8.28**) on the trunk and limbs. On the vulva, there is atrophy with loss of labium minora, stenosis of the vulval introitus and white, wrinkled skin, with a purplish rim around the perivulval and perianal skin (**Fig 8.29**, *see also* Figs 1.14, 7.39, 11.4, 11.5). Associated loss of dermal collagen leads to loss of blood vessel support and consequent purpura. These signs in childhood vulval lichen sclerosus (*see* Fig 2.36) are sometimes confused with child abuse (*see* Table 2.6). The lesions in lichen sclerosus are usually atrophic, hence the use of the alternative name 'lichen sclerosus et atrophicus'. However, as lesions may be hypertrophic, especially on vulval skin, the 'et atrophicus' part of the name is increasingly being omitted.

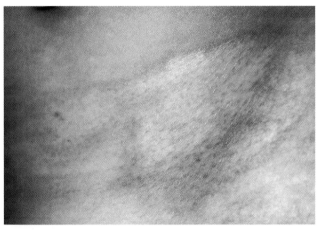

Fig 8.27 Morphoea. There is a large white plaque with surrounding red rim. The central white area feels stiffer than the surrounding skin, and hair follicles are more easily seen, suggesting that there is some loss of dermal substance. Follicles eventually shrink and disappear

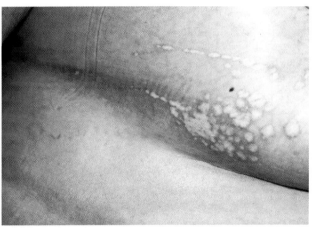

Fig 8.28 Lichen sclerosus et atrophicus. In extragenital skin, small, ivory-white shiny papules develop. These may become confluent, forming plaques. Follicular plugs (*see* 7.39, 11.4) are usually visible on the surface. Lesions may localise to trauma sites. Here, they have Koebnerised into the skin under a tight bra strap

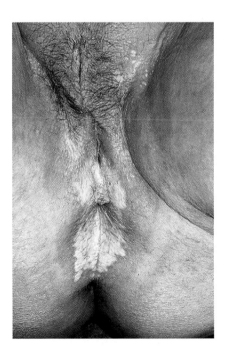

Fig 8.29 Lichen sclerosus et atrophicus—vulval changes. There is a well-circumscribed, white change around the vulva and perianal skin. Other features include vulval stenosis and atrophy of the labia majora (*see* 11.5)

147

9 Macules, papules and nodules

INTRODUCTION

Macules are discrete flat lesions of a different colour to the surrounding skin; they may have a normal skin texture or some degree of scaling but are not thickened. Macular lesions that are typically solitary or few in number are discussed in this chapter, as many of these are pigmented and enter the differential diagnosis of common pigmented papules or nodules; indeed, some nodules may develop from an initially macular lesion (e.g. compound naevi from junctional naevi) or arise within a pre-existing macule (e.g. lentigo maligna melanoma). Macules of other colours are discussed in Chapter 3, scaling macules in Chapter 7 and eruptions characterised by multiple macules in Chapter 10.

Papules and nodules (*see* 1.3) are discrete lesions, which are usually visibly raised above the skin surface but may be depressed or 'inverted'. The distinction between papules and nodules is largely artificial. A nodule is larger and characteristically very obviously raised, whereas a papule may be only slightly elevated above the surface. Small but very elevated lesions may be called nodules, although in general, a papule is usually defined as being smaller than 5–10 mm in diameter. Something between 5 and 10 mm in diameter may be called a large papule or a small nodule and anything larger than 10 mm in diameter is usually referred to as a nodule. Here, we have subdivided papules and nodules by their surface characteristics and colour as being more diagnostically useful than precise size cut-off points.

DESCRIPTIVE TERMINOLOGY

Macules

When describing a macule, it is useful to consider the following features.

History

The duration of the macule and change with time, for example rate and pattern of enlargement and changes in appearance. Most macular lesions are fixed or slowly enlarge in a radial pattern, but some may be transient or vary in size and shape. Associated symptoms include itch.

Examination

Size and symmetry—Vitiligo, for example, is typically symmetrical.

Number of lesions—This can be diagnostically useful, for example Becker's naevi (**Fig 9.37**) are typically solitary but may be confused with café au lait patches (**Fig 9.18**), which are often multiple.

Body site and distribution/pattern if multiple (*see also* Chapter 10)—Specific detail may be important, for example macular lesions in flexural sites may be due to disorders that would cause plaques elsewhere (e.g. psoriasis). Vitiligo often affects perioral, periorbital, acral or genital skin.

Shape—Most macules are essentially round or oval, but a stellate shape occurs in lesions of meningococcal infection (*see* Fig 2.12), lentigines due to sunburn or photochemotherapy (*see* Fig 1.2) or the pigmented macules in McCune–Albright syndrome. An irregular or 'geographical' outline is seen in naevus anaemicus (*see* Fig 3.19) or in Becker's naevi (**Fig 9.37**)

Other marginal or focal features—Some macules appear to be uniform apart from features that occur at the margin (for example, the marginal scaling of porokeratosis, *see* Fig 7.24). The definition of the margin is also important, for example a vascular flare, such as occurs in urticaria often has a vague border, whereas a superficial vascular birthmark such as a port wine stain is generally sharply demarcated from the adjacent skin. In vitiligo, there is often a rim of slightly hyperpigmented skin around the depigmented patches, or there may be spotty perifollicular repigmentation (*see* Fig 3.21). Some macules with a geographical border have smaller macules around the edge of the main lesion, resembling a coastal island (e.g. naevus anaemicus, *see* Fig 3.19). Alternatively, some macules may have useful diagnostic features centrally, such as the remnants of a melanocytic naevus in a circular depigmented 'halo' naevus (**Fig 9.34**).

Colour—Melanin pigmentation is a feature of many macules discussed in this chapter (**Table 9.1**). Depigmented macules and other colours of macular lesions are largely discussed in Chapter 3.

Surface characteristics—e.g. smooth or scaly, may be of particular importance. For example, small confetti-like lesions of vitiligo (normal skin texture), pityriasis alba (fine dust-like scaling), untreated pityriasis versicolor (scaly, especially when scratched) and treated pityriasis versicolor (normal texture) are depigmented macules, which are often confused in differential diagnosis (*see* Table 3.8). Finally, although macules are by definition never thickened, they may be atrophic (e.g. porokeratosis *see* Fig 7.24).

Papules and nodules

When describing a nodule or papule, it is useful to consider the following features.

History

The duration of the lesion and change with time, e.g. rate of enlargement, changes in appearance or symptoms.

Associated symptoms include pain (**Table 9.2**), itch, discharge of pus.

Table 9.1 Examples of fixed solitary or multiple discrete macules

Colour of macule	Example
Pigmented	Freckles (9.12, 9.13) Café au lait patches (9.18) Junctional naevus (9.23) Lentigo (1.2), lentigo maligna (9.41) Becker's naevus (9.37, 18.7) Naevus of Ota (9.17) Mongolian spot (6.13) Fixed drug eruption (old lesions) Tattoos
Depigmented or pale	Vitiligo (3.21) Halo naevus (9.34) Naevus depigmentosus (Achromic naevus (3.25)) Guttate hypomelanosis Ash leaf macule (3.26) Naevus anaemicus (3.19) Pityriasis versicolor (7.14) Leprosy and other infections, e.g. pinta Pityriasis alba (3.31) Porokeratosis (7.24) Traumatic (e.g. post-cryotherapy, post-radiotherapy)
Red or purple	Port-wine stain (17.50, 17.51), stork marks (6.11, 6.12) and other vascular birthmarks Telangiectatic pattern of actinic keratosis (7.33) Kaposi's sarcoma (some lesions) (9.71, 9.72) Flexural seborrhoeic dermatitis, psoriasis (8.15)

Table 9.2 Examples of painful or tender papules and nodules

Origin/Cause	Examples
Vascular	Glomus tumour (9.69) angiolipoma
Neural	Neuroma
Muscle	Leiomyoma
Appendage	Various benign neoplasms, especially eccrine spiradenoma, pilar cysts of scalp, pilomatrixoma (9.60)
Infective	Acute infection, e.g. abscess, folliculitis (14.1), carbuncle (14.9), herpetic whitlow, orf (3.33)
Inflammatory	Chondrodermatitis nodularis helicis (9.99) Erythema nodosum (17.40) Trauma, e.g. scratch, foreign-body reaction

Examination

Size and symmetry

Body site and distribution/pattern if multiple (*see* Chapters 2 and 5)—Specific detail may be important, for example, midline nodules may have deep fixation or connections, especially on the face and scalp or the lower back (e.g. neural tissue in infants, dental sinus in adults). Grouped papules or nodules are characteristic of many disorders, including syringomas, leiomyomas, localised neurofibromas and insect bite reactions. Morphology may vary depending on body site (*see* p. 156).

Shape (Figs 9.1–9.6)—e.g. dome, papillomatous, pedunculated, umbilicated, flat, etc. Most are dome-shaped (**Table 9.3**); other shapes are listed, with examples, in **Table 9.4**. In general, a square shoulder implies a superficial

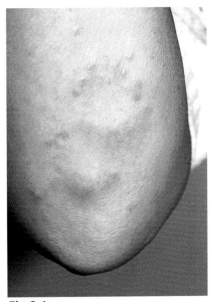

Fig 9.1

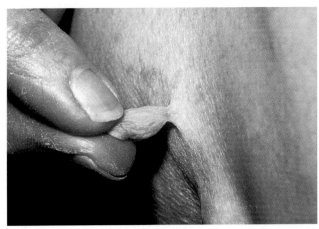

Fig 9.2

Fig 9.4

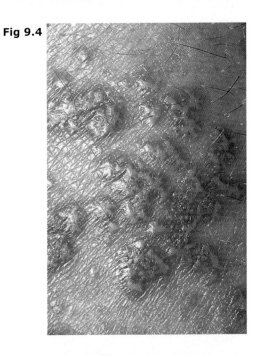

Fig 9.3

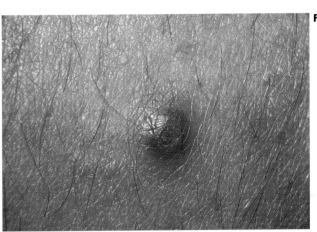

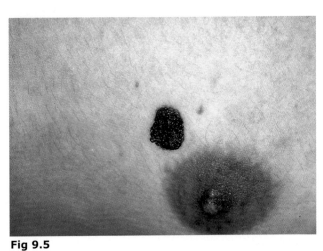

Fig 9.5

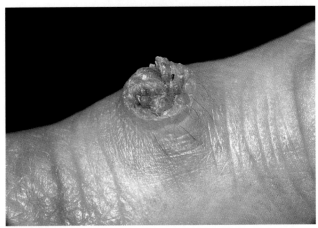

Fig 9.6

Figs 9.1–9.6 Examples of dome-shaped lesions and variations of the prototype smooth dome shape. Smooth dome (9.1), e.g. nodular granuloma annulare; pedunculated shape (9.2), like a stalk, e.g. fibroepithelial polyp ('skin tag'); umbilicate shape (9.3), with central depression, e.g. molluscum contagiosum; flat-topped lesions (9.4), e.g. lichen planus, with prominent Wickham's striae; papillomatous surface (9.5), with a cobblestoned appearance, e.g. some naevi; and warty or verrucous surface (9.6), spikier than the papillomatous appearance, e.g. viral warts (in this case with an acorn cup pattern)

Table 9.3 Examples of smooth, dome-shaped papules and nodules

Cause	Multiple	Solitary or few
Infection and infestation	Scabies (15.12) Papular urticaria Bites (2.25)	Furuncle/carbuncle (14.9) Orf (3.33)
Inflammatory	Acne Erythema nodosum Granuloma annulare (9.1) Maculopapular rashes Papular eczema Sarcoid Polymorphic light eruption	Granuloma annulare (9.1) Foreign-body granuloma
Metabolic	Xanthomata (3.35)	Calcinosis, tophi (gout)
Benign neoplasia	Naevi (9.24) Angiomas Neurofibroma (9.63) Lipomatosis (9.8) Dermatosis papulosa nigra (6.34) Syringomata (9.61) Steatocystoma multiplex	Pyogenic granuloma (9.65) Neurofibroma (9.64) Lipoma (9.8) Epidermoid cyst (9.56) Digital mucoid cyst (13.34) Lymphocytoma cutis Tuberous sclerosis Many appendage neoplasms (9.58–9.60)
Malignant neoplasm	Cutaneous secondaries (9.78)	Basal cell carcinoma (9.73) Cutaneous secondaries (9.78)

Table 9.4 Other shapes of papules and nodules*

Shape	Examples
Pedunculated (9.2)	Fibroepithelial polyps (skin tags), naevi, neurofibromas
Papillomatous (9.5)	Naevus, organoid naevi, skin tags, viral warts in flexural areas
Umbilicated (9.3)	Molluscum contagiosum, basal cell carcinoma, keratoacanthoma, punctate keratoderma
Lichenoid and flat topped (9.4)	Lichen planus, pityriasis lichenoides chronica, guttate psoriasis, Gianotti–Crosti syndrome
Warty/verrucous (9.6)	Viral wart, seborrhoeic wart, epidermal naevi, organoid naevi

*See also Table 9.2

lesion, such as a seborrhoeic keratosis (**Fig 9.7**). A shallow slope occurs in deeper nodules, such as lipomas (**Fig 9.8**), and a rolled or steeper slope of the margin occurs in between these sites. Also note the border of the lesion, e.g. sharply defined or indistinct.

Colour—e.g. flesh-coloured, erythematous, purple, yellow, brown, grey–blue. Also note features such as translucency (**Table 9.5**).

Surface characteristics—e.g. smooth, warty/verrucous, eroded/ulcerated, crusted, bleeding, scaly; also any surface or visible superficial markings (telangiectasia, striae, etc.) (**Table 9.6**).

Texture—e.g. soft, rubbery, firm, hard, compressible (**Table 9.7**).

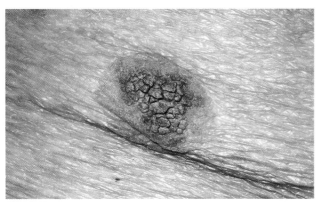

Fig 9.7

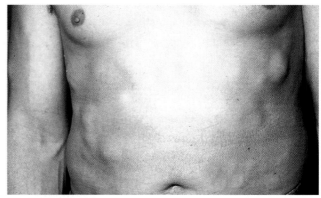

Fig 9.8

Figs 9.7, 9.8 Superficial lesions. Seborrhoeic keratoses and other superficial lesions have a square shoulder (9.7) compared with the gentle sloping edge of the lipomata (9.8), seen here in a patient with multiple lesions (9.8 *courtesy of Dr W D Paterson*)

Table 9.5 Colours of papules and nodules*

Smooth-surfaced lesions	
Colour	**Examples**
Pigmented	
Grey/blue/black	See Table 9.11
Brown	Naevus, malignant melanoma, pigmented basal cell carcinoma, mastocytoma
Non-pigmented	
Flesh	Skin tag (9.2), old naevi (9.24), neurofibromas (9.64), adenoma sebaceum, some appendage tumours (9.61)
Erythematous	Angiomas, bites, inflammatory dermatoses (e.g. erythema nodosum)
White	Calcinosis, superficial cysts, molluscum contagiosum (9.3)
Yellow	Xanthoma (3.36), sebaceous hyperplasia (6.20)
Translucent	Basal cell carcinoma (pearly colour) (9.73–9.77), granulomatous disorders (yellow–brown papules, e.g. sarcoidosis, lupus vulgaris (4.6), granuloma annulare (9.1))
Purple	Lichen planus/lichenoid eruptions, chronic sarcoidosis (5.3), vasculitis/Henoch–Schönlein purpura (17.23), Kaposi's sarcoma (9.71, 9.72)
Rough or crusted surface lesions	
Pigmented	
Grey/blue/black	See Table 9.11
Brown	Naevus, malignant melanoma (9.38–9.44), seborrhoeic warts, dermatofibroma (9.51), pigmented basal cell carcinoma (9.76), mastocytoma, old lichen planus/lichenoid eruptions
Non-pigmented	
Flesh	Old naevi (9.24), molluscum contagiosum (9.3)
Erythematous	Bites, inflammatory dermatoses (e.g. psoriasis, mycosis fungoides)
White	Calcinosis, superficial cysts, molluscum contagiosum
Translucent	Basal cell carcinoma (pearly colour), granulomatous disorders (yellow–brown papules, e.g. sarcoidosis, lupus vulgaris (4.6), granuloma annulare)
Purple	Lichen planus/lichenoid eruptions, chronic sarcoidosis (5.3), vasculitis/Henoch–Schönlein purpura (17.23), angiokeratoma (9.68), Kaposi's sarcoma (9.71, 9.72)

Table 9.6 Surface characteristics of papules and nodules

Smooth	Most dome-shaped papules and nodules (*see* Table 9.3)
Depressed or dimpled	Dermatofibroma (4.23), sinus opening (9.9)
Crusted, eroded and ulcerated	Any nodule secondary to scratch, e.g. naevi, nodular prurigo (9.10) Benign neoplasm, e.g. actinic keratosis, Keratoacanthoma (9.93) Malignant neoplasm, e.g. squamous cell carcinoma (9.95), basal cell carcinoma (9.73–9.77), malignant melanoma (9.43) Others, e.g. calcinosis
Keratotic or scaling	Inflammatory dermatoses, e.g. psoriasis (7.1), Follicular disorders: pityriasis rubra pilaris, keratosis pilaris (*see* Chapter 7) Disorders of keratinisation, e.g. Darier's disease (7.28, 7.29), porokeratosis (7.24), Flegel's disease Others, e.g. actinic keratosis (7.33), cutaneous horns (9.89–9.92), *see also* 'warty/verrucous' in Table 9.4

Table 9.7 Texture of papules and nodules

Texture	Examples
Soft or rubbery	Lipoma (9.8), neurofibroma (9.64), old naevus
Firm	Cellular infiltrates, e.g. mastocytoma (9.53), bites, cysts (9.56) Many benign or malignant tumours
Hard	Dermatofibroma (9.50–9.52), actinic keratosis (7.33), tophi, calcium
Rough	Crusted or keratotic lesions (*see* Table 9.6)
Compressible	Some cysts and lipomas (9.8) Some haemangiomas and lymphangiomas (9.70)
Associated dermal defect	e.g. anetoderma (*see* 4.21), neurofibroma ('buttonhole sign')

Depth within the skin (*see also* Chapter 4)—This is not always easy to determine. Lesions at different levels have the following characteristics:

- Epidermis and/or dermis, e.g. dermatofibroma (*see* Fig 4.23) attached or derived papules cannot be moved independently of the overlying skin.
- If there is an associated dermal defect, e.g. anetoderma (*see* Fig 4.21) and buttonhole sign in neurofibroma, a palpable depression can be detected at the base of the lesion.
- The skin can be moved freely over the underlying lesion if this arises from within the fat, e.g. lipoma.
- Deeply fixed lesions, e.g. dental sinus (**Fig 9.9**), tuberculous sinus, tumours invading bone, exostosis (see Figs 19.54 and 19.55) are palpably attached to the underlying bone.

Other features on palpation—e.g. increased temperature (infections, erythema nodosum), tenderness (**Table 9.2**) and pulsation.

Unique features—e.g. transillumination of cysts, bruits, presence of hypertrichosis. These are of particular importance in certain conditions, especially midline lesions, scalp nodules and congenital lesions.

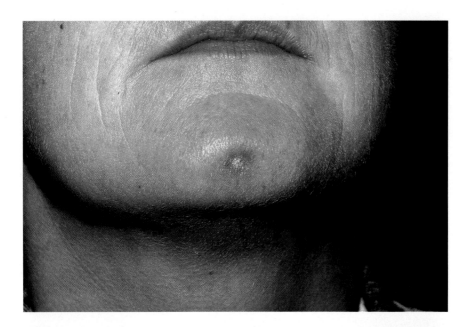

Fig 9.9 Dental sinus. A chronic nodule with history of discharge and with deep fixation. These are not always in the midline, and any lesion on the chin or submandibular region should be assessed carefully

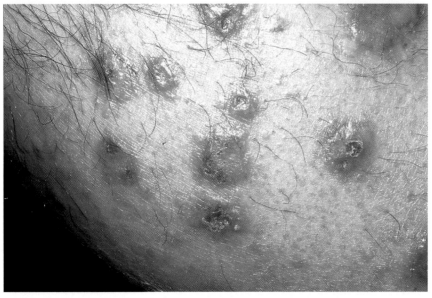

Fig 9.10 Crusted and eroded nodule. This is the result of an inflammatory disorder called nodular prurigo, in which lesions often have surface excoriation

DIAGNOSTIC TIPS AND PITFALLS

- Tumours vary in appearance depending on body site, for example, on the sole of the foot, malignant melanoma may be amelanotic or very sparsely pigmented, whereas this is rare at other body sites

- Friction and pressure alter the clinical appearance, for example, warts on the sole are relatively flat, those on the dorsum of the hand usually have a cauliflower shape, and warts on the face are usually filiform

- Body-site differences in blood flow affect appearance, for example, facial melanocytic naevi are often more telangiectatic than those on the trunk

- Fragile tumours at easily traumatised sites are often ulcerated and secondarily infected

Associated skin lesions—e.g. café au lait patches associated with neurofibromas, ash leaf macules associated with collagenomas and adenoma sebaceum in tuberous sclerosis.

BODY-SITE VARIATIONS

Papules and nodules resulting from the same disease may have different clinical appearances, depending on the body site, for various reasons, as follows (with selected examples):

Clinical patterns and behaviour

Diseases may have intrinsically different clinical patterns and behaviour at different sites.

Basal cell carcinoma (Figs 9.73–9.77)—The superficial type of basal cell carcinoma (*see* Fig 9.76), which has a broad, flat, central portion and a narrow, raised rim, is disproportionately more common on the trunk than the face, whereas a nodular (*see* Fig 9.73) or morphoeic (*see* Fig 9.75) basal cell carcinoma is seen more commonly on the face.

Malignant melanoma (Fig 9.38–9.44)—Malignant melanoma may be clinically amelanotic or very sparsely pigmented on the sole of the foot in Caucasians, although this feature is uncommon at other body sites (**Figs 9.38–9.44**)

Frictional and pressure changes

Frictional and pressure changes may alter clinical appearance.

Warts (Figs 9.83–9.85 *also see* Fig 4.37)—Plantar warts are relatively flat compared with those on the dorsum of the hand, which often have a cauliflower shape, or on the face where they may be long and narrow (filiform).

Lesions on the palms or soles

Pyogenic granulomas, fibroepithelial polyps, acquired digital fibrokeratoma, viral warts and eccrine poroma arising at these sites may be bordered by a small depression in the skin, referred to as a moat or gutter (**Fig 9.11**). This is caused by chronic compression of the harder lesion in thick palmoplantar skin. It therefore occurs in slowly enlarging (i.e. usually benign) lesions.

Differences in blood flow

Facial lesions

Nodules and papules on the face are often more telangiectatic than an equivalent lesion on the trunk, e.g. benign melanocytic naevi (**Fig 9.24**).

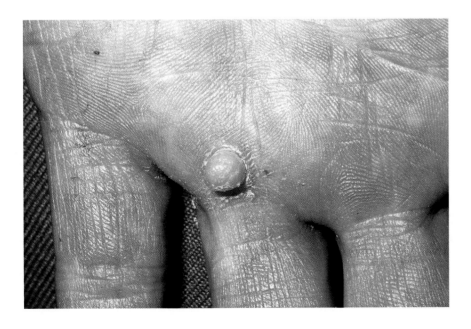

Fig 9.11 Hyperkeratotic moat.
A longstanding hard lesion arising on the palm or sole produces a depressed moat or gutter between the nodule and the adjacent hyperkeratosis as pressure pushes the papule into the thick surrounding skin

Lower leg

Seborrhoeic keratoses on the lower leg are often relatively flat and smooth but also more red than at other body sites.

Occlusion

Occlusion produces stratum corneum hydration and hence greater transparency.

Psoriasis—Flexural lesions are generally smoother and more red than equivalent lesions elsewhere, e.g. psoriasis (*see* Fig 8.15), because the surface scale is fully hydrated, and hence, the usual reflecting air–keratin interfaces are replaced by water–keratin interfaces, which transmit rather than reflect light. Thus, this disorder may present as macular erythema rather than scaly plaques, due to the different body site.

FEATURES OF COMMON MACULAR PAPULAR AND NODULAR LESIONS ACCORDING TO COLOUR AND SURFACE CHARACTERISTICS

Classification of lumps and bumps by tissue of origin does not often aid clinical diagnosis as lesions of different derivation can be clinically indistinguishable. Similarly, colours and surface characteristics may not be consistent for any given diagnosis, and lesions such as naevi or dermatofibromas may change in appearance during their lifespan. The classification used in this chapter (*see* Table 9.5) has been chosen for its clinical usefulness and is based on the typical features for each diagnosis. Although mainly concerned with papules and nodules, common discrete pigmented macules and plaques have been included in the chapter, and some localised inflammatory lesions are also discussed.

Smooth-surfaced lesions

The surface characteristics of some lesions may change as the lesion ulcerates (e.g. basal cell carcinoma) or is traumatised (e.g. pyogenic granuloma). Others lose surface roughness due to constant rubbing or pressure effects (e.g. plantar warts).

Brown and black lesions (*see also* Chapter 3)

Freckles—These are small, brown or red–brown macules, which are scattered over the skin, especially on sun-exposed areas. They result from a local increase in melanin within the epidermis, but the number of melanocytes in the basal layer remains unchanged. Usually most apparent on the cheeks, they fade in winter (**Fig 9.12**). Freckles on the upper back may be larger, rather stellate in shape and more persistent (**Fig 9.13**); these often occur in individuals who sunburn easily and should probably be considered to be a solar lentigo as they contain increased numbers of melanocytes rather than just an increase in melanin pigment. Early freckling on sun-exposed skin is a sign of xeroderma pigmentosa; these patients may not mention sun sensitivity.

DIAGNOSTIC TIPS AND PITFALLS

- Liver spots or flat brown macular lesions on the hands and forearms are either pigmented actinic keratoses, lentigo simplex or flat seborrhoeic warts. The surface texture and degree of wartyness help to distinguish these entities

- Freckles fade when protected from the sun as they are caused by increase in melanin deposition, but there is no increase in the number of melanocytes

- Lentigines do not fade in winter and are caused by increased numbers of normal melanocytes in the epidermis

- Lentigo maligna is caused by an increased number of neoplastic melanocytes in the epidermis

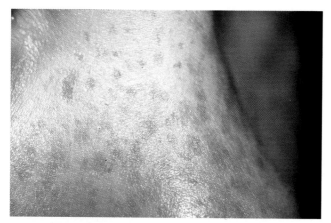

Fig 9.12 Freckles. Brown or red–brown macules on cheeks and other areas exposed to sunlight; most prominent in summer

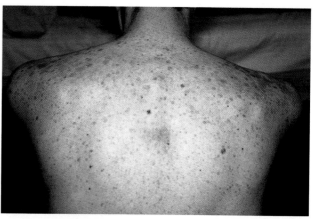

Fig 9.13 Stellate freckles. Freckles on the upper back and shoulders are larger, darker brown, more irregular in shape and more permanent than ordinary facial freckles. They may occur after sunburn

Lentigo simplex—These are small, dark brown or black macules, which occur on any body site and are not related to sun exposure (**Fig 9.14**). They may be congenital or acquired, and it may be impossible to distinguish them from junctional naevi by clinical examination. Pathological examination shows increased numbers of basal epidermal melanocytes at the tip of elongated rete ridges.

Peutz–Jeghers syndrome—patients with this condition have multiple dark brown, freckle-sized lentigos around the eyes and mouth (**Fig 9.15**) and on the fingers. They are darker than freckles and do not have the same variability in relation to sunlight but may fade with age—although the buccal lesions persist. These are a cutaneous marker for gastrointestinal polyps (**Fig 9.16**), and patients may present either in childhood because of intestinal bleeding or intussusception or in adulthood due to the development of adenocarcinoma.

Naevus of Ota—This is an acquired pigmentary abnormality, which occurs most frequently in Japanese people. It presents in childhood or young adult life as a grey or blue-coloured area of pigmentation on the cheek or eyelid (**Fig 9.17**) and may be bilateral. The pigment is intradermal but may show a notable variation during the menstrual cycle or even on a daily basis. It may be speckled in distribution and resemble freckles in mild cases.

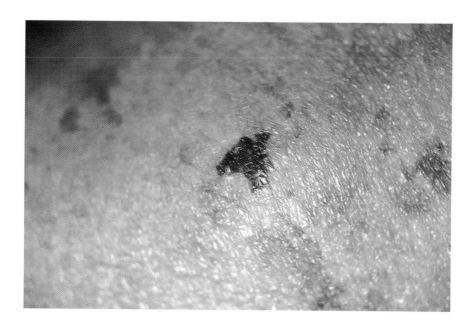

Fig 9.14 Lentigo simplex. Dark brown lesions, which look like small junctional naevi

159

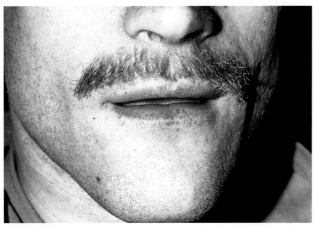

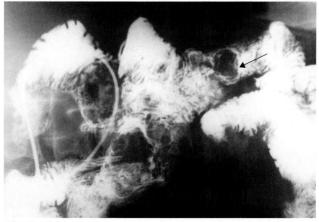

Fig 9.15

Fig 9.16

Fig 9.15, 9.16 Peutz–Jeghers syndrome. A recognisable pattern of lentigines, which affect perioral and periocular skin (9.15) (also the dorsum of the fingers and buccal mucosa). Intestinal polyps are shown by a small bowel enema in 9.16 (one is arrowed)

Café au lait patches—These are tan-coloured macules with uniform pigmentation, usually over 5 mm in diameter, and rounded or oval in shape (**Fig 9.18**). The border is sharp but is generally not a smooth circle. The alteration in pigment is due to an increase in melanocytes but also to abnormal giant pigment granules (macromelanosomes).

Although up to 20% of normal individuals have one or two small café au lait spots of a few centimetres in diameter, the importance of café au lait patches is that they are a marker for neurofibromatosis type I. More than six café au lait patches is diagnostic in about 99% of cases. This is made even more specific if axillary freckling is also present (Crowe's sign, **Fig 9.19**). Additionally, Lisch nodules may occur in the iris (**Fig 9.20**). By contrast, in patients with tuberous sclerosis, there is no increase in the number of café au lait patches compared with normal controls.

Similar lesions are seen in the Albright–McCune syndrome (pigmentation, precocious puberty and polyostotic fibrous dysplasia), but these lesions tend to be larger and more irregular or stellate in shape than café au lait patches.

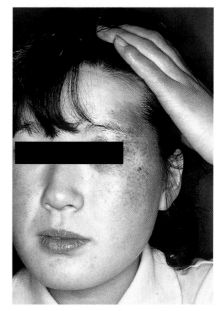

Fig 9.17 Naevus of Ota. Blue–grey pigmentation affecting the cheek and eyelid in a Japanese patient. Ocular melanosis may also occur (*photo courtesy of Dr Shingi Tamada*)

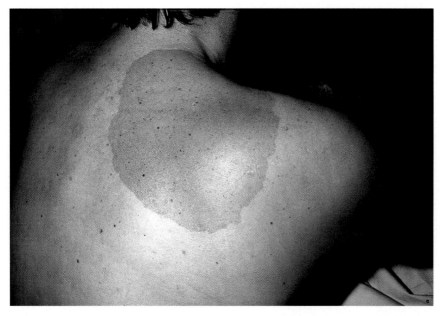

Fig 9.18 Café au lait patches. Round or oval macules, often with a rather scalloped edge. Pigmentation is uniform. One or two such lesions is a normal finding; more than six is virtually pathognomonic of neurofibromatosis type I (*see also* 9.19, 9.63)

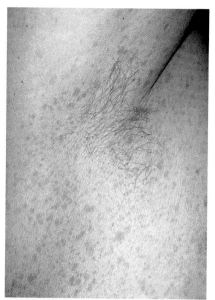

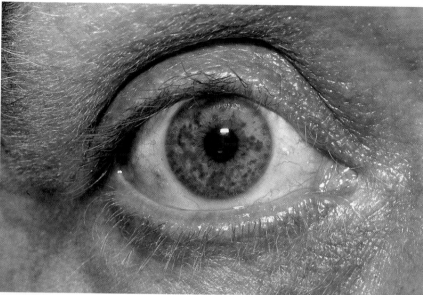

Fig 9.19   **Fig 9.20**

Fig 9.19, 9.20 Other signs of neurofibromatosis. Crowe's sign (9.19). Axillary freckling is a feature of neurofibromatosis. Lisch nodules (9.20) are raised, round, dome-shaped, brown, asymptomatic hamartomas on the iris that are present in over 90% of adults with neurofibromatosis and their apparently unaffected first-degree relatives

Lentigo senilis—These are larger, paler brown lesions (**Fig 9.21**) which are present on the sun-exposed skin of elderly people but can occur in young adults. The differential diagnosis is usually from pigmented actinic keratoses or seborrhoeic warts, which are often flatter and more uniformly brown-coloured on the face than at other sites. Lentigo maligna is considered in the section on malignant melanoma (*see* Fig 9.41).

Melanocytic naevi—Naevi are generally multiple and acquired during teenage years, although some are present at, or soon after, birth. Congenital naevi (**Fig 9.22**) often have a deep brown colour, contain darker coarser hairs than those of the adjacent skin and become thicker or cobblestoned in texture during adolescence. Some are huge and have a high malignant potential.

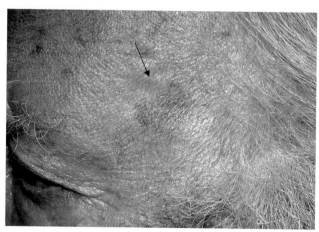

Fig 9.21 Lentigo senilis. A misleading name, as it is not restricted to elderly patients. It is related to chronic sun exposure and is seen most commonly on the face. Lesions are uniformly pigmented, sometimes slightly rough, and regular in outline

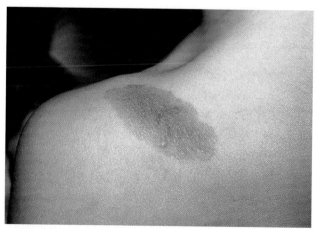

Fig 9.22 Congenital naevus. Usually a deep brown colour with cobblestoned (papillomatous) surface and coarse dark hairs

Common 'acquired' melanocytic naevi are generally flat and small, or they may be a plaque or dome-shaped papule or nodule (**Fig 9.23–9.25**). Naevi increase in number until the third decade of life and then decrease; one study showed the median number of naevi over 3 mm in Caucasians aged 20–30 years to be 24 in females and 16 in males, with only 5% of individuals in this age range having no naevi of this size. Occasionally, crops of naevi may develop after inflammatory skin conditions or associated with other stimuli, such as chemotherapy.

Most common naevi are relatively uniform and symmetrical in shape and colour. Nevertheless, it is important to recognise that they do alter in colour and shape over the years (**Figs 9.23–9.25**). Initially, the naevus cells are mainly at the lower epidermal/upper dermal zone and actively produce melanin, but naevi of longer duration have just dermal naevus cells or else a mixture of dermal and junctional components. Thus, early 'junctional' naevi are generally flat and well pigmented, whereas older ones are often more fleshy and may be either pale intradermal, or pigmented compound, naevi.

Some colour patterns and changes in naevi cause concern, although they are actually benign; examples include a speckled pattern (**Fig 9.26**), naevus spilus (**Fig 9.27**), naevus 'en cocarde' (**Fig 9.28**), spindle cell naevus of Reed (**Fig 9.29**) and halo naevus (**Fig 9.34**).

Atypical naevi—some naevi do have increased malignant potential and have been variously named as 'atypical,' 'dysplastic' and 'BK mole syndrome' (**Figs 9.30–9.32** and **Table 9.8**). The most atypical on a histological basis are sometimes relatively pale, red or tan-coloured and are usually present from

DIAGNOSTIC TIPS AND PITFALLS

- The number of naevi in an individual increases until his or her mid-20s and then decreases

- On average, white women aged 20–30 years have 24 moles larger than 3 mm in diameter and men 16

- Naevi change with time. Early 'junctional' naevi are generally flat and well pigmented, whereas older naevi are raised and either pigmented (compound naevi, with pigment cells in both the epidermis and dermis) or flesh-coloured (intradermal naevi, with naevus cells only in the dermis)

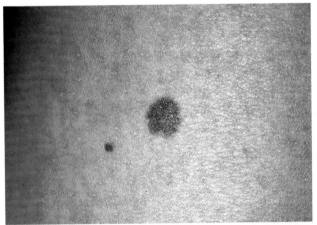

Fig 9.23

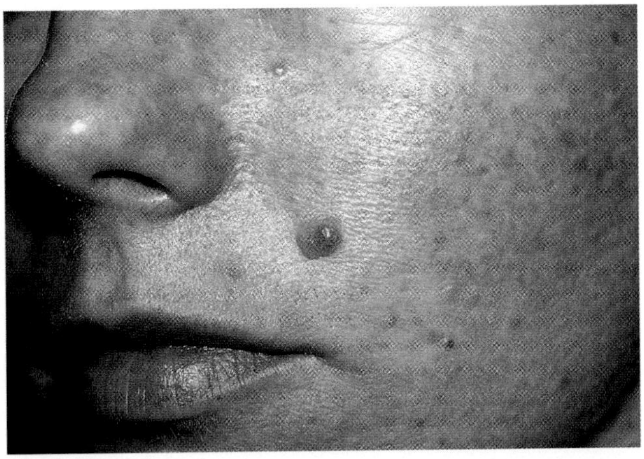

Fig 9.24

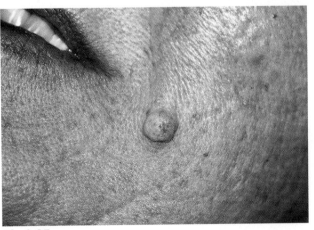

Fig 9.23–9.25 Evolution of common acquired naevi.
'Junctional' naevi are generally flat and dark brown (9.23), intradermal naevi are pale brown or flesh coloured, smooth, dome-shaped papules (9.25), and compound naevi (9.24) are intermediate between these two. (The naevi shown are in different individuals)

Fig 9.25

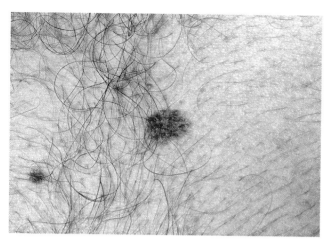

Fig 9.26 Acquired naevus. A speckled pattern of pigmentation is not uncommon. The speckles are of fairly uniform size and colour in a naevus with a smooth contour

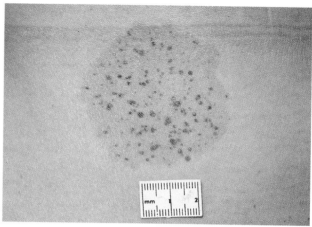

Fig 9.27 Naevus spilus. This is a macular lesion of pale brown pigment, studded with uniform darker brown papules or tiny plaques. Speckled lentiginous naevus is a more correct name

an earlier age and in greater numbers than normal. This is a confusing area, as some individuals have one or a few naevi with histological dysplasia, whereas other patients have a hundred or more. The importance of a solitary dysplastic naevus is uncertain, but those with many such naevi have an increased risk of melanoma. Other recognisable variants of naevus that may cause concern are described below.

Blue naevus—This is a deep dermal naevus (**Fig 9.33**) with spindle-shaped cells, producing large amounts of pigment. Because it is deep within the dermis, it appears blue, or even black, rather than brown. This is because longer wavelengths of light are absorbed by dermal melanin, and the shorter-wavelength blue light is scattered and reflected (Tyndall effect). The common type of blue naevus is solitary, often on the limbs rather than the trunk, and not pre-malignant.

Halo naevus—The halo naevus (**Fig 9.34**) is also known as a Sutton's naevus. This condition is most common in adolescence and consists of a ring of depigmentation around an otherwise normal naevus. It is due to an inflammatory attack on the naevus, which also damages surrounding melanocytes. Affected naevi may be transiently itchy, often become paler and may then repigment, but often disappear completely. Multiple naevi may be affected—a reassuring sign.

Meyerson's naevus—This (**Fig 9.35**) manifests as a ring of eczema around a benign naevus. It is a rare but benign cause of naevi becoming itchy and is not associated with depigmentation of either the naevus or the surrounding skin. It is usually solitary. The eczema resolves if the naevus is excised; otherwise, it may be prone to recurrence.

Spitz naevus—This (**Fig 9.36**) is also known by the confusing name of benign juvenile melanoma, which should be considered obsolete. This type of naevus is melanocytic, but the pigment is generally obscured by the high degree of vascularity, and the lesions are assumed to be angiomas unless the pigment is revealed by diascopy (*see* Fig 4.4 and 4.5). They usually arise on the face in childhood, but in adults, they may be less typical and are often darker and scaly and occur on the limbs rather than the face.

Becker's naevus—This appears as a large patch of increased pigmentation with increased hair growth (*see* Fig 18.7) and epidermal thickening (**Fig 9.37**). It usually presents in young men and often involves the upper thorax or upper arm. It normally has an irregular, jagged border and may darken in sunlight. The melanocytes, however, are normal rather than naevus cells, and the naevus is not pre-malignant.

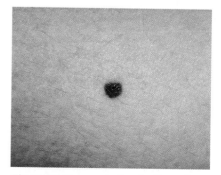

Fig 9.28 Naevus 'en cocarde.' A dark rim of pigment of uniform width around a naevus, which often also has a dark centre, is a recognised benign pattern of naevus ('*en cocarde*' means 'rosette-like')

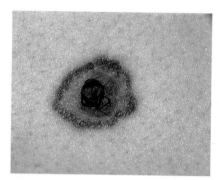

Fig 9.29 Pigmented spindle cell naevus of Reed. This benign junctional naevus can be confused histologically and clinically with melanoma. It has a characteristic deep brown or black colour and is of a small size

163

Table 9.8 Comparison of common and dysplastic naevi

Feature	Common naevus	Dysplastic naevus
Number	<30	100
Site	Any	Mainly trunk
Size	Most <8 mm in diameter	Many >8 mm in diameter
Colour	Most medium brown; if speckled, this is uniform in colour and distribution	Variable, red to black. May be tan-coloured halo around eccentrically situated raised area
Edge	Sharply defined	Irregular, merges with adjacent skin
Surface	Flat or smooth dome	May be cobblestoned
Hairs	Common on face	Not a feature

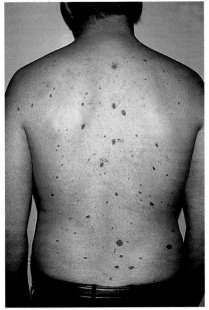

Fig 9.30

Fig 9.30–9.32 Acquired naevi.
Atypical ('dysplastic') type. Features suggestive of dysplastic naevi include greater than average numbers of naevi (9.30), irregular shapes or pigmentation (9.31), vague border and reddish tan colour (9.32). However, many naevi with these clinically atypical patterns are histologically unremarkable

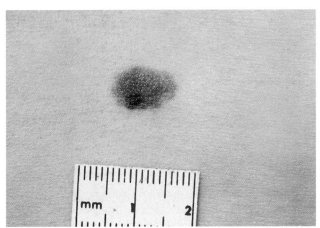

Fig 9.31

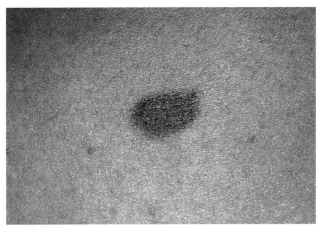

Fig 9.32

Malignant melanoma—This is a malignant tumour of melanocytes, which may arise *de novo* or from a pre-existing melanocytic naevus. There are different types, which are distinguished on the basis of histological examination and clinical features (Table 9.9).

The most important prognostic feature for all types of malignant melanoma is the depth of invasion, measured in millimetres as the Breslow thickness; adequate local excision is associated with 5-year survival rates of about 98% if the lesion is less than 0.76 mm thick. The site has some influence; for example, plantar and subungual malignant melanoma both have a

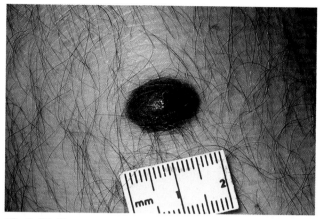

Fig 9.33 Blue naevus. The refractile properties of the dermis make deep accumulations of melanin appear blue in colour (contrast with the typical brown colour of melanin at the dermoepidermal junction in ordinary naevi and the muddy-brown colour in the upper dermis in post-inflammatory pigmentation)

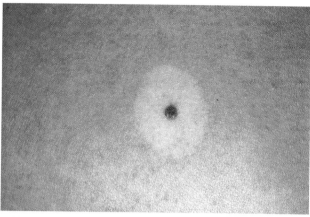

Fig 9.34 Halo naevus. Often multiple, usually in teenagers, and generally affecting naevi on the trunk, this is an acquired ring of depigmentation around a pre-existing naevus

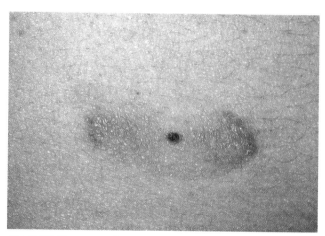

Fig 9.35 Meyerson's naevus. Halo eczema around a benign melanocytic naevus

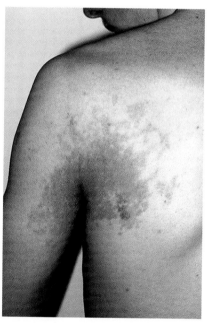

Fig 9.37 Becker's naevus. A patch of uniformly pigmented skin with increased hair growth and an irregular edge, often arising in the scapular area

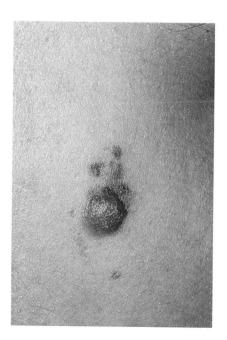

Fig 9.36 Spitz naevus. A red–brown lesion, which is very vascular—it usually occurs in childhood

Table 9.9 Features of different types of malignant melanoma*

Histogenetic type	Site	Physical signs	Frequency in Caucasians
Superficial spreading melanoma (SSM)	Any	Initially flat, expands laterally, later may develop asymmetrical nodule. Variable pigment, edge is irregular (9.39)	70%
Nodular melanoma (NM)	Any	Nodule, often with irregular rim of macular pigment. May be black, brown, pink or combination (9.44)	15%
Lentigo maligna melanoma (LMM)	Face in 90%	Nodule or plaque developing within pre-existing lentigo maligna, colour variation as SSM or NM (9.42)	10%
Acral lentiginous melanoma (ALM)	Sole and fingers	Macular pigmentation of skin of soleor nailfolds, subungual with nail pigment streaks or destruction may be amelanotic (9.43, 19.65)	5%

*Nomenclature of lentigo maligna (Hutchinson's freckle) causes a good deal of confusion. This is clarified in Table 9.10.

Table 9.10 Nomenclature of lentigo maligna and related disorders

Name	Melanocyte characteristics	Clinical correlate
Lentigo	Increased number, normal site (basal layer) and cytological appearance	Uniform pigmentation (1.2)
Lentigo maligna	Increased number, abnormal cytology, but normal site	Focal areas of darker pigmentation (9.41)
Lentigo maligna melanoma	Increased number, abnormal cytology, 'nesting' and spread from basal layer	More extreme variation in colours, development of nodules (9.42)

poor prognosis, which is at least partly because they escape detection at these sites.

Diagnosis of malignant melanoma may be easy, but it can be difficult to distinguish from other pigmented lesions with certainty, especially from some of the more unusually patterned melanocytic naevi. The most useful clinical feature is when some aspect of the lesion has changed (size, shape, colour, symptoms (**Figs 9.38–9.44**), although the time course of the change

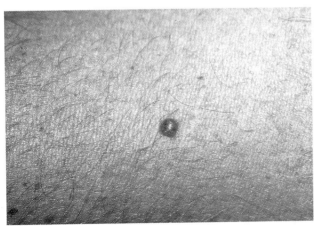

Fig 9.38

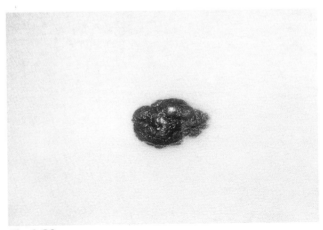

Fig 9.39

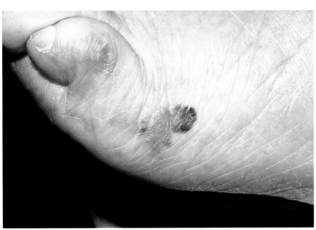

Fig 9.40

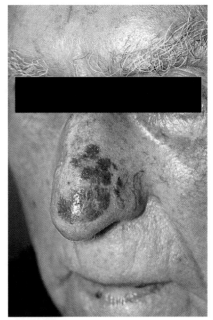

Fig 9.41

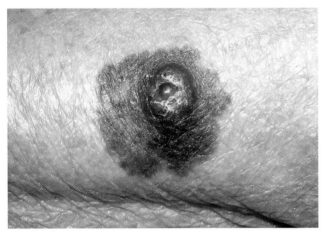

Fig 9.42

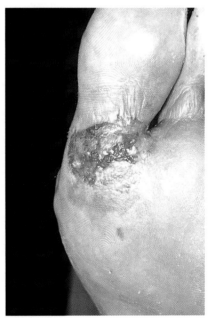

Fig 9.43

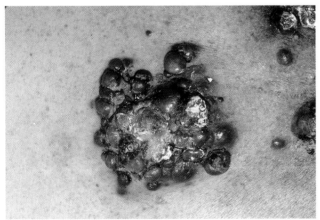

Fig 9.44

Fig 9.38–9.44 Malignant melanoma. Variable pigmentation is typical and is often grey or blue–black. An irregular or scalloped edge is a suggestive feature of this disorder. A 'new mole' (9.38), even if clinically unremarkable, should be viewed with suspicion. Superficial spreading melanoma (9.39) has an irregular shape, eccentrically placed nodule and spreading macular pigment at the periphery. Superficial spreading melanoma (9.40), showing an irregular shape; pigment varies from pink to black. Lentigo maligna is shown in 9.41. This lesion is flat and lacks an invasive melanoma component. It has developed follicular repigmentation after previous cryotherapy. Lentigo maligna melanoma (9.42) exhibits a broad area of irregular lentigo, with an eccentrically placed nodule. Acral melanoma (9.43) shows an irregular ulcer on the sole of the foot with relatively subtle pigmentation at one border. The nodular malignant melanoma (9.44), illustrated is an unusually advanced case with multiple metastases at the time of presentation

should be considered. For example, the sudden onset of itch or tenderness suggests inflammation rather than malignant change, and 'overnight' colour change is more likely to be traumatic than due to malignancy (**Figs 9.45–9.49**). New or changing pigmented lesions in adults should be viewed with suspicion. However, normal melanocytic naevi also alter with time (as indicated above), becoming less dark but often more protuberant; if doubt exists, then an excision biopsy should be performed.

The physical signs that are most helpful are (**Figs 9.38–9.44**):

- Colour—varied pigmentation, especially if it includes blue–black or greyish colours rather than the brown of most naevi.
- Irregular edge—this sign is unusual in ordinary naevi.
- Asymmetry—benign naevi are usually symmetrical.
- Irregular surface—nodules within a pigmented mole may be quite benign but should always arouse consideration of malignant change, especially if eccentrically situated.
- Large size—apart from congenital naevi, a size over 1 cm in diameter is uncommon in ordinary naevi.

Dermatofibroma—Dermatofibromas, or pigmented histiocytomas (**Figs 9.50– 9.52**), are commonly misdiagnosed lesions. They usually present as one or few asymptomatic (sometimes sore or itchy) small nodules, 0.5–1 cm in diameter. They occur most commonly on the limbs, especially the lower leg. Often initially pink/red, they generally become pigmented later, either with a uniform brown colour or as a brown rim around a pale central nodule, which is often

DIAGNOSTIC TIPS AND PITFALLS

- Breslow thickness is the single best prognostic indicator of survival in patients with a melanoma

- Melanomas on the sole of the foot can be difficult to diagnose and are often poorly or non-pigmented

Features strongly suggestive of malignant change in a mole include:

- Increase in size

- Change in colour

- Colour variation, i.e. blacks/browns/reds/greys, etc. in the same lesion

- Irregularity of the edge of the lesion

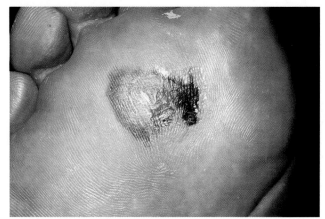

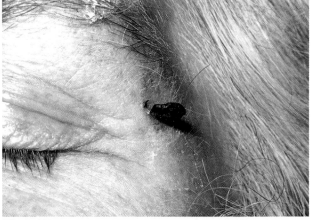

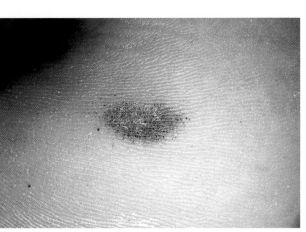

Fig 9.45

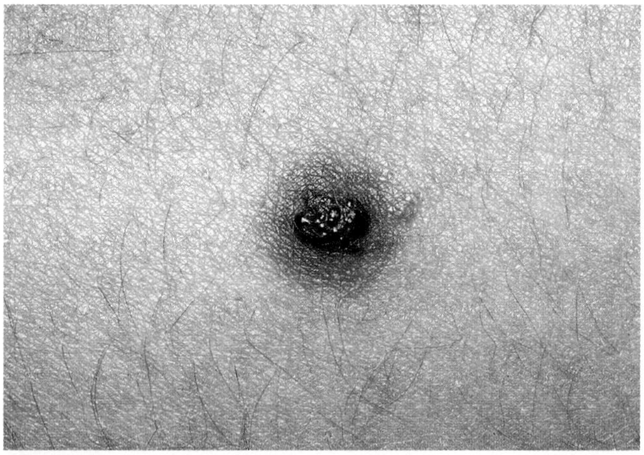

Fig 9.46

Fig 9.47

Fig 9.48

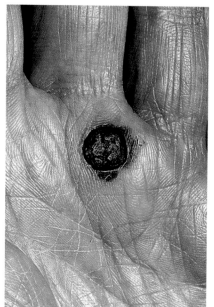

Fig 9.45–9.49 Lesions simulating malignant melanoma. Melanocytic naevi, some seborrhoeic warts, pigmented basal cell carcinoma and pigmented lesions as shown here, may be confused with malignant melanoma. Thrombosis in a fibroepithelial polyp (9.45). This showed an acute change from one day to the next, in a pedunculated lesion, so melanoma was highly unlikely. Haemorrhage within a lymphangioma (9.46) exhibited an acute change, with typical bluish colour of deep blood and a bruise-like periphery. *Talon noir* (9.47) is a lesion that often causes concern; it results from repetitive frictional damage and occurs on the heels of physically active young men mainly. If the physical signs of the individual lesion are not diagnostic the other foot should be examined, as it is usually bilateral. In cases of trauma to the sole of the foot (9.48), a haematoma on this site can appear very black and irregular. Paring the lesion shows that there is no pigment in the external shavings. Silver nitrate treatment of a wart (9.49): even with a clinical history, this lesion is worrying, but the black colour is too uniform for a typical malignant melanoma

Fig 9.49

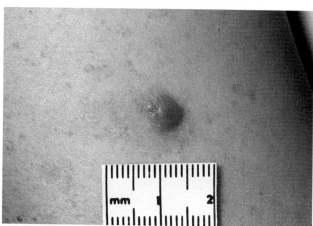

Fig 9.50

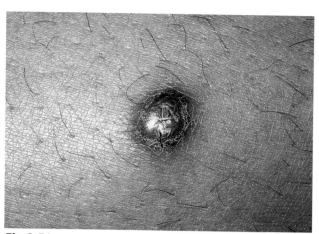

Fig 9.51

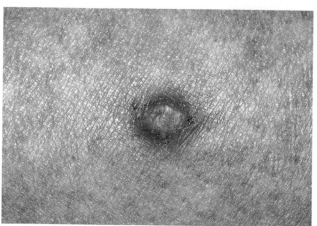

Fig 9.52

Fig 9.50–9.52 Dermatofibromas. Early lesions may be smooth red nodules (9.50), whereas older examples have brown pigmentation, either uniform (9.51) or as a rim around a paler centre (9.52). The surface of older lesions is often slightly scaly due to epidermal thickening. At all ages, the nodules are characteristically firm on palpation

slightly scaly. Other important signs are firmness on palpation, likened to feeling a button through cloth when the lesion is manipulated between the finger and thumb. Tethering of the lesion within the dermis can be shown as the 'dimple' sign (*see* Fig 4.23). Although dermatofibromas are included in the list of smooth lesions, there is often some epidermal thickening and slight scaling on the surface, but in general, they do not feel rough or develop crusting.

Mastocytosis—Focal collections of mast cells present as a solitary plaque or nodule called a mastocytoma, or as multiple localised plaques known as urticaria pigmentosa. Both occur in infants and young children and are initially itchy but gradually fade and become asymptomatic over several years. The individual lesions are shallow, dome-shaped nodules or plaques, often 2–3 cm in diameter and pale brown. They show a classic physical sign of becoming red and urticated or raised after rubbing, due to the release of histamine and other inflammatory mediators from the mast cells (Darier's sign, **Fig 9.53**, *see also* Figs 4.28–4.30). A less common variant of mastocytosis, telangiectasia macularis eruptiva perstans, is described in Chapter 17 (*see also* Fig 17.19).

Other lesions—Smooth and pigmented lesions also include skin tags, basal cell carcinoma, plane warts (**Figs 9.54 and 9.55**), seborrhoeic warts and some actinic keratoses—although these are usually rough or crusted (**Figs 9.86–9.88**, *see also* Figs 7.33 and 7.34). Angiomas are normally red but can be blue or black (**Table 9.11**); they are, however, more appropriately placed in the section on lesions that are usually red or purple (see p. 174).

White, yellow, flesh-coloured and translucent lesions (*see also* Chapter 3)

Skin tags—Skin tag is a description, rather than a diagnosis, as some skin tags are actually aged naevi or neurofibromas. The term is more appropriately applied to fibroepithelial polyps that are tiny, multiple, soft pedunculated lesions with a papillomatous surface. They occur especially in flexures, mainly the axillae, but also on the upper inner thigh and around the neck. They are either flesh-coloured or brown (*see* 5.31 and 6.43).

Cysts—Cysts arising from skin appendages are fairly common, especially on the scalp (pilar cyst) or chest. They are usually solitary or few in number, but

---

DIAGNOSTIC TIPS AND PITFALLS

Lesions commonly confused with a melanoma include:

- Benign moles: some may be difficult to distinguish from malignant melanoma
- Dysplastic naevi: clinically usually indistinguishable from a melanoma
- Seborrhoeic warts: warty greasy scale and small, cream-coloured, round keratin pearls are visible
- Haemangiomas: red rather than brown, and the blood vessel shapes can be distinguished using a dermatoscope
- Pyogenic granuloma: always look for pigment at the edge of the nodule (there should be no pigment around or in a pyogenic granuloma)
- Dermatofibroma: this feels 'like a button through a shirt', and the dimple sign is positive
- Pigmented basal cell carcinoma: the pigment is pencil-lead grey in colour and usually distributed as small pigment globules

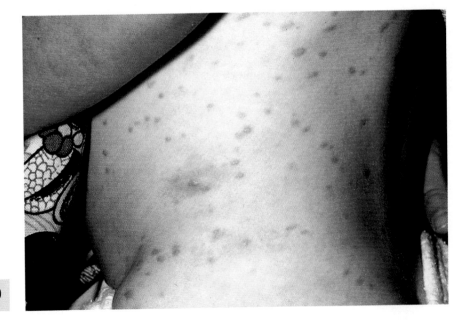

Fig 9.53 Urticaria pigmentosa.
This shows the typical brown-coloured, shallow, dome-shaped lesions. Note also the presence of an urticated rim around one lesion, after rubbing has caused release of mast-cell contents (Darier's sign *see also* Figs 4.28–4.30)

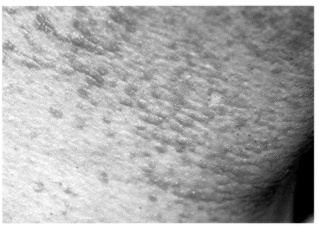

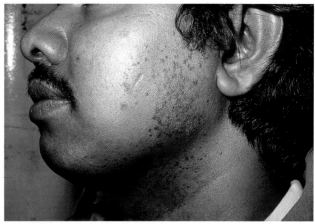

Fig 9.54   **Fig 9.55**

Fig 9.54, 9.55 Plane warts. These lesions are often a uniform pale brown (9.54) but can be very dark in racially pigmented skin (9.55). They are multiple, just palpable, small plaques, with a slightly rough surface

Table 9.11 Differential diagnosis of blue–black papules and nodules*

Melanocytic	Naevi, especially blue naevus (9.33) Malignant melanoma (9.38–9.44)
Vascular	Haematomas, e.g. subungual (19.12, 19.13), within lymphangioma (9.46) Small vessels, e.g. thrombosed vessels in warts (4.37), *talon noir* (9.47) Deep angiomas (9.69), venous lake (6.26, 9.67)
Exogenous	Dark foreign bodies (pencil point, metals)
Others	Seborrhoeic warts (9.81) 'Actinic comedone' (6.16) Cystic lesions, e.g. apocrine hidrocystoma Pigmented basal cell carcinoma (9.77), orf (3.33)

* *See also* Table 3.7 regarding other blue–black-coloured skin lesions.

multiple cysts can occur in some patients. Multiple cysts also present in acne, in some specific disorders, e.g. steatocystoma multiplex, and at specific body sites, e.g. multiple scrotal cysts. Individually, the lesions are smooth and firm (**Fig 9.56**), and visibly yellowish white. In thin skin areas, there may be telangiectasia in stretched skin over the cyst. The overlying skin is mobile except near the punctum, although a punctum cannot always be identified and is not characteristic of all cysts. Deep fixation is not a feature, although it may occur after rupture or inflammation around a cyst. Mobility of the skin over a cyst may be very difficult to show on the scalp.

Milia are tiny epidermoid cysts that do not have a punctum and are too superficial and small to be recognised by the above criteria; they are firm white papules, about 1–2 mm in diameter, arising spontaneously on the cheeks (*see* Fig 6.48) or eyelids or at other sites after subepidermal blistering (*see* Fig 13.51).

Nodules arising from appendages—In addition to cysts, other relatively common lesions related to skin appendages are organoid naevi and benign tumours.

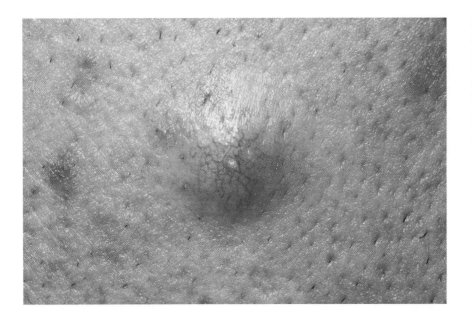

Fig 9.56 Epidermoid cyst.
A smooth swelling with normal or stretched skin over the surface, a white colour if visible through thin skin and a noticeable punctum where it attaches to the surface. This may allow entry of bacteria or expulsion of the cheesy content, which is keratin not sebaceous gland secretions

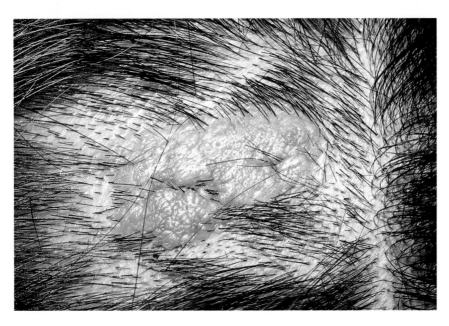

Fig 9.57 Organoid naevus (naevus sebaceous of Jadassohn).
A hamartoma, which is typically orange in colour, usually occurs on the scalp and often presents in later childhood as it tends to become more verrucous at puberty

An organoid naevus is also known as naevus sebaceous of Jadassohn (**Fig 9.57**). This is a hamartoma, which occurs most commonly as a solitary lesion on the scalp and should not be confused with melanocytic naevi. It may present as a localised area of alopecia, usually with scanty rather than absent hairs, or in teenage years when it becomes more papillomatous or warty. The lesions are softer than viral warts and more orange–yellow than either viral warts or scalp naevi. Nodules with histological features of a wide variety of benign appendage neoplasms may develop within a naevus sebaceous. Basal cell carcinomas also occur within these lesions.

Benign appendage neoplasm—Benign appendage neoplasms (**Figs 9.58–9.60**) are moderately common but generally cannot be diagnosed clinically as they often present as smooth, domed, sometimes telangiectatic nodules that may resemble naevi or basal cell carcinoma. Some, arising from hair follicles, may have a crusted centre. The lesions most likely to be diagnosed clinically are those with a striking clinical feature, such as pilomatricomas, which often occur in children as stony, hard lesions that may extrude calcium. Diagnosis

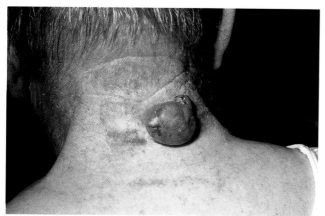

Fig 9.58

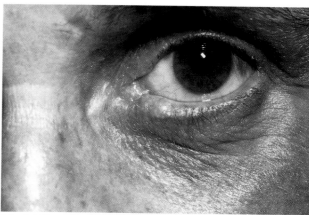

Fig 9.59

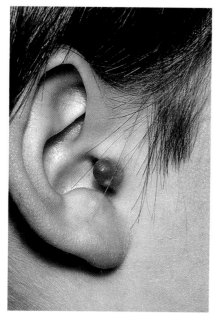

Fig 9.60

Fig 9.58–9.60 Appendage neoplasms. Most are benign, smooth, dome-shaped papules or nodules. 9.58 shows a cylindroma on the nape of the neck. The scalp and head or neck are typical sites, and the nodules often appear pink or vascular. A hidrocystoma (9.59) is a greyish translucent tumour, which clinically may resemble a basal cell carcinoma. A pilomatrixoma (9.60) is usually a solitary lesion, which may be quite purple but can often present as just a hard lump on the face or arm in children—the hardness is due to calcification. The eponymous name for this tumour is calcifying epithelioma of Malherbe

DIAGNOSTIC TIPS AND PITFALLS

- Stretching the tumour edge between the finger and thumb excludes blood from the skin and makes it easier to see the pearly component of a basal cell carcinoma

- Sebaceous hypertrophy are yellowish, usually multiple and have a small central depression, even in the smallest lesions

- Other adnexal tumours, e.g. cylindroma, trichoepithelioma, are rarely ulcerated, pearly papules

- Bowen's disease presents as a crusted and scaly plaque with no rolled edge

- Squamous cell carcinoma produces keratin, hence the surface scale or keratinous surface. They are not pearly and not obviously telangiectatic

may also be suggested by a characteristic distribution in some cases, e.g. syringomata, which arise from eccrine sweat ducts and appear as multiple small papules on the lower eyelids (**Fig 9.61**).

Sebaceous hypertrophy—This is a common disorder that may cause solitary or multiple lesions on the face, especially in elderly skin (*see* Fig 6.20). Its importance is that it shows a clinical resemblance to basal cell carcinoma, although lesions of sebaceous hypertrophy are usually multiple and distinguished by their yellow colour.

Keloid and hypertrophic scars—Diagnosis of keloid and hypertrophic scars is usually straightforward if there is a recent surgical scar but may be less apparent initially if there is spontaneous development of a keloid. Minor injury can cause development of keloids, e.g. vaccinations or ear piercing (**Fig 9.62**). Keloids occur especially in African–Caribbean and young people and especially in the mantle area of the upper trunk, neck and upper arms. Individual lesions are asymptomatic, very firm, smooth, dermal plaques or nodules.

Neurofibromas—These are typically multiple in von Recklinghausen's disease (**Fig 9.63**); this should be suspected if other signs such as café au lait

173

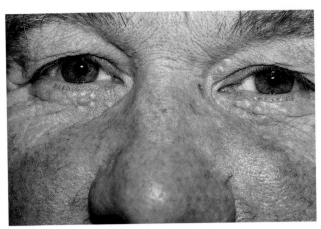

Fig 9.61 Syringomata. Some appendage tumours are typically multiple, the most common being syringomata, which are small, smooth, brownish or skin-coloured papules, often on the lower eyelids

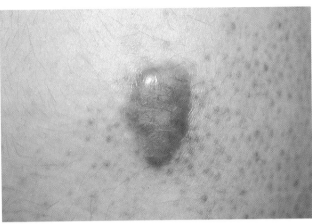

Fig 9.62 Keloid. Smooth firm dermal nodule, in this case caused by trauma of minor surgery

patches (**Fig 9.18**), axillary freckling (Crowe's sign (**Fig 9.19**)) or Lisch nodules (**Fig 9.20**) are also present. However, solitary neurofibromas also occur as a sporadic, non-inherited feature and cause greater problems of clinical differential diagnosis. Individually, these lesions are soft, domed or pedunculated, smooth or papillomatous, flesh-coloured or slightly blue–brown and may have mild surface telangiectasia (**Fig 9.64**).

Xanthomas—these are characterised by their pale yellow colour and are summarised in **Table 3.10**.

A yellow–brown colour is also seen in juvenile xanthogranulomas, which occur as solitary or multiple nodules in children but are not associated with hyperlipidaemia.

Red and purple lesions (*see also* Chapter 17)

Angiomas—These are lesions composed of abnormal blood vessels; however, they are more usefully described here than in Chapter 17, although some angiomas, such as spider naevi (*see* Fig 17.17), present as telangiectasia or punctate lesions rather than as nodules and are discussed later (*see* p. 306).

Haemangiomas—These are tumours of blood vessels, which may have a red, purple or blue colour (*see* Chapter 17 for discussion of colours of vascular

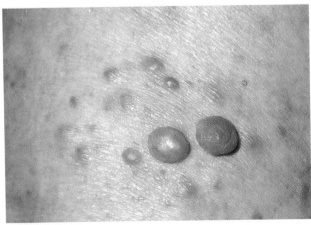

Fig 9.63 Neurofibromatosis. Multiple pale flesh-coloured, soft or rubbery nodules in neurofibromatosis

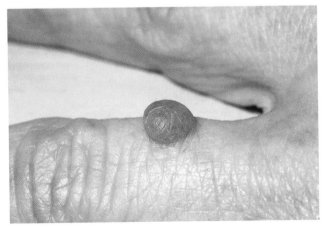

Fig 9.64 Neurofibroma. A solitary neurofibroma, which is clinically similar to the individual nodules shown in 9.63

lesions). Many different types occur, the commonest being cherry angiomas or Campbell de Morgan spots (*see* Figs 6.24 and 6.25), which may be confused with vasculitis when multiple small lesions are present (*see* Fig 6.25). They occur in adults and are generally said to have no importance, although their characteristic bright red colour does become dusky in patients with cyanosis and may therefore be considered a useful physical sign.

Pyogenic granuloma—This is an alarming lesion (**Fig 9.65**), which is found mainly in adults, usually on the hands, and commonly during pregnancy; the lesions are solitary, grow rapidly and are very vascular, with frequent and copious bleeding because there is a deep arteriolar blood supply. Although the lesions are initially smooth and bright red, the tendency to bleeding means that they often present as a scabbed (dried blood) or crusted nodule.

Strawberry naevi—In children, strawberry naevi (**Fig 9.66**) present as solitary angiomatous lesions, which generally appear in the first month of life, enlarge over several months and then slowly involute. They are bright red but develop central grey–white areas during involution.

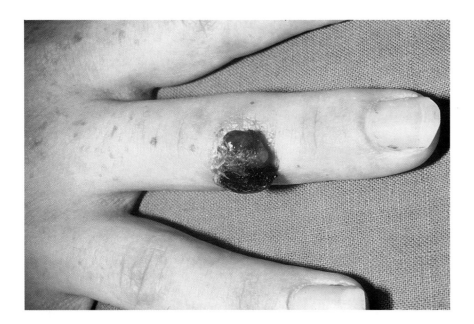

Fig 9.65 Pyogenic granuloma. A very vascular rounded nodule, sometimes pedunculated, and often with dried blood or crusting on the surface

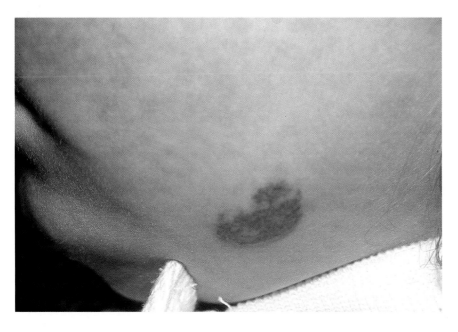

Fig 9.66 Strawberry naevus on the cheek of a child. This is an angioma, which appears soon after birth and gradually involutes. The grey colour is typical of established lesions undergoing regression

Venous lakes—These (Fig 9.67) are soft, compressible, blue-coloured, flat-topped papules, which present as a solitary lesion on the lips (*see* Fig 6.26) but occasionally may be multiple and occur on other areas such as the cheeks.

Angiokeratomas—These are considered here for ease, as they have a similar colour and appearance to venous lakes but are often palpably rough on the surface. They may be solitary and sometimes quite deep, but can also occur as multiple grouped papular lesions (Fig 9.68).

Other angiomas that are usually blue in colour include multiple glomus tumours (Fig 9.69) and blue rubber bleb naevi.

Lymphangiomas—These are localised lesions derived from lymphatics. They typically present as tightly grouped, clear, vesicular papules, likened to frog spawn (Fig 9.70). There may be focal haemorrhage, which can cause alarm. The lesions may have deep lymphangiomatous caverns associated with a relatively innocuous appearance at skin level.

Kaposi's sarcoma—The range of appearances of Kaposi's sarcoma will not be covered in depth here. The classic form is of multiple grouped lesions,

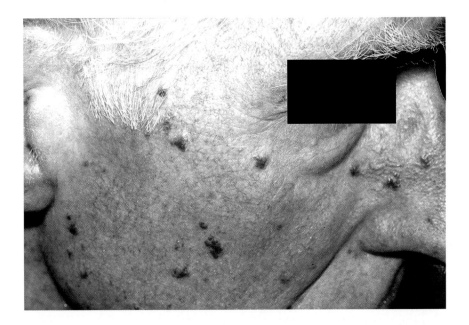

Fig 9.67 Venous lakes. Most are solitary lesions on the lip, but multiple lesions may occur, as shown here. They have a deep blue colour and are soft compressible lesions

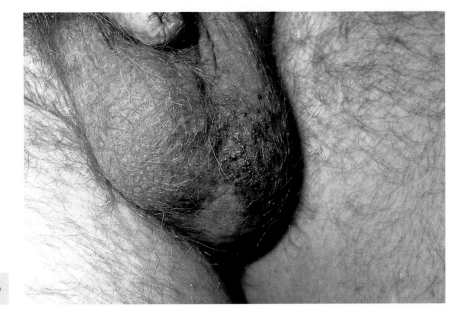

Fig 9.68 Angiokeratoma of Fordyce. Multiple small papular lesions with typical dusky blue–purple colour

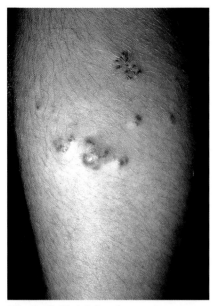

Fig 9.69 Multiple glomus tumours. These are painless vascular tumours that are inherited as an autosomal dominant trait; these show the typical deep blue colour. Compare with the exquisitely tender solitary type of glomus tumour (*see* 19.59)

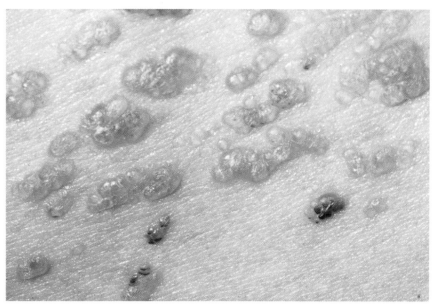

Fig 9.70 Lymphangiomas. The presence of clusters of dilated lymphatic vessels with clear or milky fluid content causes the typical 'frog-spawn' appearance. Note the haemorrhage in some lesions

usually on the lower leg, the individual nodules being a purple–red colour (**Fig 9.71**). Now, multiple disseminated AIDS-related Kaposi's sarcoma is the more common form; the lesions may be apparent as purple–red plaques or nodules (**Fig 9.72**) but may also be much more subtle grey 'bruise-like' patches, including intra-oral lesions.

Basal cell carcinoma—This has many different morphological variants, but is included here, as the most common type is a dome-shaped or slightly umbilicated nodule that has a slightly translucent 'pearly' colour and surface telangiectasia (**Fig 9.73**). Most are 5–10 mm in diameter and arise on the face from later middle age onwards; differential diagnosis on the cheeks may be difficult as there is often some degree of background telangiectasia, which will therefore be present on the surface of any nodule at this site, e.g. benign

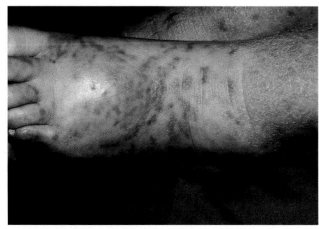

Fig 9.71 Classic Kaposi's sarcoma. Multiple grouped purple nodules on the leg

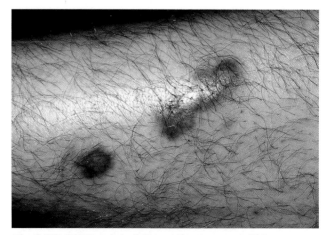

Fig 9.72 AIDS-related Kaposi's sarcoma. This relatively late lesion is a smooth purple nodule

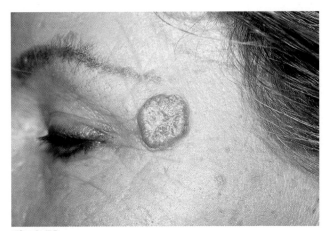

Fig 9.73

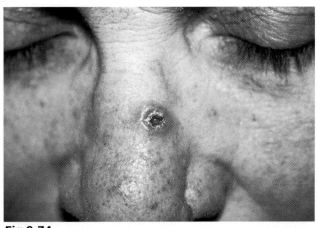

Fig 9.74

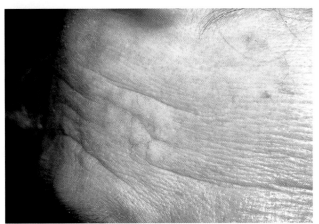

Fig 9.75

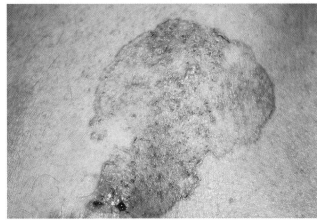

Fig 9.76

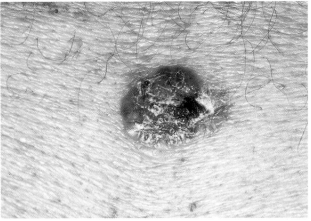

Fig 9.77

Fig 9.73–9.77 Basal cell carcinoma. Several different morphologies are shown. 9.73 shows a typical slightly umbilicated dome-shaped nodule with translucent or gelatinous pearly grey colour and fine surface telangiectasia. The central ulceration with a 'rolled' edge is evident in 9.74; the border is recognisable as a typical basal cell carcinoma. The morphoeic variety (9.75) is less well defined, with a grey or white scar-like appearance. On palpation, it feels hard or stiff compared with the surrounding skin; telangiectasia is also visible in this example. The superficial type (9.76) occurs on the trunk and has a thin, raised, pearly rim, and the centre may be scarred or crusted. In the pigmented basal cell carcinoma (9.77), the pigmentation may obscure some of the typical features but is itself suggestive of the diagnosis when it exhibits this speckled 'pencil lead-like' appearance, which is coarser and more grey than that seen in pigment cell naevi

naevi. The umbilication may become more prominent as size increases, and ulceration with a 'rolled' edge is another characteristic feature. Several variants are shown in **Figs 9.73–9.77**.

Secondary tumour—Although cutaneous metastases from internal tumours are uncommon, large deposits may be very characteristic. They may be solitary or multiple, usually red–purple–brown in colour, and may be predominant in vascular areas such as the scalp (**Fig 9.78**). Multiple nodules or plaques may occur in lymphomas, myelomonocytic leukaemia and carcinomas.

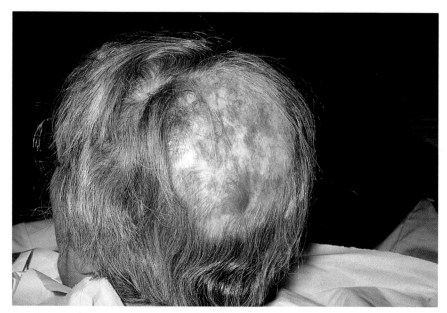

Fig 9.78 Metastatic carcinoma. The scalp is a relatively common site for cutaneous metastases, which cause plaques or nodules. These are usually erythematous or skin–coloured and may cause alopecia

> ### DIAGNOSTIC TIPS AND PITFALLS
>
> Variants of basal cell carcinoma include:
>
> - Pearly nodular type
> - Ulcerated tumour with a raised or rolled edge and crusted bleeding centre
> - Pigmented basal cell carcinoma: the pigment is pencil-lead grey in colour and usually distributed as small pigment globules. The pearly appearance and telangiectasia can usually also be distinguished
> - Superficial basal cell carcinoma: these usually occur on the trunk as large (>5 cm in diameter) plaques. They are commonly confused with eczema but have a raised edge on close examination

Abscess—An abscess is a deep localised collection of pus, which may have various causes (infective, inflammatory, degeneration of tumours, etc.); it is considered here because, in the skin, it generally presents as a tender erythematous nodule.

Sinus—A sinus is a channel leading from an abscess or hollow viscus to a site of drainage. It may have a simple external opening but is sometimes associated with a nodule at the skin surface. In skin, the most common example is hidradenitis suppurativa, an inflammatory disorder of apocrine glands in the axillae, groin and perineal region. Smooth, red, dome-shaped nodules, which are clinically similar to nodular acne lesions, may occur in this disorder.

Sinuses may arise from developmental lesions, especially on the face, scalp and neck. This possibility should always be considered if a sinus emerges in the midline of the neck or at the umbilicus.

Deep inflammation can cause sinus formation, for example a dental sinus from a root abscess (*see* Fig. 9.9). Some sinuses may have surface crusting due to inflammation or discharge of pus.

Rough (crusted, warty) or ulcerated lesions

Brown and black lesions (see also Chapter 3)

Seborrhoeic wart or keratosis (basal cell papilloma)— Seborrhoeic warts usually occur as multiple lesions and are most common on the trunk and face (**Fig 9.79–9.81**). They range from thin plaques to warty dome-shaped nodules and from yellowish tan to deep brown. The surface keratin is soft, crumbly, easily squashed or greasy compared with the sharper verrucous hyperkeratosis of a viral wart, although some facial seborrhoeic warts are virtually flat. Diagnostic problems occur if there are unusual features, such as very dark or variegated colouring or occurrence at an unusual site, such as the lower leg. The most difficult diagnostic problem is inflamed or 'irritated' seborrhoeic warts, which are often itchy and crusted rather than hyperkeratotic and may have surrounding inflammation. Plane warts and actinic keratoses may also be pigmented (*see* below).

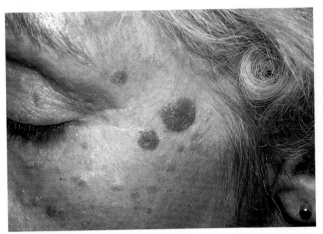

Fig 9.79

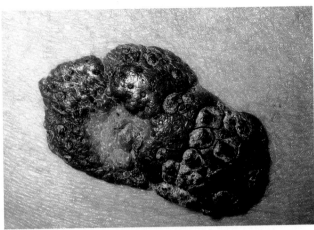

Fig 9.80

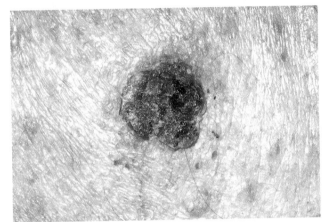

Fig 9.81

Fig 9.79–9.81 Seborrhoeic warts (keratoses). These lesions are often multiple, typically having a greasy or rough yellowish brown or greyish brown surface (9.79). Unusually large and dark seborrhoeic keratoses (9.80) may cause confusion, but 'pseudofollicles,' which are actually small areas of focal keratinisation, are a typical feature, as shown here. The other variant that causes concern is a more inflammatory and non-specifically crusted variety known as an 'irritated' seborrhoeic keratosis (9.81)

Warty pigment cell naevus—Clinically, these benign compound moles are easily confused with seborrhoeic warts. Their papular component is made up of fleshy tissue rather than thickened keratin, and large dark brown keratin plugs are studded into their surface (**Fig 9.82**).

White, yellow, flesh-coloured and translucent lesions

Viral warts—These generally occur as multiple lesions on the hands or soles of feet in children and young adults. Several patterns occur (**Figs 9.83–9.85**). Common warts are dome-shaped lesions with a rough keratotic or filiform verrucous appearance. Elongated filiform warts are relatively more common on the face, occurring around the nostrils and on the lips. Genital warts may be softer and smoother, with a papillomatous rather than a verrucous surface. Warts on the feet (verrucae) are less sharply defined and less nodular; plane warts are generally multiple, brownish coloured and are barely palpable plaques rather than nodules. Differentiation between a plantar wart and a corn is discussed in Chapter 4 (*see* Figs 4.36 and 4.37).

Actinic keratosis—These (**Figs 9.86–9.88**) occur on sun-exposed skin on a background of solar or actinic elastosis. The plaques are generally multiple and reddish with a hard, usually conical spike of keratin, so that they often appear more like papules than plaques (*see also* Figs 7.33 and 7.34).

Cutaneous horn

The term cutaneous horn describes an appearance rather than a diagnosis. It is used to describe the presence of a column of hard keratin or keratosis, also

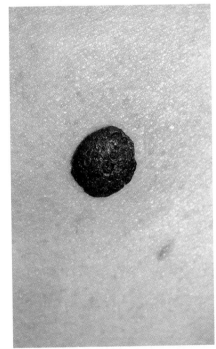

Fig 9.82 Warty pigment cell naevus. These are easily confused with seborrhoeic warts. The papule is fleshy with large pigmented keratin plugs studded into the surface

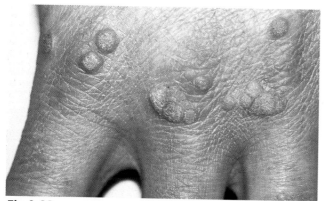

Fig 9.83

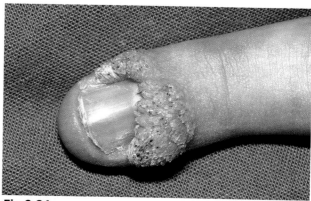

Fig 9.84

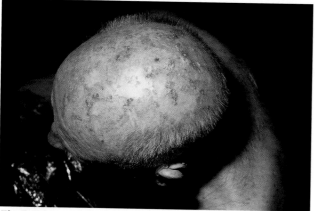

Fig 9.85

Fig 9.83–9.85 Viral warts. Common warts on the dorsum of the hand (9.83) and the fingertip (9.84) and 'kissing' warts on the toes (9.85)

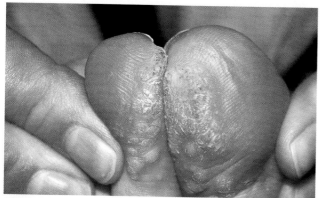

Fig 9.86

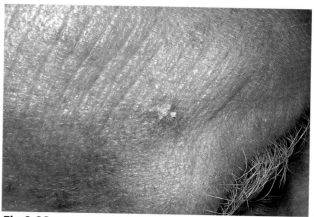

Fig 9.88

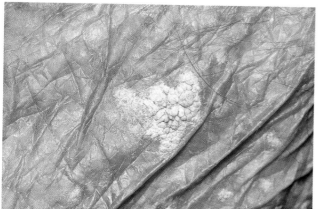

Fig 9.87

Fig 9.86–9.88 Actinic keratosis. 9.86 illustrates the typical distribution of actinic keratoses on the scalp. A white hyperkeratotic actinic keratosis is shown in 9.87. The most important clinical feature is often the quality of the keratosis, which is typically very hard and spiky (9.88)

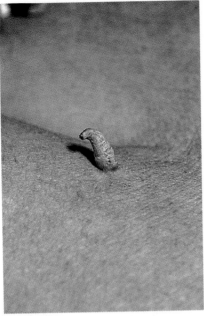

Fig 9.89

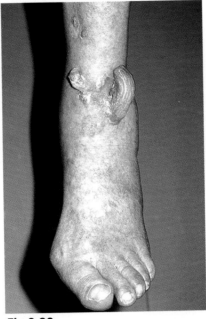

Fig 9.90

Fig 9.89–9.92 Cutaneous horns.
The horn shown in 9.89 is arising as though stuck on to normal skin and is unlikely to be of serious importance. Although there is no overt fleshy base (9.90), a large horn such as this is likely to have at least *in-situ* dysplasia of the underlying epidermis. The presence of a fleshy nodule, although small, at the base of a cutaneous horn (9.91) is a warning that it may be malignant. This lesion on the nose was a squamous cell carcinoma (9.91). 9.92 shows a cutaneous horn of reasonably large size and with a fleshy base, arising on a squamous cell carcinoma

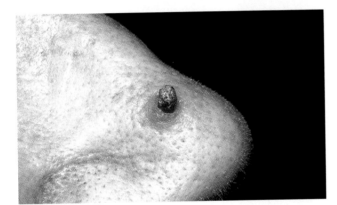

Fig 9.91

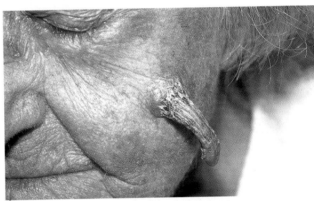

Fig 9.92

a descriptive rather than a diagnostic term. Cutaneous horns may be a feature of viral warts, seborrhoeic warts, benign squamous papillomas, actinic keratoses, digitate keratoses, keratoacanthomas and squamous cell carcinomas (**Figs 9.89–9.92**). The important physical sign is how the horn arises from the skin surface; a 'stuck on' appearance is usually benign, but a fleshy papular or nodular base is suggestive of malignancy.

Keratoacanthoma—These have an alarmingly rapid growth phase, but their final behaviour is benign in that they gradually involute without metastasis. However, they may be very destructive locally and can be indistinguishable from squamous cell carcinoma, to which they are clearly closely related. The vast majority are solitary, symmetrical, broad, rounded, yellowish-coloured nodules; the edge of the lesion forms a distinct shoulder with a telangiectatic surface, which overhangs a central crater filled by a broad horn or with keratinous debris (**Figs 9.93 and 9.94**).

Squamous cell carcinoma—These usually occur on sun-exposed sites such as the face, bald scalp, ears, lips, dorsum of the hand and lower leg. They range from having a fairly banal appearance early in their evolution to irregularly shaped and often poorly defined nodules or plaques at a later stage, with crusting or an eroded surface (**Figs 9.95–9.97**). The usual differential diagnosis is large actinic keratoses, sometimes basal cell carcinomas or amelanotic

DIAGNOSTIC TIPS AND PITFALLS

A cutaneous horn can be produced by:

- Viral warts: fine delicate keratin horn
- Seborrhoeic warts: the broad-based rather greasy keratinous horn is usually easily removed
- Actinic keratoses: well-formed keratin but arising on a thin non-indurated base
- Keratoacanthomas: when present the keratin horn arises from a symmetrical nodule
- Squamous cell carcinoma (SCC): well-differentiated (SCC) may produce a hard keratin horn arising on an indurated base

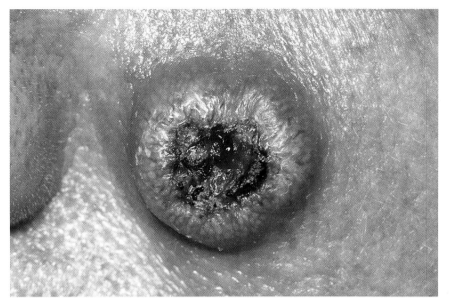

Fig 9.93

Fig 9.93, 9.94 Keratoacanthoma. A typical lesion (9.93) is a symmetrical, uniformly circular, broad nodule with a yellow telangiectatic shoulder of stretched normal skin. This overhangs a central crater in which there is a hard, centrally placed horn or keratin debris. These lesions gradually involute (9.94), as shown here 10 weeks later in the same patient, but only the most typical should be observed rather than actively treated. The residual scar of spontaneous resolution is characteristically crateriform and may be ugly but can be excised more easily than the primary lesion because it is much smaller

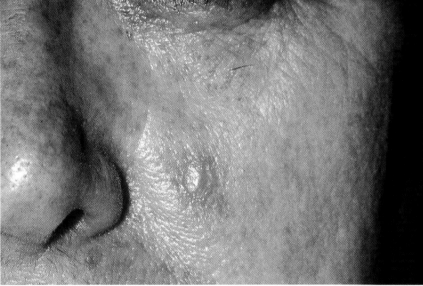

Fig 9.94

DIAGNOSTIC TIPS AND PITFALLS

- Keratoacanthoma are best considered to be self-resolving squamous cell carcinoma
- Clinically and histologically, keratoacanthomas may be indistinguishable from squamous cell carcinoma
- A true keratoacanthoma should have the following features:
  - Be solitary
  - Be symmetrical
  - Have a broad, rounded shape
  - Possibly contain yellowish-coloured nodules
  - The edge of the lesion forms a distinct shoulder with a telangiectatic surface that overhangs a central crater filled by debris or a keratin horn
  - The sides of the tumour nodule are covered in normal skin, which is stretched over the central tumour

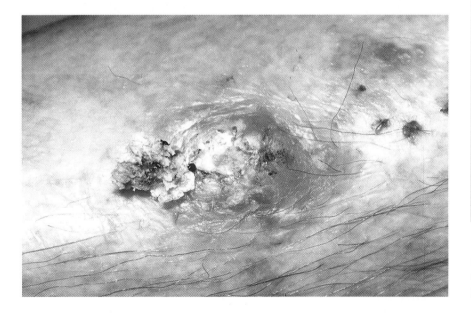

Fig 9.95 Squamous cell carcinoma. An irregularly shaped, poorly defined, crusted nodule

183

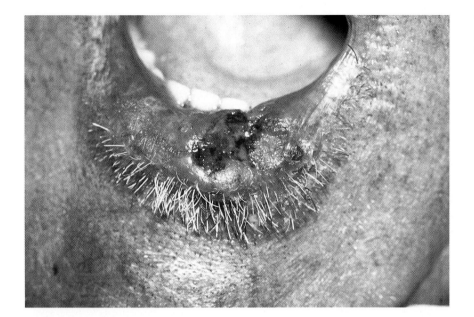

Fig 9.96 Squamous cell carcinoma. The lower lip is a characteristic site

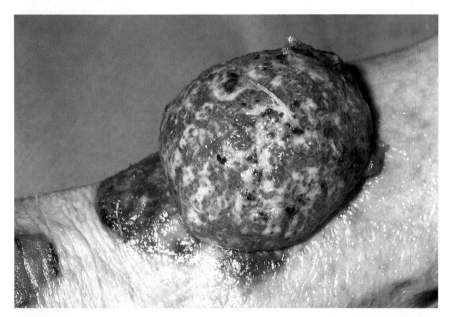

Fig 9.97 Squamous cell carcinoma. A more rapidly growing, less well-differentiated tumour, which is ulcerated and does not form an identifiable horn

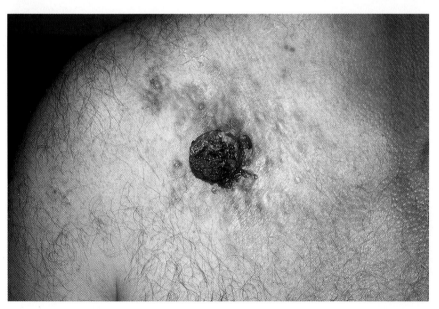

Fig 9.98 Dermatofibrosarcoma protuberans. A rapidly enlarging, crusted nodule, which can appear identical to a squamous cell carcinoma in some cases

malignant melanoma. Occasionally, fibrous tumours, which are usually smooth-surfaced when small, may enlarge rapidly and have a crusted surface similar to squamous cell carcinoma (**Fig 9.98**). Removal of the surface crust reveals a gelatinous or velvety red eroded surface.

Chondrodermatitis nodularis helicis—This is a not uncommon lesion, which occurs on the pinna of the ear and often presents as a differential diagnosis of a 'keratosis' or cutaneous tumour. It is actually the result of inflammation of the underlying cartilage, probably due to friction or pressure, and is characterised by the sites affected and by the symptoms caused (sharp pain, which often disturbs sleep). In women, the most common site is the antihelix; in men, it is the lateral aspect of the upper part of the helix (**Fig 9.99 and 9.100**). The lesion itself is a firm, tender, variably crusted nodule, about 5 mm in diameter.

Acquired digital fibrokeratoma—These are papular lesions, which occur on the dorsum or sides of the fingers. They are firm to the touch, off-white or flesh-coloured and slightly rougher than the adjacent skin; a collarette of hyperkeratosis may be present (**Fig 9.101**). They may be confused with accessory digits, although accessory digits generally present on the ulnar border of the palm and may be bilateral (**Fig 9.102**).

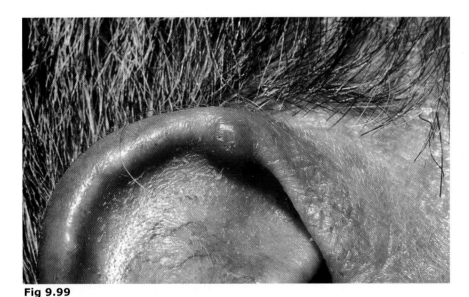

Fig 9.99

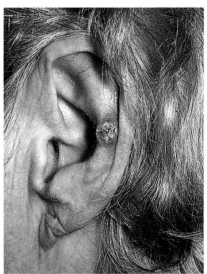

Fig 9.100

Fig 9.99, 9.100 Chondrodermatitis nodularis helicis. Lesion on the lateral rim of the helix (9.99), the most typical site in men, and on the antihelix (9.100), a common site in women

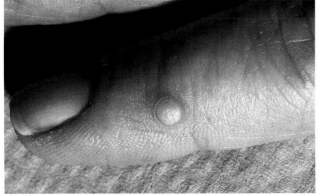

Fig 9.101 Acquired digital fibrokeratoma. A pale flesh-coloured papule on the finger, which may be columnar in shape. The usual differential diagnosis is of accessory digits

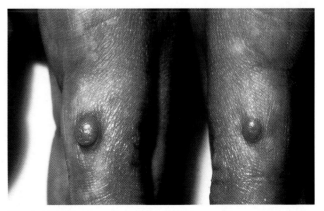

Fig 9.102 Accessory digits. These usually occur on the ulnar border of the hand and may be symmetrical

185

10 Macular and maculopapular rashes

DEFINITION

A macule is a flat *discrete lesion* with a different colour from the surrounding skin but without any difference in texture or thickness; it may be fixed or transient. The fundamentals of examination of discrete macules are discussed in Chapter 9. Atrophic macules are discussed in Chapter 12.

Macules with a diameter larger than 10 mm are usually called patches. This chapter concentrates on multiple transient macules and maculopapular eruptions that are usually the result of viral infection or drug reactions (**Table 10.1**). Examples of fixed discrete macules are discussed in Chapters 3 and 9.

CLINICAL PATTERNS OF GENERALISED ERYTHEMAS

Persistent multiple macules are usually relatively fixed in position, e.g. vitiligo, and may also have associated scaling as a constant feature, e.g. pityriasis versicolor and guttate psoriasis. Multiple transient, usually red-coloured, macules are a feature of numerous systemic, toxic or idiosyncratic drug reactions or occur as a response to several infective agents, particularly viral exanthemata (**Table 10.2**). Some such eruptions are entirely macular, due to changes in local blood flow resulting from the skin inflammation, whereas others are entirely papular due to local oedema (both of these being transient phenomena). Most commonly, there is a mixture of macular and papular

---

Table 10.1 Causes of multiple transient macules and maculopapular eruptions

Drugs
Ampicillin, barbiturates, sulphonamides, thiazide diuretics, phenytoin, gentamicin, etc.

Viral exanthem
See Tables 10.2 and 10.3

Bacterial
Staphylococcus aureus—toxic shock syndrome
Streptococcus pyogenes—scarlet fever (10.10)

Physiological
Erythema neonatorum (6.5, 6.6)

Table 10.2 Synonyms for common infectious diseases

Historical disease number*	Common (other name)	Infectious agent
First	Measles (10.4)	Paramyxovirus
Second	Scarlet fever (10.10)	Group A streptococcus
Third	German measles (rubella) (10.5)	Rubella virus (unclassified)
Fourth	Duke's disease (this is no longer accepted as an entity)	Probably a coxsackie virus or echovirus
Fifth	Slapped cheek disease (erythema infectiosum) (10.9)	Parvovirus B19
Sixth	Roseola (roseola infantum; exanthem subitum = sudden rash)	Herpesvirus-6

*Historical name refers to the order in which these infections were recognised as distinct disease entities.

elements; hence, these varied conditions can be grouped together under the term 'maculopapular eruptions'. In all cases, there may be large or small macules or a mixture of the two. However, the description of eruptions as maculopapular is often poorly applied and may be used for transient or chronic dermatoses. More precise descriptions are more valuable although not always helpful. For example, there is good evidence that the differences in the appearance of the rash in acute infectious erythemas in children do not enable the clinician to identify the infective cause, as the same features may be caused by a range of infectious agents.

Some infections, e.g. measles, rubella, fifth disease or rheumatic fever (**Fig 10.1**), can produce characteristic patterns of exanthem, with only occasional atypical rashes. Unfortunately for the diagnosing clinician, other infectious agents can produce virtually identical eruptions to the classic viral exanthemata (**Table 10.3**). Many exanthemata occur in individuals treated with

Fig 10.1 Erythema marginatum. This rash is not pathognomonic for rheumatic fever; it occurs in 10–20% of cases, but has also been reported in healthy individuals and in those with serum sickness. It is a very rapidly changing figurate macular or papular erythema, usually on the trunk. Lesions typically last 2–3 hours but may persist for days. It is difficult to distinguish from an annular urticaria, although histological differences may be helpful (*photo courtesy of Dr Andrew Cant*)

Table 10.3 Infectious causes of generalised erythemas in children*

Erythema	Cause
Macular, papular and maculopapular	Measles, group A streptococcus, rubella, roseola, echo viruses, mycoplasma pneumonia, respiratory syncytial virus, Epstein–Barr virus (infectious mononucleosis) (10.6–10.8), hepatitis A. Others: adenovirus, parvovirus, rotavirus, etc.
Sheeted macular erythema and scaling	Group A streptococcus, Epstein–Barr virus
Urticarial	Echo viruses, mycoplasma pneumonia, Coxsackie A16, enterovirus, Epstein–Barr virus
Vesicular and papulovesicular**	Varicella (chicken-pox), coxsackie virus type A9 (hand-foot-and-mouth disease)
Papular acrodermatitis of childhood (Gianotti–Crosti syndrome) (10.16, 10.17)	Hepatitis B, group A streptococcus, rubella, coxsackie virus A16, Epstein–Barr virus, cytomegalovirus, respiratory syncytial virus, parainfluenza virus

*Given in order of frequency.
**Herpes simplex and orf also produce blisters, but if these occur with a widespread rash, this is due to erythema multiforme (see Table 13.3) rather than being an integral part of the underlying infection.

antibiotics, who also have a presumed viral infection. In this situation, it may be impossible to determine whether the rash is due to the drug, the infection or a combination of both (e.g. rash due to ampicillin in patients with infectious mononucleosis). Provided a drug allergy has been excluded, precise diagnosis is usually not required as symptoms will settle spontaneously. However, it is important to exclude a group A streptococcal (i.e. *Streptococcus pyogenes*) infection because of the risk of glomerulonephritis and rheumatic fever, so throat swabs are helpful. In some circumstances, e.g. an immunocompromised patient or a pregnant woman, specific diagnosis may be required, in which case, a rise in specific IgM antibody titre in paired acute and convalescent serum samples should be looked for. For example, rubella or, especially, parvovirus infections can both cause varied eruptions, and both have important effects on the developing fetus.

Peeling or annular scaling (**Fig 10.2**) as the rash fades, similar to the peeling seen after sunburn, is a late and relatively common minor feature of measles, rubella and other viral or drug-induced causes of maculopapular eruptions. By contrast, sheets of peeling on hands and feet is an important late feature of scarlet fever, Kawasaki disease and toxic shock syndrome.

The following five patterns of macular and maculopapular eruptions with or without scaling can be distinguished clinically and provide a useful way of recognising some of the more important infectious causes of this type of eruption.

Small plaque with or without scaling (papulosquamous disease)

This pattern of scaly small plaques is seen in psoriasis (*see* Figs 8.9–8.13), pityriasis rosea (*see* Fig 7.21) and secondary syphilis (**Fig 10.3**); these papulosquamous disorders are dealt with more fully on pp. 123–126.

Maculopapular erythema with or without scaling

This is the largest group. The whole range of macular, papular and maculopapular erythema with small and large lesions is included. Apart from a few

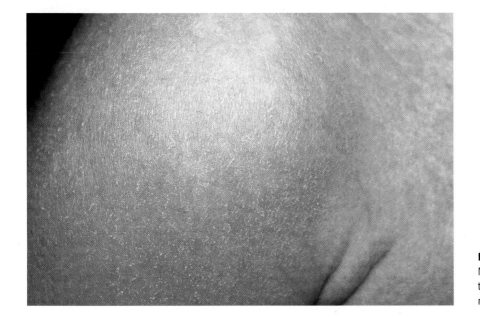

Fig 10.2 Maculopapular erythema. Mild scaling is apparent on the skin of this child with a feverish illness and macular rash

189

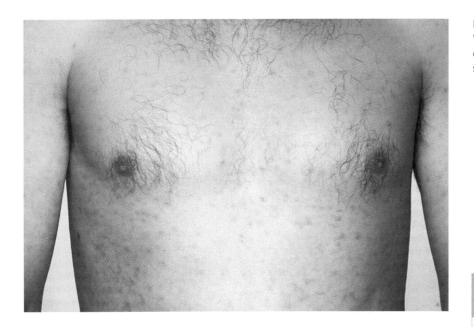

**DIAGNOSTIC TIPS
AND PITFALLS**

- Purpura may be present in
  any severe maculopapular
  erythema, particularly on the
  lower legs, due to
  gravitational effects

---

exceptions, for example the pink macules or rose spots of typhoid fever, these subgroups are not specific to any causative agent or as a reaction pattern in any one individual.

In measles (**Fig 10.4**), the typical rash consists of erythematous papules, which join up or become confluent, producing net-like or reticulate red areas. This appearance is so distinctive that the term morbilliform (measles like) is used to describe similar appearances when this occurs in other maculopapular erythemas such as rubella (**Fig 10.5**), pityriasis rosea (*see* Fig 7.21) and secondary syphilis (**Fig 10.3**).

Purpura may be present in any type of severe maculopapular erythema and is usually most prominent on the lower legs due to gravitational effects (*see* p. 28). Purpura is a common feature of the rash of infectious mononucleosis (**Figs 10.6–10.8**) and in particular the rash that occurs 7–10 days after inadvertently giving ampicillin to a patient with infectious mononucleosis.

Sheeted (confluent) erythema and scaling

This describes the development of sheets or confluent areas of skin redness, sometimes with associated surface change. The following four important infectious diseases can present with this type of eruption, although each has some unique features.

Fifth disease (slapped cheek disease)—Fifth disease is characterised by the sudden onset of coalescing red papules on the face, followed 2–3 days later by net-like red maculopapules on the arms (*see* Fig 17.6) and legs (**Fig 10.9**).
Scarlet fever—In scarlet fever, a streptococcal disorder, the rash starts approximately 48 hours after the onset of fever, pharyngitis and nausea. The face is flushed, with sparing of the skin around the mouth. Other areas are covered in numerous pinpoint red papules, which give a rough texture to the skin (**Fig 10.10**). Linear petechiae (Pastia's sign) are found in the groin and axillae. The desquamation that follows the acute illness is much more pronounced than that which occurs in other viral exanthems; this starts on the face and then involves the hands and feet.

Scarlatiniform (meaning like scarlet fever) is a term used to describe similar appearances with punctate, slightly elevated, areas without evidence of pharyngeal group A streptococcal infection.

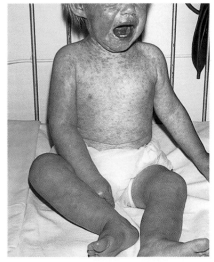

Fig 10.4 Measles. The small red spots start on the face and spread to the trunk. After 3–4 days, they increase in size (as shown here) and become confluent. Fine scaling follows at this stage. Koplik's spots appear 1–2 days before the rash as blue–white spots surrounded by a red halo on the buccal mucosa (*photo courtesy of Dr Andrew Illchyshyn*)

Toxic shock syndrome—Toxic shock syndrome (TSS) due to *Staphylococcus aureus* infection presents as a scarlatiniform eruption with diffuse or palmar redness followed by peeling, mediated by the toxic shock syndrome toxin-1 (TSST-1). This disease is associated with a fatality rate of approximately 4%. The causative staphylococcal infections have been described in association with using high-absorbency tampons, skin infection, surgical wound infection, childbirth and as a complication of influenza.

Streptococcal TSS may arise in isolation or be associated with deep streptococcal soft tissue infection, usually due to group A or G streptococci of M1 or M3 type and producing type A streptococcal pyrogenic exotoxin (SPE-A). Acute renal failure and hypotension occur, and there is a 30% mortality. Survivors may have typical skin peeling, similar to that of scarlet fever.

Kawasaki disease (mucocutaneous lymph node syndrome)—Early diagnosis of Kawasaki disease is very important. If not detected early, affected children may die from coronary artery aneurysm or thrombosis, which can be prevented by aspirin and high-dose intravenous gamma globulin therapy. The diagnosis is considered in children with an unexplained fever lasting more than 5 days and when staphylococcal or streptococcal infection, measles, leptospirosis and rickettsial disease have been excluded. Children must present with four of the following: bilateral conjunctival injection; changes in the upper respiratory tract, such as injected pharynx, cracked lips or strawberry tongue; changes in the peripheral extremities including oedema (**Figs 10.11** and **10.12**), erythema or late desquamation; a polymorphous rash; and lymphadenopathy. Thus, the cutaneous features are non-specific, apart from the late appearance of peeling on the extremities (**Fig 10.11**), which is similar to that seen after scarlet fever. An increase in white cell count, platelet count and erythrocyte sedimentation rate also occurs.

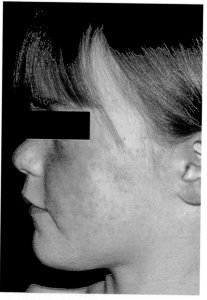

Fig 10.5 Rubella. The rash may be very mild in rubella; when present, it is similar to measles, with maculopapular erythema starting on the face and spreading to the trunk. The spots are 1–2 mm in diameter and slightly raised. In rubella, there is also enlargement of the cervical and occipital lymph nodes

Fig 10.6

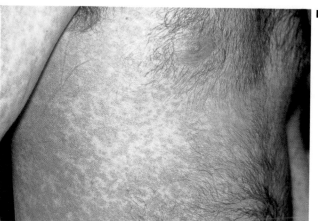

Fig 10.8

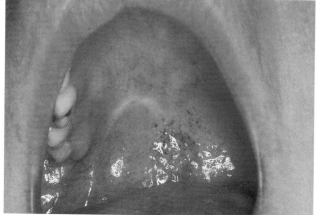

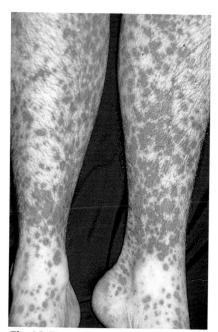

Fig 10.7

Figs 10.6–10.8 Infectious mononucleosis. Generalised slightly elevated erythema (10.6) that is purpuric on the lower limbs (10.7). The patient had enormous tonsils, lymphadenopathy and splenomegaly. Petechiae on the hard palate (10.8) appear with the lymphadenopathy and are shown here in a different patient (*10.8 courtesy of Dr S Natarajan*)

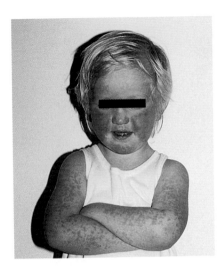

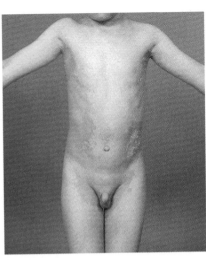

Fig 10.9 Fifth disease. Slapped cheek disease is an apt name for this parvovirus infection. Reticulate erythema is visible on the forearms (*photo courtesy of Dr Andrew Illchyshyn*)

Fig 10.10 Scarlet fever. There are sheets of red skin on the flanks in this child with scarlet fever. The red areas are made up of multiple small papules that give the skin a rough sandpaper-like texture (*photo courtesy of Dr Andrew Illchyshyn*)

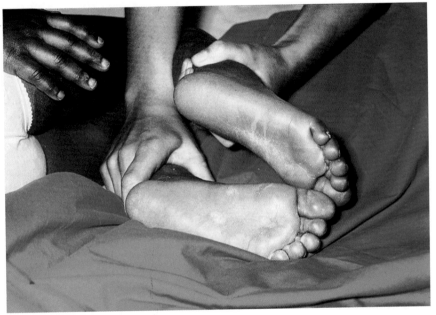

Fig 10.11

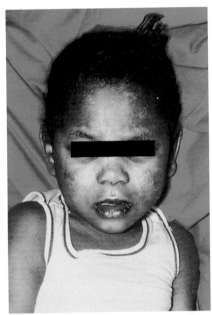

Fig 10.12

Figs 10.11, 10.12 Kawasaki disease. The rash of Kawasaki disease is not specific and is variously described as urticarial or maculopapular. Red oedematous feet (10.11) and hands develop within 3–4 days of onset of fever and are useful early cutaneous features. Scaling of the skin in the extremities is usually pronounced but a late feature and therefore of little help in early diagnosis. Cherry-red fissured crusted lips (10.12) are recognised features (*photos courtesy of Dr Andrew Cant*)

Urticaria and urticated reactions

Viral infections and drug eruptions of various types may present with true urticarial lesions, i.e. weals that last less than 24 hours. This is dealt with in more detail in Chapter 15. By contrast, urticated lesions are red and oedematous and hence palpable, but unlike urticaria, they persist for longer than 24 hours and have associated features such as scaling or blistering.

DIAGNOSTIC TIPS AND PITFALLS

- Sheeted or confluent erythema occurs in three important infectious diseases, i.e. the toxic shock syndromes, Kawasaki disease and scarlet fever

Toxic urticated erythema (**Fig 10.13**) is a term used to describe widespread oedematous red plaques, usually without scaling. Occasionally, the palpable urticated papules may become purpuric centrally. This type of eruption may be due to a drug reaction (**Fig 10.14**) or virus infection, although commonly, no cause is found (**Fig 10.15**). Toxic urticated erythema is used synonymously with maculopapular eruptions by some authors.

Other characteristic patterns

Papular acrodermatitis of childhood (Gianotti–Crosti syndrome)—Although originally described in Italian children with hepatitis B infections, it is now clear that this type of eruption is the result of a wide range of infectious agents (**Table 10.3**). The rash is characterised by widespread development of reddish brown papules on the thighs and buttocks, which then spread to the arms and face (**Figs 10.16** and **10.17**) over the space of 3–4 days. The eruption is unusual in that it lasts for at least 2–3 weeks and sometimes longer. A variant with multiple small umbilicated pink–brown papules, which are reminiscent of mollusca contagiosa, has also been described.

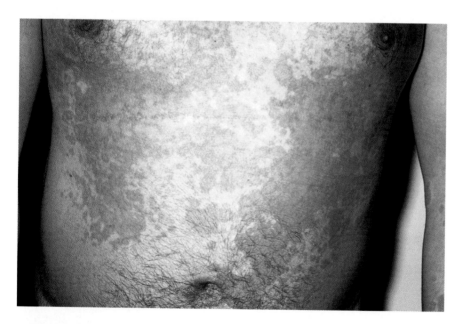

Fig 10.13 Toxic urticated erythema. Toxic urticated erythema is a pattern of acute eruption that has some histological features of erythema multiforme. The lesions are rounded with a greyish central colour and have a tendency to coalesce

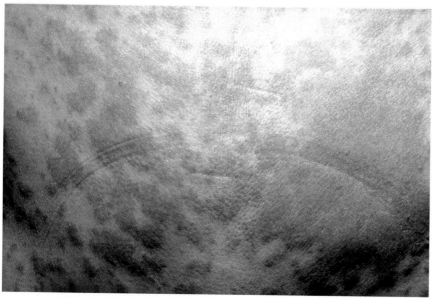

Fig 10.14 Ampicillin eruption. Maculopapular drug eruptions develop first on the limbs and then spread to the trunk, in contrast to viral maculopapular erythema. This patient has developed an urticated reaction to ampicillin

Purpuric gloves and socks (stockings) syndrome—This relatively recently described exanthem is closely linked with parvovirus B19 infection (which also causes erythema infectiosum (**Fig 10.9**)). It is described in more detail in the section on acral erythema (*see* Chapter 17).

Unilateral laterothoracic exanthem—Also known as asymmetrical periflexural exanthem, this disorder occurs mainly in young children, although adult cases (some associated with parvovirus B19) have been reported. It is distinctive due to the asymmetry, usually occurring on one flank or axillary region, but can become bilateral over the couple of weeks before it resolves.

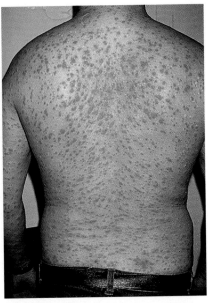

Fig 10.15 Papular viral exanthem. Scattered papules on the trunk in a non-specific exanthematous pattern

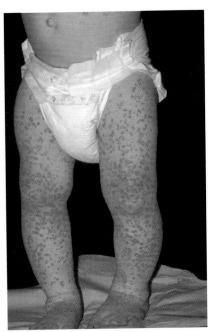

Fig 10.16

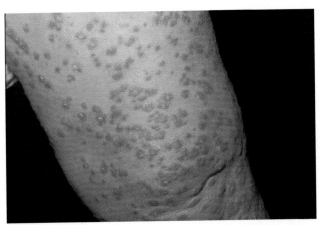

Fig 10.17

Figs 10.16, 10.17 Gianotti–Crosti syndrome. Clustered discrete papular lesions affect the legs (10.16), hands, elbows and face. The individual lesions (10.17) have central umbilication

DIAGNOSTIC TIPS AND PITFALLS

- Papular acrodermatitis of childhood (Gianotti–Crosti syndrome) may last for up to 8 weeks

INTRODUCTION

Appreciation of changes in texture requires familiarity with the qualities of normal and pathological skin. Dermatologists routinely feel rashes and localised lesions, even when visual inspection has already suggested a probable diagnosis, because textural changes add an extra dimension to the appearance. Indeed, many textural changes in the skin are actually diagnosed by both vision and palpation, the eye assessing quality of scale, prominence of skin markings, wrinkling, vascular changes and tissue swelling before the skin is palpated. The importance of palpation of the skin is discussed in general terms in Chapter 4 and in relation to localised papules and nodules in Chapter 9. Palpation is also relevant to scaling disorders, described in Chapter 7.

This chapter covers some of the more diffuse changes in skin thickness and texture. There is no simple way to present these disorders, for a variety of reasons:

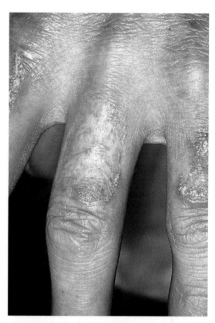

Fig 11.1 Discoid lupus erythematosus. Typical features of atrophy (white shiny centre) and follicular hyperkeratotic 'plugging'

- Pure epidermal atrophy without any alteration in the dermis is probably very rare and not clinically detectable as a change in skin thickness. Most disorders in which there is epidermal atrophy include changes in quality of at least the upper part of the dermis, e.g. lichen sclerosus et atrophicus and actinic damage.
- Some disorders may have epidermal thinning but dermal or deeper swelling. For example, the skin is often stretched over dermal or deeper nodules, such as epidermoid cysts, and the epidermis may seem thin on histological examination. The effects of stretching the epidermis are easily observed in patients with a prominent recent onset of oedema of the lower leg. The skin appears slightly shiny due to stretching and thinning of the epidermis, although the deeper swelling makes it more difficult to pick up a fold of skin. If the oedema is cleared rapidly, the skin appears slightly wrinkled for a while afterwards.
- Features may change with time. Discoid lupus erythematosus is a good example of this; in the early stages, the lesions may be quite thickened due to inflammation and scaling (*see* Figs 7.40 and 8.21), but old lesions are atrophic (**Fig 11.1**).
- Some causes of atrophy may vary in their effects. For example, topical steroids may cause epidermal atrophy or dermal atrophy (stronger agents or longer duration), predominantly dermal atrophy (intralesional administration), profound fat atrophy (depot preparations) or skin atrophy with increased fat deposition (systemic).

- Although increased firmness generally implies thickening by infiltration or fibrosis, there are occasions when notable atrophy of the skin can feel firm. These occur especially in some localised forms of scleroderma, where there is an element of fibrosis as well as atrophy of subcutaneous tissue, so that the lesional skin can feel firm and apparently bound down to underlying bony structures (**Fig 11.32**).
- Conversely, atrophy or degeneration can cause apparent swelling. This occurs in some dermal defects, such as anetoderma, a defect of elastic tissue, where the deeper tissues bulge through the dermal defect to produce a soft swelling (*see* Figs 4.21 and 4.22).
- Skin texture is due to more than simple thickness. The degree of surface scaling influences appreciation of texture, as does hydration of the skin (note the difference in feel between wet and dry skin). Absence of sweating causes the skin to feel smooth, and hyperhidrosis increases the sensation of friction.

This chapter is therefore divided into two sections, dealing with disorders where the overall impression is of thinning or thickening.

SKIN THINNING

Epidermal atrophy

The epidermis comprises less than 10% of the thickness of the skin, and atrophy of the epidermis in the absence of some degree of dermal change is rare. Palpation is not sensitive enough to detect the condition, the physical signs of which are visual; these include increased visibility of vessels and fine wrinkling of the skin surface (known as cigarette paper wrinkling), which can be shown by gently squeezing the skin. Such signs suggest epidermal atrophy but are generally accompanied by dermal changes, such as atrophy, sclerosis or other changes in quality. By contrast, because the dermis is thicker and firmer than the epidermis, alterations in dermal quality are more striking. Examples of disorders with a prominent component of epidermal atrophy are listed in **Table 11.1**.

Aging changes

Aging changes are a complex mixture of the dermal and epidermal changes discussed in Chapter 6. The epidermis is thinned (*see* Figs 6.14 and 6.15), and the dermal tissues become altered, with the development of 'solar elastosis,' which causes a yellowish cobblestoned appearance of the skin (*see* Fig 6.17).

Table 11.1 Disorders of skin thinning: epidermal atrophy

Aging changes and actinic damage

Topical corticosteroid effects (11.3)

Lichen sclerosus (11.4)

Poikilodermas (11.6)

Subacute cutaneous lupus erythematosus (11.8)

Discoid lupus erythematosus (11.1)

Post-radiotherapy (11.9)

Necrobiosis lipoidica (11.10)

Topical corticosteroid use

Regular application of potent topical corticosteroids (**Figs 11.2** and **11.3**) causes atrophy, which may be apparent as prominent telangiectasia, especially of the face, or as striae due to dermal atrophy. Striae are most noticeable in thin areas of skin, such as at the axillae and on the inner thighs. Similar changes can occur as a result of systemic steroid administration or in Cushing's syndrome.

Lichen sclerosus

Lichen sclerosus (**Fig 11.4**) is characterised by sharply demarcated, ivory white atrophic patches, which have preserved or even accentuated follicles (*see* Fig 7.39). This latter feature contrasts with morphoea in which skin appendages are lost (*see* Fig 8.27). The quality of the upper dermal collagen is altered, which decreases the support of the capillary vessels and may cause purpura, especially in areas such as the penis, where there is also frictional damage. Absent or vanishing labia minor are a useful sign of lichen sclerosus of female genitalia (**Fig 11.5**), where the disorder typically produces a figure-of-eight shape of affected skin around the vulva and anus.

DIAGNOSTIC TIPS AND PITFALLS

- Morphoea and lichen sclerosus may be confused, as both cause white plaques. However, morphoea lesions are thickened and sclerotic rather than atrophic, and there is loss of follicular structures compared with the accentuation of follicles that occurs in lichen sclerosus

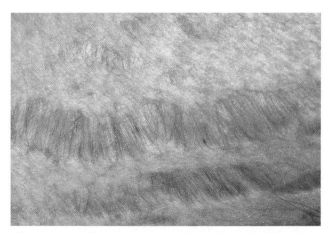

Fig 11.2 Atrophy due to topical corticosteroids. This stretched area shows wrinkling and visible vessels. Similar striae occur in pregnancy and during periods of rapid increase in height in adolescents (horizontally on the back) (*see* 6.35)

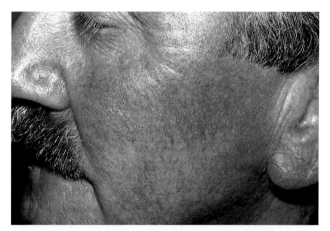

Fig 11.3 Atrophy due to topical corticosteroids. Awareness of the effects of prolonged use of potent topical steroids has made this pattern of red telangiectatic atrophy of the facial skin uncommon now

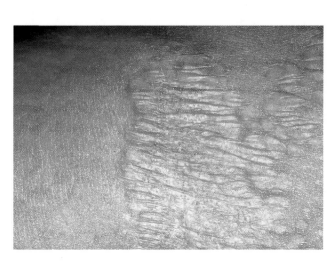

Fig 11.4 Lichen sclerosus. Typical white lesions with follicular prominence

Table 11.2 Causes of poikiloderma

T-cell lymphoma and pre-mycotic eruptions	Poikiloderma vasculare atrophicans, mycosis fungoides, granulomatous slack skin
Genodermatoses	Rothmund–Thomson syndrome Bloom's syndrome, Goltz syndrome
Collagen vascular disease	Discoid lupus erythematosus, dermatomyositis, graft versus host disease
Physical injury	Radiotherapy, actinic damage
Unknown	Poikiloderma of Civatte

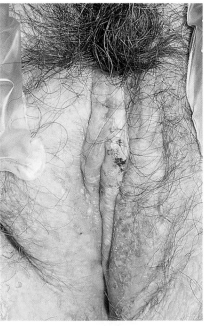

Fig 11.5 Lichen sclerosus. Fusion of labia minora to labia majora is a typical occurrence in female genital skin (*see also* 1.14). Note the presence of purpura

Poikiloderma

Poikiloderma is really a description rather than a diagnosis, defining the combination of mottled pigmentation with atrophy and telangiectasia. It occurs in several disorders (**Table 11.2**), including some genodermatoses, as a precursor of mycosis fungoides (**Fig 11.6**), in collagen vascular diseases such as lupus erythematosus (**Fig 11.1**) and dermatomyositis (**Fig 11.7**) and as a common form of pigmentary disturbance on the neck in women, when it is known as poikiloderma of Civatte.

Discoid lupus erythematosus/subacute cutaneous lupus erythematosus

Lupus erythematosus is a disorder that is very variable in appearance. Damage to the dermo-epidermal junction causes atrophy (**Fig 11.1**) which is often associated with inflammation and hyperkeratosis of follicles, causing the appearance of 'follicular plugging' (*see* Figs 7.40 and 7.41). Note, however, that initial inflammation may produce thickening in the acute phase, whereas atrophy is the more typical late change. In subacute cutaneous lupus erythematosus (**Fig 11.8**), a variant with prominent photosensitivity and often arthritis, the skin lesions may be psoriasiform or sometimes noticeably

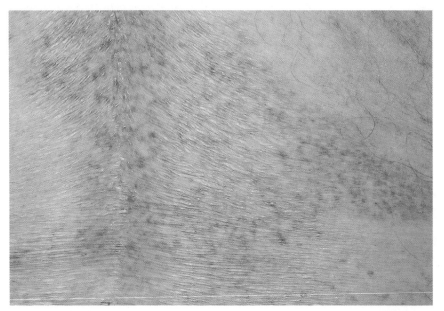

Fig 11.6 Poikiloderma. This pre-mycotic lesion has typical atrophy (seen as wrinkling), varied pigmentation and telangiectasia (*see also* 1.15)

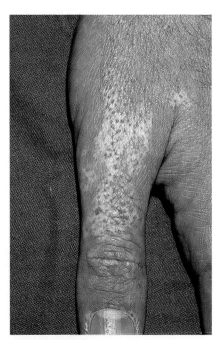

Fig 11.7 Poikilodermatous change on the thumb in a patient with dermatomyositis.

annular (*see* Fig 2.8). The combination of epidermal thinning and pigment disturbance at the dermo-epidermal junction may lend a characteristic grey colour to the central part of the lesions.

Radiotherapy

Although less common with present day radiotherapy regimens, radiation damage may produce a characteristic white patch of atrophy, with telangiectatic vessels clearly visible (**Fig 11.9**, *see also* Fig 12.6).

Necrobiosis lipoidica

Necrobiosis lipoidica (**Fig 11.10**) is often associated with diabetes mellitus, possibly in up to 50% of cases. Small, early lesions are inflammatory plaques, but the typical established lesion is yellow–orange in colour (due to visible fat, both in the subcutis and dermis), with fine-wrinkled epidermal atrophy and prominent telangiectasia (especially at the edge of the lesions, which are generally redder in colour than the central part).

Dermal atrophy

Dermal defects are varied because of the different tissues present and the pathological processes that can occur (**Table 11.3**).

Abnormal elastic tissue

Abnormal elastic tissue can cause a variety of changes, not all of which are clinically atrophic; for example, elastosis perforans serpiginosa is characterised by annular inflammatory crusted papules in which fragmented elastic tissue is extruded through the skin surface. In general terms, the 'anelastic' disorders cause sagging, wrinkled skin when a broad area is affected (e.g. cutis laxa, **Fig 11.11**) but protruding soft nodules of subcutaneous tissue if the elastic defect is localised (e.g. anetoderma, *see* **4.21, 4.22**). This may affect specific sites, e.g. the eyelids (a disorder known as blepharochalasis). Other examples are discussed below.

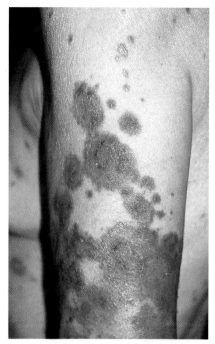

Fig 11.8 Subacute cutaneous lupus erythematosus. Annular lesions with a slightly grey central colour due to the combination of atrophic epidermis and pigmentary disturbance (*see also* 7.20)

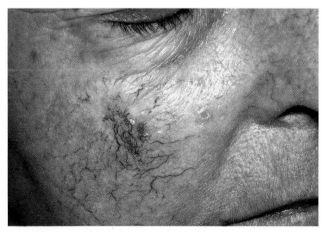

Fig 11.9 Radiotherapy scar. White dermal scar and prominent telangiectasia. A small new basal cell carcinoma is also present adjacent to, but distinct from, the nasal margin of the previously treated area

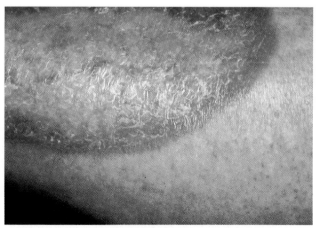

Fig 11.10 Necrobiosis lipoidica. Typical atrophy, telangiectasia and a central yellow–orange colour

Table 11.3 Disorders of skin thinning: dermal atrophy

Abnormal elastic tissue	Blepharochalasis Cutis laxa (11.11) Anetoderma (4.21)
Collagen defects	Ehlers–Danlos syndrome (11.12, 11.13) Atrophoderma of Pasini and Pierini (11.15) Scars (11.14) and striae Focal dermal hypoplasia Atrophodermas (11.16, 11.17)

Cutis laxa

Cutis laxa (**Fig 11.11**) may be generalised or localised and can be very dramatic, with rapid onset and appearance of premature aging. The skin feels soft and doughy and shows noticeable wrinkling. Abnormal neural tissue, such as the plexiform neuroma of von Recklinghausen's disease (neurofibromatosis) can exhibit a similar quality on palpation.

Anetoderma

Anetoderma (*see* Fig 4.21) is a localised defect of elastic tissue, which allows herniation of the underlying fat.

Other causes of herniating lesions include:

- Piezogenic papules (painful nodules on the feet) (*see* Fig 6.51).
- Neurofibroma (buttonhole sign).
- Follicular atrophoderma (**Fig 11.16**) and focal dermal hypoplasia (*see* p. 201).

Collagen defects

Collagen defects have a wide spectrum of expressions.

Ehlers–Danlos syndrome

Ehlers–Danlos syndrome embraces a group of disorders all exhibiting an abnormal quality of collagen. This factor leads to 'hyperelastic' tissue, which

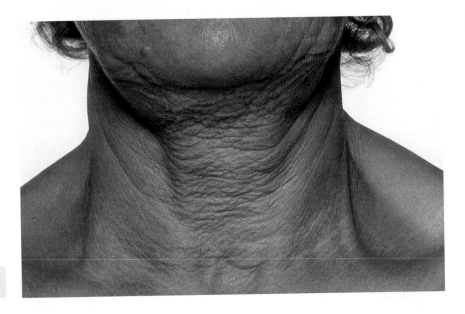

Fig 11.11 Cutis laxa. Soft wrinkled tissue with a doughy feel is present due to loss of normal elasticity

stretches much more than normal (**Fig 11.12**), but then recoils to its original position; the cause is not an increase in elastic tissue but an abnormality of the usually stronger collagen. Poor-quality collagen also leads to the formation of patulous scars (**Fig 11.13**). The deficient quality of collagen supporting blood vessels and, in some variants, actually forming part of the blood vessel wall, leads to another typical feature of this syndrome, which is an easy bruising tendency (**Fig. 11.13**). Increased joint laxity is also a feature, and in some variants, rupture of large blood vessels is a major cause of morbidity.

Scars

Any scar contains deficient collagen. Ill-advised skin surgery, in areas of high tension, produces a stretched scar (**Fig 11.14**). Other notable shapes of scars are the 'ice-pick' scar of acne (*see* Fig 6.36) and varioliform scars, which are broad and depressed (*see* Fig 6.39). Scars in so-called malignant atrophic papulosis (Degos disease), an endarteritis, are typically sharply demarcated and 'porcelain white,' with marginal hyperpigmentation. Scars associated with major dermal loss or necrosis (such as those secondary to some leg ulcers or vasculitis) are usually depressed below the skin surface.

Note, however, that scar tissue is formed by fibroblast proliferation and formation of dermal collagen and ground substance, and thus may be thickened and firm in texture.

Focal dermal hypoplasia

Focal dermal hypoplasia implies a quantitative defect in the dermis, which, being thinner than normal, allows focal herniation of the underlying fat. In practice, the dermal atrophy has a streaky pattern and occurs in a rare disorder known as Goltz syndrome.

Atrophodermas

Atrophoderma of Pasini and Pierini—This (**Fig 11.15**) is a relatively uncommon but characteristic variant of morphoea, in which there is a sharply localised depression within the dermis and hyperpigmentation. Follicles may be apparent within this but are lost in the more typical sclerotic type of morphoea.

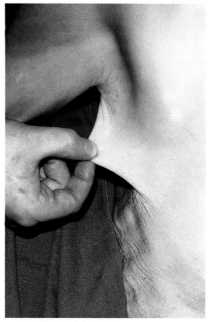

Fig 11.12 Ehlers–Danlos syndrome. Skin can be stretched easily but returns to its normal position

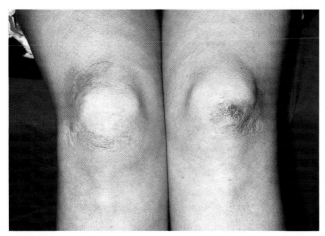

Fig 11.13 Ehlers–Danlos syndrome. Easy bruising and atrophic patulous scars are often apparent on the knees

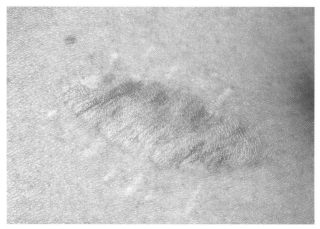

Fig 11.14 Stretched scar. In this broad scar, the elongated freckles are clear evidence that stretching has occurred after healing of the epidermis

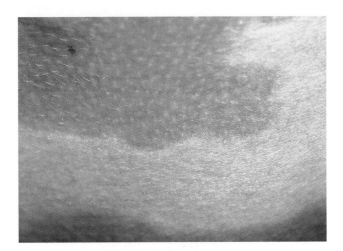

Fig 11.15 Atrophoderma of Pasini and Pierini.
Sharply demarcated, hyperpigmented, depressed dermal atrophy on the trunk

Atrophodermas—These (**Fig 11.16** and **11.17**) are a group of disorders, which combine abnormal keratinisation, inflammation and atrophy. These often affect the face and are associated with hair abnormalities, such as sparse scalp hair or loss of eyebrows. The pattern of atrophy involves the dermis and epidermis as well as the follicles and appears in a typical vermiculate or honeycombed arrangement of tiny atrophic depressed scars known as atrophoderma vermiculatum or honeycomb atrophy (**Fig 11.16**). A rarer follicular atrophoderma is shown in **Fig 11.17**.

Perifollicular atrophy—This may also occur as more scattered and discrete lesions, which are sometimes protuberant and resemble anetoderma (*see* Figs 4.21 and 4.22) but are not due to abnormal elastic tissue. The most common cause is as an end result of inflammation in an infective folliculitis or acne.

Fat atrophy (lipoatrophy)

This is simpler to diagnose than many of the disorders discussed so far, as it is usually an isolated rather than a mixed atrophy and because the skin feels normal in thickness and elasticity. It may present in three main forms, which are described below.

(1) Localised lipoatrophy—This was a feature of subcutaneous injection of older types of insulin but is less common now (**Fig 11.18**) and is more

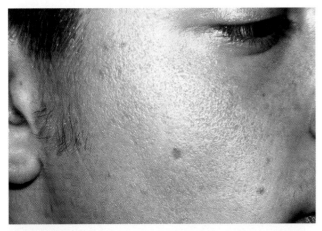

Fig 11.16 Atrophoderma vermiculatum (honeycomb atrophy). This occurs on the cheeks, usually in children or young adults

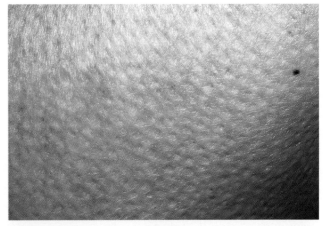

Fig 11.17 Follicular atrophoderma. This shows typical shallow-delled lesions in a patient with Basex syndrome (an autosomal dominant disorder with follicualr atrophoderma, multiple basal cell carcinoma and hair thinning)

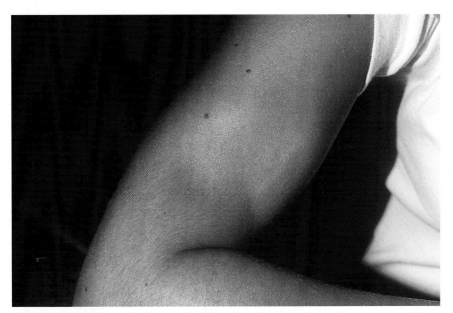

Fig 11.18 Lipoatrophy due to insulin. The depressed area is more rounded and less sharply defined than dermal atrophy

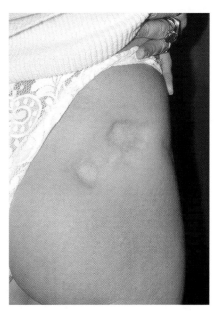

Fig 11.19 Lipoatrophy due to a depot steroid preparation

commonly seen after depot injections of corticosteroids (**Fig 11.19**). Fat atrophy also occurs at sites of pressure, such as that caused by shoulder straps (**Fig 11.20**), and sometimes results from injury. Semicircular atrophy is an interesting pattern of fat atrophy that occurs on the thighs, in which pressure from the edge of seats has been suggested to be the aetiological factor.

(2) Partial lipodystrophy—There are various forms of partial lipodystrophy, the most important of which is associated with deficiency of complement C3 and glomerulonephritis (**Fig 11.21**). The typical gaunt appearance is due to the loss of facial fat. The trunk may seem to be very muscular, and hypertrophy of fat may affect the legs.

(3) Panatrophy—This is a rare disorder associated with atrophy of cutaneous and subcutaneous tissue (**Fig 11.22**). As all levels of skin and subcutaneous tissue are reduced in thickness, there is prominence of underlying bony structures.

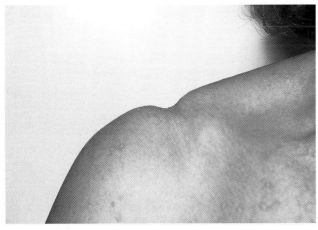

Fig 11.20 Fat atrophy. This has occurred at the superior aspect of the shoulder owing to the effect of prolonged pressure from a bra strap

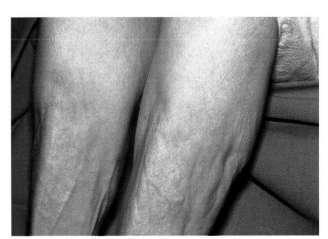

Fig 11.21 Local panatrophy. There is total loss of subcutaneous fat with associated atrophic skin, through which the veins can be seen

203

SKIN AND SUBCUTANEOUS THICKENING

Epidermal thickening

Histological evidence of epidermal thickening (acanthosis) is a feature of numerous localised nodules (Chapter 9), lichenification (Chapter 7) and many rashes, such as psoriasis (Chapter 8) and ichthyoses (Chapter 7). Other physical signs are often present, and in the context of this chapter, the disorders considered are those where the thickening is not notably associated with scaling (i.e. the thickening is due to increased epidermal cells rather than increased stratum corneum). Examples are described below.

Acanthosis nigricans

This disorder causes thickened, brown, warty plaques in flexural areas, especially axillae (*see* Fig 3.17). The thickening is presumably generalised, but less easy to demonstrate at other sites; in extreme forms, there is a generalised wartiness, including the mucous membranes, and a characteristic thickening of the palms known as 'tripe hands' (**Fig 11.23**).

Acanthosis nigricans is characteristically associated with internal malignancy (over 50% of cases occur in gastric adenocarcinoma) but is actually much less common than the variant associated with insulin-resistant states and hyperandrogenism (*see* Table 3.6).

Finger pebbling in diabetes

Exaggeration of the normal cobblestoned pattern of the skin over the knuckles and on the dorsal aspect of the terminal phalanges of the fingers has been described as finger pebbling (**Fig 11.24**). It is due to a mixture of epidermal thickening with hyperkeratosis and enlarged dermal papillae containing thickened collagen bundles. A similar pattern of skin thickening is seen on the dorsum of fingers and toes in Down's syndrome.

Knuckle pads

Knuckle pads are a much circumscribed thickening, probably of epidermis and dermis, usually over the proximal interphalangeal joints (**Fig 11.25**).

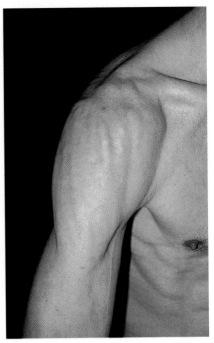

Fig 11.22 Partial lipodystrophy.
This man shows partial lipodystrophy associated with renal disease. The deltoid muscle is easily visible owing to loss of overlying fat

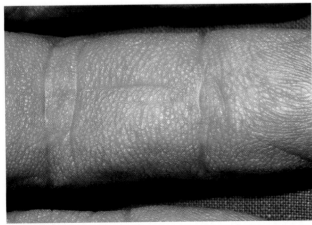

Fig 11.23 Acanthosis nigricans. Exaggerated epidermal ridge pattern on fingertip is a manifestation of 'tripe palms'

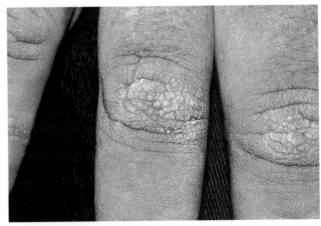

Fig 11.24 Finger pebbling in diabetes. (*photo courtesy of Dr G M White*)

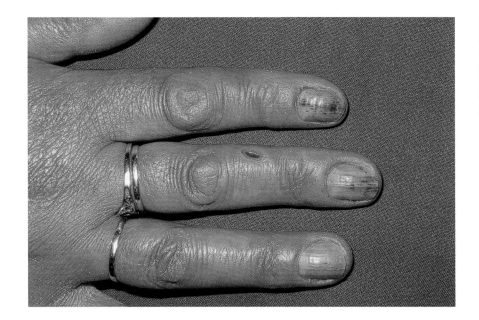

Trauma of picking or chewing is the important cause; similar lesions occur in bulimia, when the fingers are regularly inserted into the mouth to provoke self-induced vomiting.

Dermal thickening

Dermal thickening embraces a large group of disorders (**Tables 11.4** and **11.5**). Some groups have innumerable examples, a few of which are discussed here to illustrate the physical signs of the various different patterns of the condition.

Smooth dome-shaped lesions or plaque of swelling

Any disorder where an acute increase in tissue fluid occurs can produce skin thickening, e.g. urticarias (*see* Chapter 15).

Inflammatory, cellular and other infiltrates cause smooth swelling. Applying pressure to the skin may sometimes help to distinguish between a swelling due to fluid and a purely cellular infiltrate; the latter is not compressible, but fluid may be.

Calcification or bone formation may cause localised nodules or more diffuse changes and is palpable as a stony consistency (**Figs 11.26** and **11.27**).

Cobblestone appearance

A cobblestone appearance can occur as a result of almost complete confluence of closely grouped papules (**Fig 11.28**). It is also a feature of some diffuse alterations of connective tissue, such as pretibial myxoedema (*see* below). Lichen amyloidosis (due to deposition of amyloid protein, *see* Fig 8.25) and lichen myxoedematosus (a disorder associated with paraproteinaemias) can both cause cobblestoned areas of skin.

Altered collagen

Granuloma annulare—This (**Fig 11.29**) presents as flesh-coloured, yellowish or erythematous lesions, which are annular in overall shape; the raised border has the appearance of coalesced papules, and the central skin in larger lesions has an almost normal clinical appearance, which may cause confusion

Table 11.4 Causes of dermal thickening and altered texture

Appearance	Cause	Examples
Smooth swelling (dome/plaque)	Fluid	Urticaria (16.1)
		Oedema
	Cellular infiltrate (many others with epidermal change also, or cells and fluid)	Jessner's lymphocytic infiltrate
		Polymorphic light eruption
	Other	Bone or calcium (osteoma cutis (11.26), dystrophic calcification, etc.)
Cobblestoned appearance	Altered connective tissue	Granuloma annulare (11.29) (also contains cellular infiltrate)
		Pretibial myxoedema (11.31)
		Elastosis
		Connective tissue naevi
		Pseudoxanthoma elasticum (11.30)
		Lichenification (mainly epidermal) (15.27)
	Infiltrates	Xanthomas (some) (3.35)
		Lichen amyloidosis
		Lichen myxedematosis
	Closely grouped papules (various causes)	Sarcoidosis
		Some eczemas, psoriasis (11.28)
		Actinic reticuloid
		Diffuse granuloma annulare
		Tuberous sclerosis
Sclerotic disorders (see Table 11.5)	Altered connective tissue	Scleroderma (11.39)
		Morphoea (11.36)
		Keloids (9.62)
		Diabetic thick skin
Peau d'orange (11.33) appearance	Altered connective tissue	Connective tissue naevi
		Scleredema (11.34, 11.35)
		Pre-tibial myxoedema (11.31, 11.32)
	Cellular infiltrate	Neoplastic
	Fluid	Localised oedema
		Intradermal injections

Table 11.5 Disorders causing sclerosis

Genodermatoses and paediatric	Progeria, Werner's syndrome
	Infantile and juvenile fibromatoses
Collagen-vascular disorders	Systemic sclerosis
	Morphoea and variants (linear, 'en coup de sabre')
	CREST, mixed connective tissue disease
	Graft versus host disease
	Vinyl chloride disease
Metabolic and endocrine	Porphyria cutanea tarda
	Diabetes (stiff skin, cheirarthropathy)
	Carcinoid tumour
	POEMS syndrome
	Scleromyoedema
Inflammatory	Sclerosing panniculitis, lupus profundus, eosinophilic fasciitis
Physical	Injury, surgery, radiotherapy
Others	Lymphoedema, bullous disease (cicatricial pemphigoid, epidermolysis bullosa dystrophica), drugs (vitamin K injection sites, pentazocine)

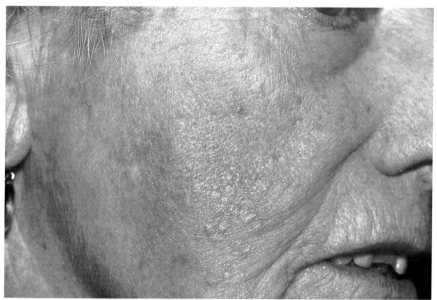

Fig 11.26

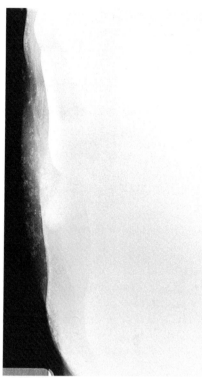

Figs 11.26, 11.27 Osteoma cutis. Stony, hard, creamy white lesions on the face (11.26) are visible on an oblique X-ray film of the cheek as multiple small calcified papules (11.27)

Fig 11.27

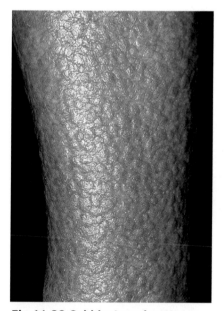

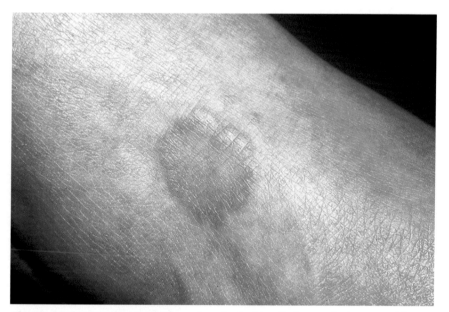

Fig 11.28 Cobblestoned pattern. This patient has chronic psoriasis of the lower legs, treated with topical corticosteroids

Fig 11.29 Granuloma annulare. Annular lesions that seem to be caused by a ring of confluent papules, having a cobblestoned pattern. The abnormality is due to altered dermal collagen

with ringworm. However, granuloma annulare does not have the scaling that is characteristic of ringworm (*see* Fig 7.18). The disorder has been associated with diabetes mellitus (although this is present in less than 2% of cases), but the association is much stronger (up to 30%) in some atypical forms, such as generalised or perforating granuloma annulare. It usually occurs on hands and feet in children and is often misdiagnosed as a wart but has a smooth surface (compare with warts, *see* Figs 9.83–9.85).

Connective tissue naevi—These may include abnormal collagen and elastic tissue. Most are smooth-surfaced plaques, cobblestoned in appearance, or with a peau d'orange texture (**Fig 11.33**).

Abnormal elastic tissue

Pseudoxanthoma elasticum—This (**Fig 11.30**) is a group of inherited disorders producing a yellow-coloured cobblestoned pattern of dermal thickening, which is most apparent on the neck and in axillae. Its diagnosis can be critical, as there may also be cardiac and vascular abnormalities, including those of the retinal vessels.

Solar (actinic) elastosis—This is discussed on p. 103.

Infiltration/deposition of abnormal materials

Pre-tibial myxoedema—Although a smooth swelling is a feature in the early stage of pre-tibial myxoedema (**Figs 11.31** and **11.32**), it is generally apparent by its cobblestoned or peau d'orange appearance. It is caused by deposition of mucin in the dermis.

Peau d'orange appearance—A peau d'orange appearance is seen when dermal swelling causes patulous prominent follicular openings at the skin surface. Causes include:

- Intradermal injections.
- Connective tissue naevi (**Fig 11.33**)
- Pre-tibial myxoedema (**Figs 11.31** and **11.32**).
- Scleredema (**Figs 11.34** and **11.35**).

Scleredema (which is totally separate from scleroderma) is rare and comes on acutely. Reported cases have an association with diabetes mellitus as well as with acute streptococcal infections. Mucin deposition occurs, often most prominently on the upper back, where a peau d'orange appearance and pitting can be shown (**Figs 11.34** and **11.35**).

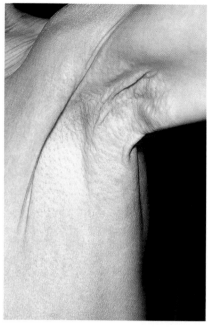

Fig 11.30 Pseudoxanthoma elasticum. Cobblestoned 'plucked chicken' appearance of yellow papular lesions

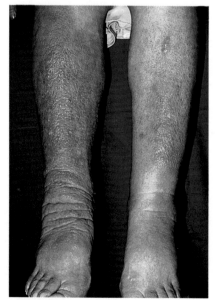

Fig 11.31

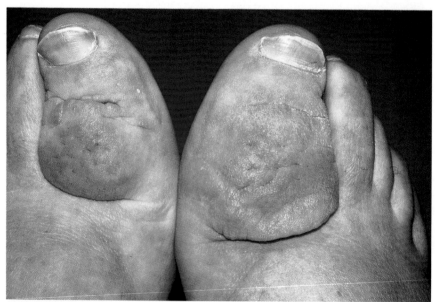

Fig 11.32

Figs 11.31, 11.32 Pre-tibial myxoedema. Typical distribution. (11.31) dimpling and peau d'orange appearance on the toes (11.32). Affected areas may be flesh-coloured but more often are a purplish-red, as shown here

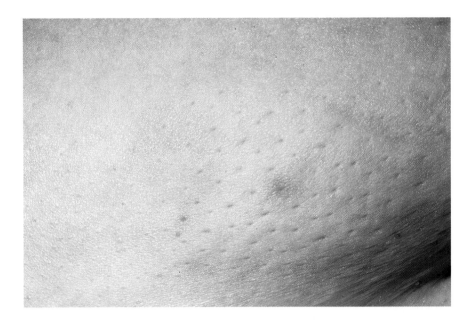

Fig 11.33 Connective tissue naevus. The peau d'orange appearance of swelling with follicular prominence (compare with adjacent normal skin) is clearly evident here. This lesion was on the breast and caused concern because of the differential diagnosis of neoplastic infiltration. However, the lesion illustrated is paler than the normal skin, whereas a neoplastic infiltrate is usually associated with erythema due to inflammation

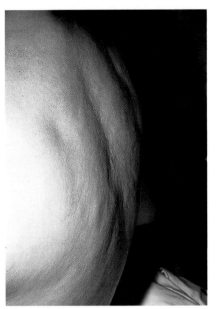

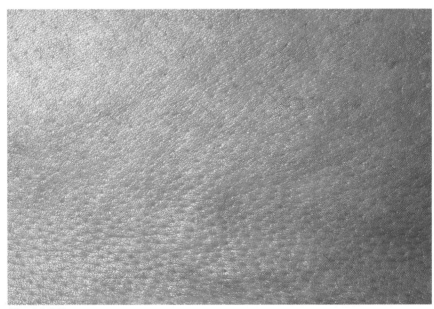

Fig 11.34   **Fig 11.35**

Figs 11.34, 11.35 Scleredema. Pitting oedema of the upper back, the typical distribution, is seen here. Several shallow depressions produced by fingertip pressure are apparent (11.34), as is the peau d'orange appearance (11.35), which is not associated with erythema. This disorder was associated with streptococcal infection

Sclerosis (hard skin)

Sclerosis implies a scar-like quality and may be the result of surgery, injury or burns or the end result of an inflammatory process (**Table 11.5**). Traumatic or surgical scars may be thickened, when they are known as hypertrophic scars, but in general scar tissue is thinner than the adjacent skin. Keloid scars are those in which active scar thickening extends beyond the area of injury, usually in the few months after the skin is damaged; spontaneous keloids mainly affect the upper trunk.

The essential physical signs of sclerosis can be appreciated only by palpation; the skin feels firm, and the ability to pick up a fold of skin by pinching is decreased. However, it should be appreciated that a thin scar may be bound

Fig 11.36 Morphoea. A typical lesion

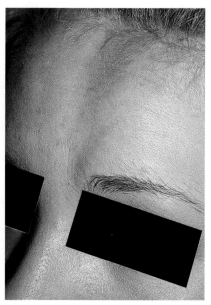

Fig 11.37 Morphoea en coup de sabre. A typical vertical forehead lesion

down and tethered to underlying fat or deeper structures, so that a fold of skin cannot be picked up easily. Examples of sclerotic disorders are described below.

Morphoea—This (**Fig 11.36**) causes diagnostic problems. The typical acute lesion is smooth, firm, raised, shiny, ivory white and has a violaceous rim (*see* Fig 8.27). The follicular orifices shrink and become invisible, a useful clinical feature in the differential diagnosis between morphoea and lichen sclerosus et atrophicus (*see* Fig 7.39). Lesions of morphoea gradually soften with time, often with a residual, slightly shiny appearance and sometimes with noticeable hyperpigmentation around the lesions. Two variants are characteristic in their distribution. Linear morphoea extends along a limb (and may cause joint contractures), whereas morphoea 'en coup de sabre' (**Fig 11.37**) runs vertically across the forehead and adjacent scalp (usually as a single band, but sometimes more than one). The latter is most apparent when frowning, as the area of dermal abnormality does not move normally.

Scleroderma—The term scleroderma (**Figs 11.38–11.40**) is used as a description of the appearance of the skin in several disorders, particularly

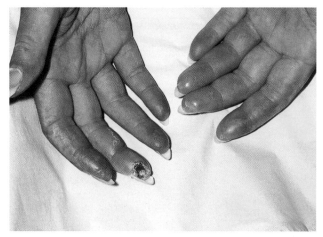

Fig 11.38 Sclerodactyly. Tight shiny skin of the fingers, with ulceration, healed fingertip infarcts and cyanosis

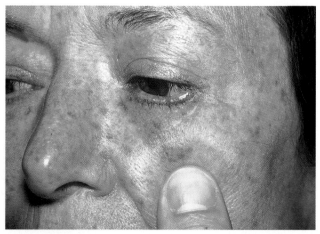

Fig 11.39 Scleroderma (systemic sclerosis). Note telangiectasia and inability to evert the lower eyelid by firm traction

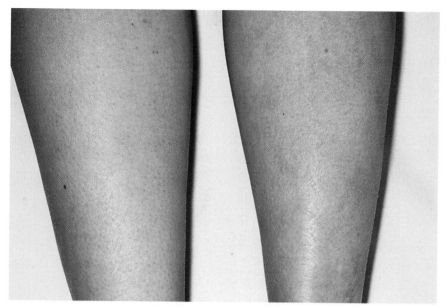
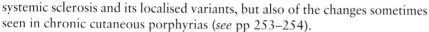

Fig 11.40 Scleroderma. This shown atrophy of the affected leg, with shiny skin and absent hair follicles—compare with the unaffected side

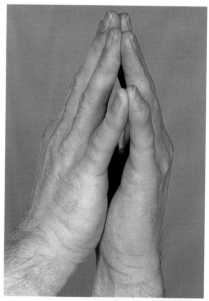

Fig 11.41 Prayer sign in diabetes. Cheirarthropathy causing the 'prayer sign' in a patient with diabetes (*Photo courtesy of Dr S Russell*)

systemic sclerosis and its localised variants, but also of the changes sometimes seen in chronic cutaneous porphyrias (*see* pp 253–254).

The skin lesions of progressive systemic sclerosis are pathologically similar to morphoea, although the sites affected and therefore the clinical features are different. Systemic sclerosis may involve the lungs, gut and kidneys. The usual dermatological manifestation is a tightness of the skin of the fingers in association with Raynaud's phenomenon (*see* Fig 17.13); nailfold telangiectasia (*see* Fig 19.42 and 19.43) and a ragged cuticle are typical, and the affected skin is tight, cool, shiny, variably hypopigmented and hyperpigmented, with loss of hairs and sometimes fingertip ulceration (**Fig 11.38**). On the face, telangiectasia is an early feature, and there is often tightness of the skin of the nose (with a beaked appearance) and impaired opening of the mouth, with radiating skin creases ('radial furrows'). Follicular openings disappear (**Fig 11.40**), as in morphoea.

Generalised morphoea can appear very similar but tends to involve the trunk and proximal limbs rather than the face and hands and typically spares the periareolar region of the breast.

Scleroderma is often clinically limited in extent, especially in a disorder termed the CREST syndrome on the basis of the combination of Calcinosis, Raynaud's phenomenon, Esophagus (motility disorder), Sclerodactyly and Telangiectasia. The features of sclerodactyly are as described for systemic sclerosis.

Diabetes—A disorder known as diabetic thick skin has been described in which the usual clinical sign that can be demonstrated is due to associated limited joint mobility (cheirarthropathy). This manifests as the so-called prayer sign; affected individuals are unable to press the palms and fingers flat together when the hands are in the praying position with the wrists extended (**Fig 11.41**). The skin may appear waxy in extreme examples. This abnormality is due to increased cross-linking of collagen by long-term changes in glycosylation.

Keloid scars—Hypertrophic scars that arise spontaneously are called keloids (*see* Fig 9.62).

Other localised sclerotic nodules—Dermatofibromas (pigmented histiocytomas) have a typical tethered feel on palpation (*see* Fig 4.23 and p. 169).

DIAGNOSTIC TIPS AND PITFALLS

● The prayer sign occurs in disorders where there is sclerotic collagen of the hands or where the hands are puffy due to soft tissue swelling. Affected individuals are unable to press the palms and fingers flat together when the hands are in the praying position with the wrists extended to 90 degrees. It is a feature of scleroderma, mixed connective tissue disease, diabetic thick skin and disorders of the fascia in the hands

Subcutaneous thickening: fat and fascia

Fat can undergo two main processes that cause thickening: hypertrophy and inflammation (panniculitis). The latter may lead to fibrosis. It is clinically very difficult to distinguish the fibrotic stage of panniculitis from a primary fasciitis.

Fat hypertrophy

Fat hypertrophy is distinguished from the inflammatory disorders of fat by the fact that it is soft or only moderately firm and not clinically inflamed. Apart from localised lesions (lipomas), the main disorders are:

* Localised fat hypertrophy. This occurs in some patients in relation to insulin injection (**Fig 11.42**).
* Widespread fat hypertrophy, for example on the lower limbs in some patients with partial lipodystrophy.

Panniculitis

There are numerous causes of panniculitis and an overlap with disorders causing inflammation of the overlying lower dermis (e.g. erythema nodosum) or the underlying fascia. Panniculitis usually presents as tender nodules or plaques, often on the legs, which are firm and inflamed (**Fig 11.43**). Ulceration and discharge of fatty material may occur as a result of fat digestion following release of lipase from pancreatic carcinomas (**Figs 11.44** and **11.45**) and as a result of acute, chronic and traumatic pancreatitis. Some forms of panniculitis, such as that associated with venous disease, may 'burn out' to leave residual firm nodules or plaques in the deeper tissues.

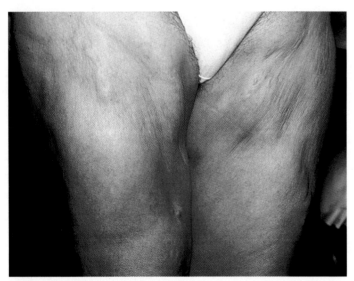

Fig 11.42 Fat hypertrophy and atrophy. Fat hypertrophy, as well as fat atrophy, associated with insulin injection sites in a diabetic patient

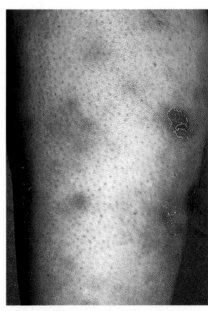

Fig 11.43 Panniculitis. This shows typical inflamed lesions on the legs, which are dimpled due to tethering by deep inflammation. Some post-inflammatory pigmentation is also apparent

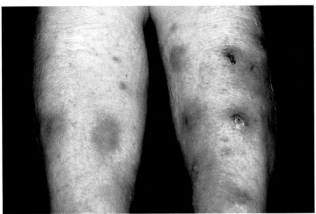

Fig 11.44

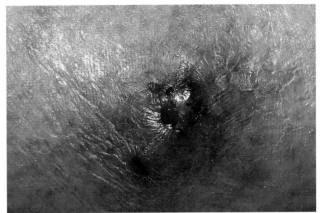

Fig 11.45

Figs 11.44, 11.45 Fat necrosis in a patient with adenocarcinoma of the pancreas. This patient had multiple red and relatively non-tender nodules on her arms and legs and later on her trunk. Many of these nodules discharged yellowish oily material, characteristic of lipase-induced panniculitis

Fasciitis

Fasciitis may be impossible to distinguish from panniculitis, but is generally a more diffuse process rather than a localised lesion. Thus, scleroderma spectrum disorders are also in the differential diagnosis. Fasciitis has a tendency to produce a contracted appearance as it heals, in which case the resulting contracture pulls the overlying skin downwards, leading to a guttering appearance around larger subcutaneous veins and delineation of the underlying muscle groups by depression of the skin between them. The latter is one of the physical signs known as the groove sign (the other is the depression between inguinal 'pseudobuboes' in donovanosis) and is best seen in the upper arm when the arms are raised above the head.

Ulcers

INTRODUCTION

An **ulcer** is an area of loss of epidermis and dermis, which in some cases extends as deep as muscle or bone (**Fig 12.1**).

An **erosion** is an area of superficial skin loss, limited to the epidermis. The underlying dermis is exposed as a red oozy surface, but the area heals without scarring. Erosions occur after superficial injury, for example after scratching in eczema or after a blister roof is shed (*see* Fig 13.36).

A **fissure** is a deep narrow crack in the skin. Fissures commonly occur in chronic eczema and intertrigo and occasionally in psoriasis. They form when the skin loses flexibility because of a thick hyperkeratotic scale (**Fig 12.2**) or when it becomes brittle due to changes in the water content of the stratum corneum. Fissures are most prominent in areas that are stretched by movement, e.g. feet (*see* Fig 7.46), lips (**Fig 12.3**) and hands (**Fig 12.4**).

An **excoriation** is a superficial erosion or ulcer caused by scratching or rubbing and so will usually be linear or have a geometric outline. Occurring in any itchy skin condition (*see* Tables 15.1 and 15.2) and in artefactual skin disease (*see* p. 288), excoriation does not therefore identify a specific depth of damage but describes a cause of tissue loss. The cause of skin ulceration can often be determined by a careful history and examination. The following points need to be taken into account.

SPEED OF PROGRESSION

There are a limited number of causes of acute skin ulceration (**Table 12.1**). Virtually any of these ulcers may become recurrent or chronic if not treated

215

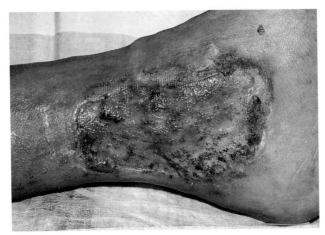

Fig 12.1 Venous ulcer. This usually first develops on the medial aspect of the lower leg. With repeated ulceration and scar formation, recurrent ulcers may appear anywhere around the ankle. There is surrounding hyperkeratosis, pigmentation, haemosiderin staining and eczema

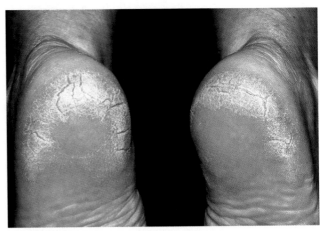

Fig 12.2 Fissures in hyperkeratotic eczema of the heels (keratoderma climactericum). Thick hyperkeratotic scaling eczema localised to the heels, with fissuring at the heel margins

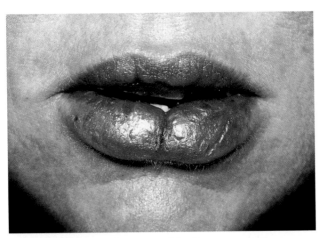

Fig 12.3 Fissured lip. Central lip fissures may be very persistent and often unresponsive to topical steroids. Fissures also develop at the corners of the mouth in angular cheilitis

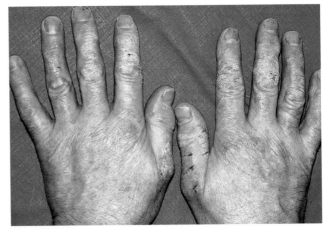

Fig 12.4 Fissured hand eczema. There are several deep fissures in the affected sites on the back of the hands in this man with a chronic irritant eczema

correctly. However, in general, chronic ulcers are neoplastic, infective, vascular or inflammatory. Neoplastic ulceration is typically progressive, whereas ulcers that heal and then recur locally are usually inflammatory, artefactual or infective rather than neoplastic.

TRAUMA

Many ulcers occur after trauma, including common problems such as venous ulceration. However, there are relatively few causes of rapidly progressive ulceration after minor injuries—the most important are infections (e.g. streptococcal) and pyoderma gangrenosum.

Pyoderma gangrenosum

Pyoderma gangrenosum produces a typical deep, painful, ulcer with an undermined purple edge. The lesions usually present on the legs (**Figs 12.17**

Table 12.1 Possible causes of acute-onset skin ulceration

Trauma, excoriation

Blister necrosis

Infections
  Viral
    Herpes simplex and herpes zoster
  Bacterial
    Streptococcus pyogenes—ecthyma (12.8), cellulitis (12.31) or necrotising
      fasciitis
    Clostridium welchii—feel for crepitus
  Endemic areas
    Amoebic ulcer, tropical ulcer
  Immune compromised patient
    Bacterial sepsis, e.g. pseudomonas (ecthyma gangrenosum), atypical
      mycobacteria (2.16)
    Fungal sepsis, e.g. sporotrichosis, cryptococcosis, blastomycosis,
      coccidiomycosis and other deep fungal infections

Vascular
  Vasculitis (12.7)
  Venous and arterial ulcer (12.1, 12.23)
  Temporal arteritis (12.26)

Drugs
  Warfarin (12.5)
  Heparin
  Extravasation at chemotherapy injection sites
  Intramuscular phenylbutazone

Pyoderma gangrenosum (12.17, 12.18)

DIAGNOSTIC TIPS AND PITFALLS

- Neoplastic ulceration is typically progressive, whereas ulcers that heal and then recur locally are usually inflammatory, artefactual or infective rather than neoplastic

- Rapid skin ulceration can be due to vasculitis, vascular occlusion or pyoderma gangrenosum or in association with streptococcal cellulitis; occult exotic infections must always be excluded in an immune compromised patient

and **12.18**), although they can occur at all body sites, including the face. The patient presents with sudden, usually painful, skin necrosis, sometimes associated with blister formation (*see* Fig 13.44), followed by ulceration. Other variants include pustular pyoderma (*see* Fig 14.23), seen usually on the back with multiple deep, painful pustules that ulcerate and scar. Scars arising in healed pyoderma gangrenosum produce a characteristic cribriform appearance (*see* Fig 2.24). This disease occurs in association with a variety of conditions, the most common being ulcerative colitis (**Table 12.2**). Before treatment with steroids begins, it is essential to exclude other possible infective causes, including anaerobic infections (*see* above) and deep fungal infections due to coccidiomycosis and blastomycosis.

SYMPTOMS

Most ulcers are painful either continuously or intermittently. Some are extremely painful even when the ulcer is small (**Table 12.3**). In a few circumstances ulcers are always painless, this is the case in neuropathic ulcers

Table 12.2 Associations with pyoderma gangrenosum

Ulcerative colitis
Crohn's disease
Rheumatoid arthritis
Monoclonal gammopathy
Leukaemia, myeloproliferative disease, polycythaemia
Chronic active hepatitis
Behçet's disease

Table 12.3 Painful and painless ulcers

Painful	Painless
Infected varicose or mixed ulcers	Neuropathic ulcers
Behçet's disease	Neoplastic ulcers
Orogenital aphthous ulcers	Varicose ulcers, occasionally
Arterial ulcers	Syphilitic gumma
Pyoderma gangrenosum	
Hypertensive ulcers	
Atrophie blanche ulcers	

(**Figs 12.34** and **12.36**), where the sensory deficit causes the ulcer by allowing trauma to occur without the warning sensation of pain. The tertiary-stage syphilitic gumma is invariably pain free. The well-defined, hard primary chancre of syphilis is commonly painful when examined but may not be so at other times.

Neuropathic ulceration

On the face, particularly around the nose, the trigeminal trophic syndrome following trigeminal ganglion injection for intractable facial pain may produce an area of altered or absent sensation, which is repeatedly picked at or damaged by the patient, resulting in a steadily increasing ulcer (**Fig 12.36**).

On the hands, neuropathic ulcers usually follow sensory loss caused by a peripheral nerve injury (**Fig 12.33**) or syringomyelia. In carpal tunnel syndrome, blisters and ulceration of finger tips may occur.

Neuropathic ulceration of the feet is a major problem if there is unnoticed trauma from footwear. This occurs most commonly in diabetic peripheral neuropathy but also in several types of nerve root damage.

PRECEDING SKIN CHANGES

In all blistering disorders, blisters burst, leaving erosions that—through infection or trauma—may become deeper, forming ulcers. In blisters resulting from skin necrosis (*see* pp. 249–253), e.g. vasculitis, vascular occlusion and pyoderma gangrenosum (**Figs 12.17 and 12.18**), or in association with streptococcal cellulitis (**Figs 12.30 and 12.31**), large ulcers may appear as soon as the blister roof sloughs off. In these cases, ulceration is alarmingly rapid. In the immunocompromised patient, opportunistic and unusual infections must be considered (**Table 12.1**).

SPECIFIC FEATURES OF ULCERS

Ulcer edge

The ulcer edge can be soft or hard. A firm, rubbery or hard edge (**Fig 12.20**) suggests ulceration within a tumour whether it is secondary or primary. A soft edge is a consequence of an inflammatory lesion or healing in a vascular ulcer.

> **DIAGNOSTIC TIPS AND PITFALLS**
>
> - Neuropathic ulcers are painless

Ulcer profile

An **undermined edge** is created by an ulcer being wider at the deep margin than it is superficially (**Figs 12.17** and **12.18**). As a consequence, the ulcer margin is poorly vascularised and appears bluish. An undermined edge is characteristic of pyoderma gangrenosum and tropical ulcer.

In a **punched-out ulcer,** the sides are vertical (**Fig 12.19**), and the base is flat, so that the ulcer appears to have been cut out using a leather punch or pastry cutter. Punched-out ulcers occur in arterial disease, ecthyma and secondary syphilis.

A **rolled or elevated edge** is characteristically seen at the edge of an ulcerated basal cell carcinoma (**Fig 12.20**).

Ulcer shape

Facticial ulcers

Facticial or traumatic ulcers usually have a **straight-edged** or geometric outline (**Fig 12.21**). Such ulcers are seen most commonly on the face and breast (**Fig 12.10**), although any site can be affected. This includes the limbs, where ulceration or intermittent oedema, due to the use of a tourniquet (*see* Fig 17.45), is well recognised. They may be induced by mechanical means or irritant chemicals, but the patient rarely admits details of the method.

Ulcer colour

The colour of an ulcer or ulcer edge is occasionally of diagnostic value. This is distinct from the colour of adjacent skin changes, such as the brown colour of venous stasis disease.

One of the more characteristic colour changes is the blue colour of the ulcer edge of pyoderma gangrenosum (**Fig 12.17, 12.18**).

A purplish or brown colour is typical of repeated fixed drug eruptions, which may ulcerate due to blistering, with epidermal necrosis (*see* Figs 3.10, 3.11).

Ulcer scarring

The presence of scarring after ulceration is rarely specific, although some disorders cause characteristic patterns, notably the cribriform scarring (colander-like) of pyoderma gangrenosum (*see* Fig 2.24). Ulceration due to chronic radionecrosis is typically surrounded by rather sclerotic yellowish white scar tissue, usually with prominent telangiectasia and sometimes some brown pigmentation. Erosions without dermal damage (e.g. due to impetigo (*see* Fig 13.15) or sunburn) may cause transient pigmentary disturbance but do not cause scars.

ASSOCIATED SKIN CHANGES

Abnormalities of the skin around the ulcer or at distant sites may provide important clues as to the cause of skin ulceration. These changes often reflect the nature of the preceding insult (*see* above).

Changes confined to adjacent skin

Ulcers secondary to an abnormality of the surrounding skin will be surrounded by the changes of the primary disorder, e.g. venous ulcers, necrobiosis lipoidica

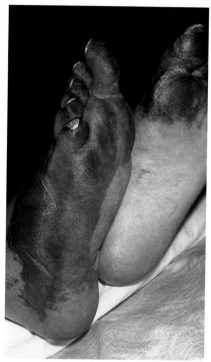

Fig 12.5 Coumarin necrosis. A sheet of vasculitis affected the feet of this patient 2 days after starting warfarin. Involvement of the extremities has been described, although necrosis usually affects fatty sites such as buttocks, breast and abdomen. It is associated with heterozygote protein C or S deficiency or acquired protein C deficiency, for example in disseminated intravascular coagulation

DIAGNOSTIC TIPS AND PITFALLS

- Facticial or traumatic ulcers usually have a straight-edged or geometric outline

219

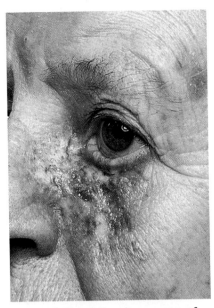

Fig 12.6 Ulceration in an area of radiotherapy-treated skin. Note the atrophy, telangiectasia and scarring of the skin around the ulcerated area. Radiotherapy was originally given to treat a basal cell carcinoma. There was no evidence of recurrent or new tumour formation when the damaged skin was excised

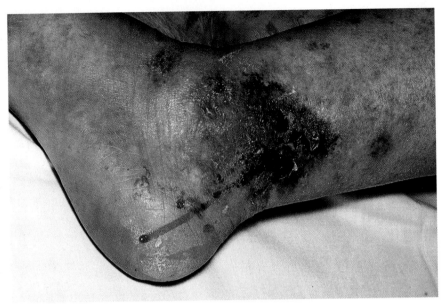

Fig 12.7 Ulcerated vasculitis. In areas of vasculitis, blisters may form initially (*see* 13.45), but ultimately, ulceration develops at these sites

(*see* **Fig 12.37**), radiotherapy-damaged skin (**Fig 12.6**, *see also* Fig 11.9), vasculitis (**Fig 12.7**) or deep streptococcal infection (**Fig 12.30**). Occasionally, significant abnormalities of the surrounding skin may seem irrelevant to the inexperienced, for example, local hyperhidrosis is sometimes seen in association with ulceration caused by an arteriovenous fistula of the foot.

Generalised skin changes

Ulcerated excoriations or erosions arising as a result of a blistering disorder will almost invariably be associated with skin changes at other sites. One exception to this is mucous membrane ulceration associated with blistering disorders (*see* Table 5.4). In cicatricial pemphigoid and pemphigus, and occasionally in bullous pemphigoid, patients may present with mouth or genital symptoms before other skin features develop.

No skin abnormalities

Normal surrounding skin suggests that the process is localised to the ulcer. This occurs in ecthyma (**Fig 12.8**), a streptococcal infection localised to the epidermis, herpes simplex, pyoderma gangrenosum (**Figs 12.17** and **12.18**) and syphilitic gumma. In neoplasia, the entire tumour may be ulcerated so that the ulcer seems to be arising in normal skin (**Fig 12.9**); more commonly, only part of it is affected, the rest of the tumour being visible around the ulcer (**Fig 12.20**).

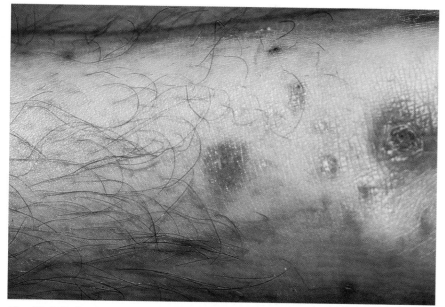

Fig 12.8 Ecthyma. This term is used to describe skin infections with *Streptococcus pyogenes* that cause crusting and ultimate scarring. Lesions are multiple and discrete, and removal of the crust reveals an oozy base. The lesions heal with crateriform scarring. On the leg at the centre of the picture, there is a healed area of white shiny scarred skin with multiple pinpoint capillaries similar to those seen in atrophie blanche (*see* 12.22, 17.21)

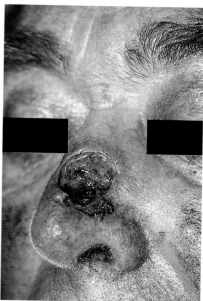

Fig 12.9 Ulcerated tumour. This man had an ulcer on his nose for 1–2 years. Biopsies on two occasions showed no evidence of tumour, but the ulcer failed to heal completely, although the size reduced with repeated dressings. After full excision, histology showed this to be a poorly differentiated squamous cell carcinoma. Note the depth and irregularity of the base of the ulcer compared with that seen in the neuropathic ulcer in 12.37

MULTIPLE VERSUS SOLITARY ULCERS

Solitary or grouped ulcers arising within a single area of abnormal skin are common and occur in a range of conditions (**Table 12.4**), the most important of which is the ulcerated primary skin tumour.

Multiple disseminated ulcers with intervening areas of normal skin are unusual but are seen in ecthyma, dermatitis artefacta, vasculitis and, occasionally, in pyoderma gangrenosum (**Figs 12.17** and **12.18**).

In vascular disease, the pattern of ulceration may reflect the pattern of blood supply to the skin, so that a reticulate pattern of skin ulceration or broken livedo (**Fig 12.14**, *see also* Figs 17.16 and 17.28) appears.

In generalised blistering disorders, rupture of blisters may produce multiple erosions (*see* Fig 13.36), which may become deeper due to infection or trauma. The presence of generalised bullous disorder is usually apparent, but patients with just a few lesions of a bullous drug eruption may cause diagnostic problems.

In patients receiving methotrexate for psoriasis, erosions appearing within plaques of psoriasis may be due to methotrexate toxicity, producing plaque skin necrosis (**Figs 12.15** and **12.16**).

SITE

Most types of skin ulceration can occur at various sites, including the mucous membranes (*see* Table 5.4). However, in a few instances, the ulcer site is characteristic of the ulcer type. Some of these are listed in **Table 12.5**.

Table 12.4 Causes of leg ulcers

Vascular
Venous ulcers (12.1)
Arterial insufficiency (12.23)
Vasculitic ulcers (12.7)
Diabetic ulcers
Atrophie blanche (12.22)
Hypertensive ulcers
Collagen vascular disease—chilblain lupus, scleroderma, rheumatoid arthritis
(12.25)
Arteriovenous fistula

Haematological
Chronic haemolytic anaemia, sickle-cell anaemia, hereditary spherocytosis
Cryoglobulinaemia (17.39)
Polycythaemia

Infection
Streptococcus pyogenes—ecthyma (12.8), cellulitis (12.30), necrotising
fasciitis
Anaerobic—streptococcus, *Clostridium welchii*
Treponema—syphilis, yaws
Tuberculosis—erythema induratum
Amoebic ulcer
Deep fungal infections—sporotrichosis, blastomycosis

Pyoderma gangrenosum (12.17, 12.18)

Neoplastic ulcers
Bowen's disease and squamous cell carcinoma—ulcerated tumour on the lower
leg especially in women (12.27)
Squamous cell carcinoma arising in a longstanding venous ulcer (12.28)

Metabolic
Necrobiosis lipoidica (12.37, *see also* 11.10)
Ulcerated gouty tophi (12.24)

Neuropathic (12.34)

Traumatic
Facticial ulceration (12.10)
Corrosive chemical, e.g. cement burns inside a shoe or boot
Venomous snake or insect bite

Pressure sore (12.11)

Table 12.5 Specific sites of skin ulceration

Site		Cause
Scalp		Temporal arteritis (12.26)
Ear	Helix and antihelix	Chondrodermatitis nodularis (9.99, 9.100)
	Behind the ear	Granuloma fissuratum (12.12, 12.13)
Face	Midline	Wegener's granulomatosis
	Nose	Neuropathic ulceration after trigeminal ganglion ablation (12.36)
Fingers		Syringomyelia with dissociated loss of pain sensation
		Carpal tunnel syndrome (12.33)
Foot	Pressure area	Neuropathic ulcer (12.33, 12.34)
	Dorsum	Arterial ulcer (12.23)

Scalp

Temporal arteritis

Patients with temporal arteritis usually present with severe headache, visual loss and tenderness on the scalp over the temporal and facial arteries, with loss of pulsation of these vessels. Pain on chewing occurs because of ischaemia of the muscles of mastication. Ischaemia can occur in any organ supplied by the internal carotid artery, including the tongue and scalp (**Fig 12.26**), where redness, hair loss and blistering may occur initially.

Pressure areas

Pressure areas such as the heel (**Fig 12.11**) and sacrum are liable to ulcerate because they are sites of repeated trauma and thus pressure necrosis. 'Coma blisters' (historically associated with barbiturates because overdose caused prolonged coma) are also due to prolonged pressure over bony prominences, leading to skin necrosis.

Neuropathy or other nerve damage that causes loss of pain sensation means that warning of imminent skin damage is lost, such that injury to the skin may lead to the development of neuropathic ulceration. On the feet, neuropathic ulcers may occur secondary to peripheral neuropathy, for example due to diabetes or alcohol misuse. Diastematomyelia may produce an area of sensory loss in adolescence on the sole of the foot (**Fig 12.34**). The patient should be examined for an area of increased hair growth, a 'faun tail', over the lower spine (**Fig 12.35** *see also* Fig 18.6).

Pressure from poorly fitting spectacles may cause ulceration behind the ear in granuloma fissuratum (**Figs 12.12 and 12.13**).

Mucous membranes

Ulcers affecting mucous membranes may be specific to the mouth or the genital skin or may affect any mucous membrane surface (**Table 12.6**). Many immunobullous disorders first present with mouth ulceration because fragile bullae are easily damaged in the mouth. Most ulcerating disorders of the mucous membrane present with multiple ulcers; acute solitary genital ulcers can occur in Behçet's disease, but infections should always be excluded. Solitary chronic oral or genital ulcers should arouse suspicion of neoplasia.

DIAGNOSTIC TIPS AND PITFALLS

- Spontaneous scalp ulceration associated with headache, visual loss and tenderness strongly suggests temporal arteritis

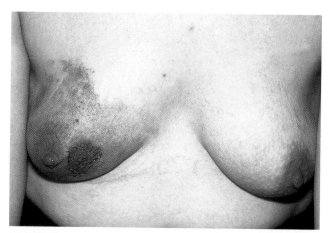

Fig 12.10 Dermatitis artefacta. A facticial erosion of the breast was created by this woman. Other causes were excluded, and the ulcer healed when the area was occluded

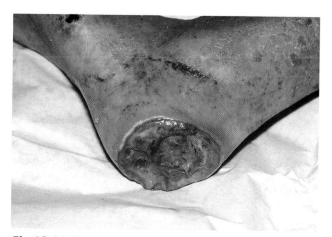

Fig 12.11 Pressure sore. A deep pressure sore on the heel of a man immobilised due to dementia complicated by a toxic confusional state

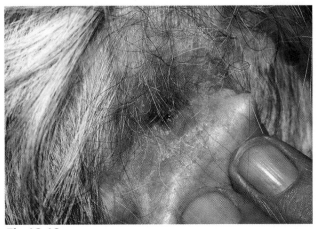

Fig 12.12

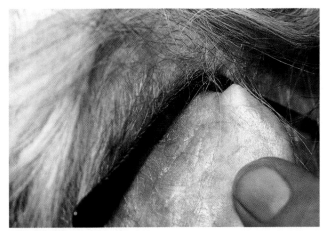

Fig 12.13

Fig 12.12, 12.13 Granuloma fissuratum. This man presented with a small persistent ulcer behind his ear (12.12). It was clearly related to rubbing from his poorly fitting spectacles (12.13) and healed when dressings were applied and his spectacles refitted

Table 12.6 Common causes of mucous membrane ulceration

Acute

- Infection
  Veneral
    Syphilis**
    Gonorrhoea**
    Lymphogranuloma venereum**
    Anaerobic streptococci**
  Non-veneral
    Hand-foot-and-mouth
    Chickenpox
    Herpes simplex
- Erythema multiforme (13.32)
- Trauma

Chronic

- Blistering diseases
  Cicatricial pemphigoid
  Bullous pemphigoid
  Pemphigus (13.48)
  Epidermolysis bullosa aquista
- Lichen planus* (2.22)
- Lichen sclerosus** (11.5, 17.30)
- Neoplasia (5.36)

Recurrent

- Aphthosis* (5.17)
- Erythema multiforme (13.32)
- Herpes simplex
- Bechet's syndrome
- Plasma-cell vulvitis and balanitis (5.34)

*Occurs principally in oral ulcers
**Occurs principally in genital ulcers

DIAGNOSTIC TIPS AND PITFALLS

- Arterial leg ulcers are typically solitary painful ulcers on the anterior leg or dorsum of the foot
- Venous leg ulcers are characteristically situated on the medial lower third of the leg overlying the site of the perforating veins that connect the deep and superficial venous systems of the leg

Table 12.7 Differences between arterial and venous leg ulcers

	Arterial	Venous
Symptoms	Painful	Often painless
Site	Toes, dorsum of the foot, shins	Around the ankle
Surrounding skin	Dry, scaling skin, pale or cyanosed	Pigmentation, eczema, pink warm skin, subcutaneous calcification, lipodermatosclerosis
Associated changes	Hair loss, nail changes, absent foot pulses	Hair and nails normal, pedal pulses present

Leg ulcers

Leg ulcers are a special case because, although most are vascular, a huge variety of disorders may be responsible (**Table 12.4**). Distinctions between the commonest causes of leg ulceration (venous and arterial disease) are given in **Table 12.7**.

Vascular ulceration

Venous ulcers—Longstanding venous insufficiency causes oedema, red-cell extravasation with haemosiderin staining, eczema—which may also be due to a contact allergy—and, ultimately, ulceration (*see* **Fig 12.1**). With repeated infection and chronic oedema, scarring occurs, particularly in the lower third of the leg, resulting in an inverted champagne-bottle appearance. The skin above the ankle becomes as hard as wood and is sometimes referred to as lipodermatosclerosis.

Arterial ulcers—These are solitary painful ulcers on the upper leg or dorsum of the foot (**Fig 12.23**). Associated features of arterial insufficiency are usually present (**Table 12.7**, *see also* Tables 17.12 and 17.13). In chronic tophaceous gout, tophi sited around finger and toe joints may ulcerate (**Fig 12.24**) and can be confused with ischaemic or neuropathic ulcers.

Hypertensive ulcers (Martorell's ulcer)—Hypertensive arterial ulcers present as exquisitely painful punched-out lesions on the calf, usually in older women with hypertension. Prompt diagnosis is important, since sympathectomy, which commonly helps to control the pain and aid healing, can then be employed.

Rheumatoid ulcers—In rheumatoid arthritis, leg ulceration can result from a variety of causes, including vasculitis, venous or arterial disease, pyoderma gangrenosum and trauma (**Fig 12.25**).

Atrophie blanche—This is commonly seen on the lower legs of patients with venous insufficiency. There are patches of shiny white scarred skin in which there are multiple tiny red capillary loops, oriented perpendicularly to the surface of the skin (**Fig 12.22**, *see also* Fig 17.21). Any scarring process on the leg results in a similar appearance. In most instances, because the injury is limited in extent, the resulting area of atrophie blanche type of change is much smaller than that found in venous insufficiency. This appearance is seen in biopsy scars and healed vasculitic ulcers and ecthyma (**Fig 12.8**).

Neoplastic ulcers

Primary skin tumours ulcerate as the tumour outgrows its blood supply or the fragile tumour is traumatised and then becomes secondarily infected (**Fig 12.27**). In these instances, ulceration occurs in association with other signs; in particular, features at the ulcer edge may enable a diagnosis to be made (*see* **Fig 12.20**). Squamous cell carcinoma arising within a chronic venous ulcer

DIAGNOSTIC TIPS AND PITFALLS

- Multiple disseminated ulcers with intervening areas of normal skin are seen in ecthyma, dermatitis artefacta, vasculitis and pyoderma gangrenosum

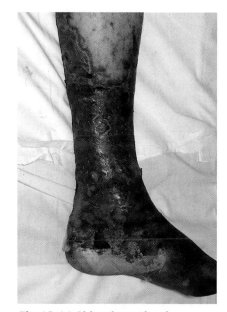

Fig 12.14 Skin ulceration in cryoglobulinaemia. This shows skin necrosis arising as the result of precipitation of cryoglobulin in skin venules at the sites of least blood flow in the skin. This man with a cryoglobulinaemia became cold while travelling on a plane. He developed areas of reticulate purpura, which became confluent and ulcerated (same patient as in 17.28)

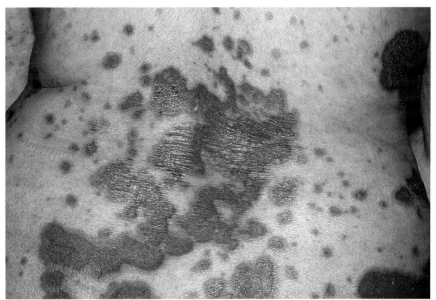

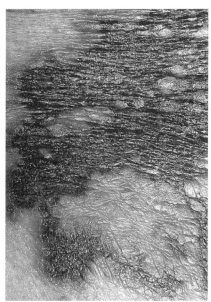

Fig 12.15

Fig 12.16

Fig 12.15, 12.16 Methotrexate skin ulceration. This patient's psoriasis had been partially controlled with methotrexate 7.5 mg weekly for 3 years, when she suddenly developed painful eroded psoriatic plaques (12.15). The eroded centre and purple edge of these plaques are well seen on close-up (12.16). There were no other features of methotrexate toxicity and the erosions healed 2 weeks later. The patient was restarted with methotrexate 5 mg weekly. No precipitating causes, including drug interactions, were identified

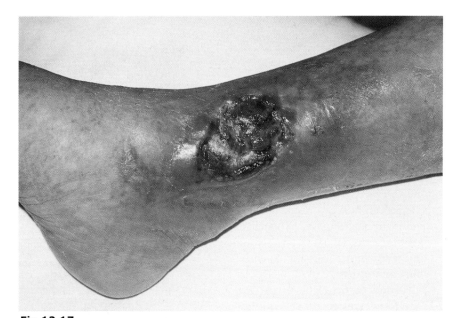

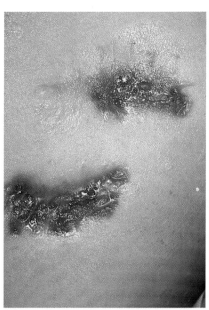

Fig 12.17

Fig 12.18

Fig 12.17, 12.18 Pyoderma gangrenosum. A typical ulcer in pyoderma gangrenosum (12.17) arising within a boggy-blue-coloured area of intense inflammation. This patient had a myelodysplastic syndrome: a well-recognised association. There are two large ulcers (12.18), one of which has recurred after a mistaken attempt to excise and suture the original ulcer. The patient has ulcerative colitis. The ulcer edge is not undermined as this lesion is beginning to heal. Note the beginnings of a cribriform scar (*see* 2.24) appearing in the lower ulcer

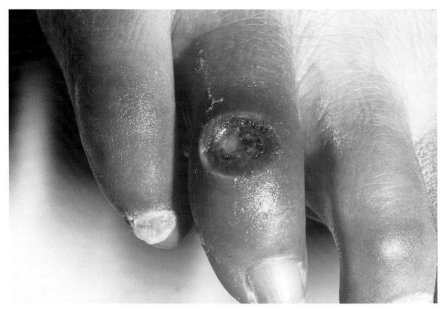

Fig 12.19 Punched-out ulcer. This occurred in a patient with severe nutritional deficiency due to anorexia nervosa and was associated with cyanosed extremities

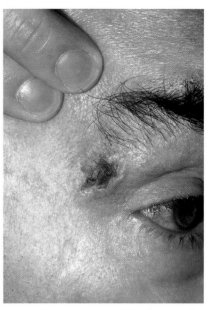

Fig 12.20 Rolled edge in basal cell carcinoma. There is a large basal-cell carcinoma on the corner of the eye, with a crusted centre and rolled edge. Gentle traction of the skin allows these features to be seen more easily

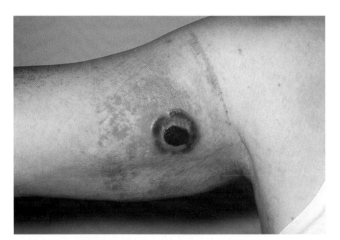

Fig 12.21 Caustic ulcer. A perfectly circular ring of ulceration on the arm, possibly due to contact with a caustic material on a contaminated work surface

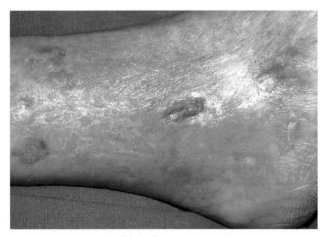

Fig 12.22 Atrophie blanche. There are extensive areas of scarring on this woman's leg, within which are multiple small dotted capillaries. In the centre is a small but painful ulcer

may sometimes be difficult to distinguish from an exuberant healing ulcer edge (Fig 12.28). A gradual increase in ulcer size in association with a raised and granulating ulcer edge should suggest the diagnosis (Fig 12.9).

Spontaneous ulceration in multiple skin secondaries is a very unusual event, although this is typical of late-stage mycosis fungoides (Fig 12.29). When patients present with multiple ulcerated skin nodules, the underlying condition is usually due to vasculitis, pyoderma gangrenosum or lymphomatoid granulomatosis (there is now evidence that the last is primarily a vasculitic lymphoma).

DIAGNOSTIC TIPS AND PITFALLS

- An ulcer with an undermined edge is characteristic of pyoderma gangrenosum and tropical ulcer

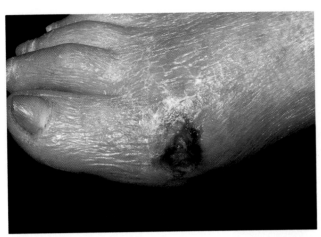

Fig 12.23 Arterial ulcer. A relatively small ulcer on the foot within an area of shiny skin due to chronic arterial disease. The ulcer is painful, well circumscribed and lacks any of the eczematous changes typical of venous ulcers

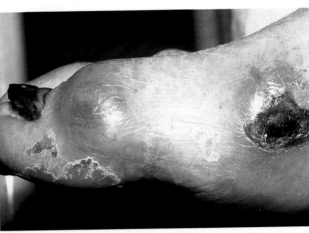

Fig 12.24 Ulcerated gouty nodule. In tophaceous gout, the tophi appear around finger and toe joints. These may ulcerate and can be confused with ischaemic or neuropathic ulcers. There are tophi of the interphalangeal and metatarsophalangeal joints. The latter has ulcerated. (Same patient as in 12.11)

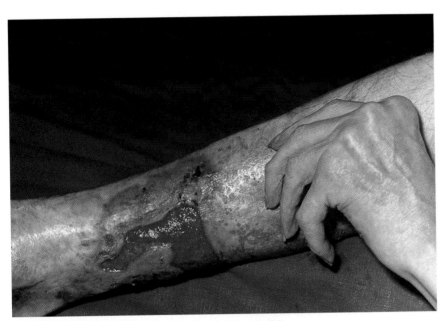

Fig 12.25 Leg ulceration in rheumatoid arthritis

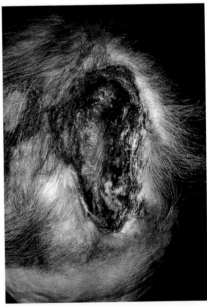

Fig 12.26 Temporal arteritis. Full-thickness scalp necrosis due to temporal arteritis (*photo courtesy of Dr Andrew Illchyshyn*)

Haematological

Vasculitic ulcer—Ulcers presenting in vasculitis always occur on a background of palpable purpuric change. In cryoglobulinaemia and other hyperviscosity syndromes, the purpuric changes may localise to the normal vascular markings on the leg, producing a reticulate broken livedo (*see* Figs 17.28 and 12.14).

Infection

Streptococcus pyogenes—Infections of the skin with *Streptococcus pyogenes* produce different clinical features depending on the depth of the infection.

> ### DIAGNOSTIC TIPS AND PITFALLS
>
> ● Leg ulceration in rheumatoid arthritis can result from rheumatoid vasculitis, venous or arterial disease, pyoderma gangrenosum or trauma

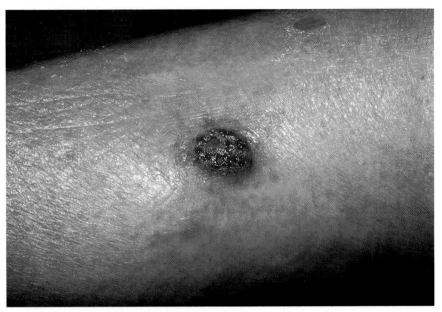

Fig 12.27 Bowen's disease on the leg. Intra-epidermal carcinoma of the skin below the knee is common in women after chronic sun exposure. The tumour often ulcerates

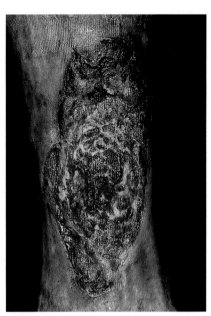

Fig 12.28 Marjolin's ulcer. Squamous cell carcinoma arising in a longstanding venous leg ulcer. This type of neoplastic change occurs only occasionally at this site

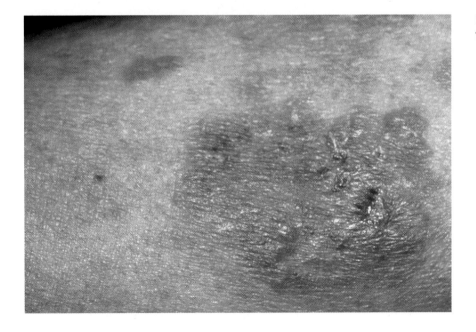

Fig 12.29 Ulcerated mycosis fungoides

Superficial or subcorneal infection results in impetigo (*see* Fig 7.4). Infection causing death of the entire epidermis results in ecthyma, which presents as crusting over an oozy punched-out ulcer (**Fig 12.8**).

Infection of the dermis produces extensive redness and swelling. If the dermal involvement is relatively superficial, the redness is well demarcated, as occurs in erysipelas (*see* Fig 17.1). Involvement of deeper dermal levels causes cellulitis with a more indistinct, irregular red border with swelling, blisters, and sometimes skin necrosis (**Fig 12.30**), lymphangitis and lymphadenopathy. *Streptococcus pyogenes* infections of the fat and deep fascia cause necrotising fasciitis (type II or streptococcal necrotising fasciitis,

229

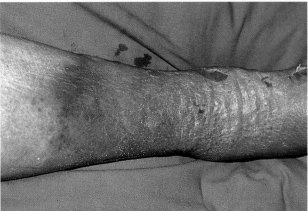

Fig 12.30

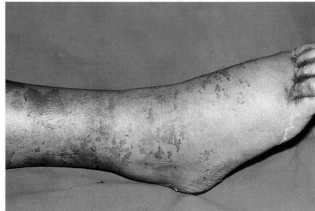

Fig 12.31

Fig 12.30, 12.31 Cellulitis before and after treatment. At presentation (12.30) there was oedema, redness obvious around the ankle but also extending to the knee, blistering and crusting. After 14 days of intravenous and oral antibiotic therapy (12.31), all signs of inflammation settled, but the oedema persists because of lymphatic damage caused by the infection. Fissures in the toe webs have been treated with magenta paint

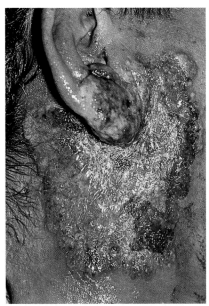

Fig 12.32 Pustular pyoderma. This man with myelofibrosis presented with sudden onset of a painful, pustular blistered plaque on the side of his neck. Culture and virology were negative. The histological changes were consistent with the superficial variant of pyoderma gangrenosum. The superficial and bullous variants of pyoderma gangrenosum are more commonly associated with underlying leukaemia and myeloproliferative disease

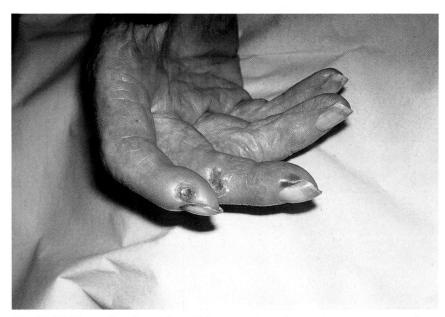

Fig 12.33 Fingertip ulceration. This occurs in patients who are unaware of thermal or mechanical injury. In the case illustrated, the patient has a sensory deficit, thenar muscle wasting and autonomic neuropathy, in a pattern suggestive of carpal tunnel syndrome; he also has peripheral vascular disease and persistently cold hands

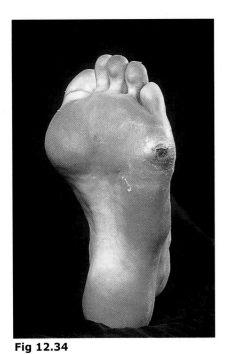

Fig 12.34

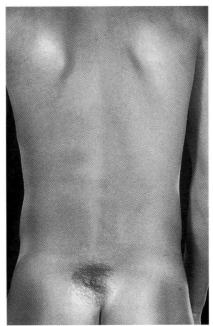

Fig 12.35

Figs 12.34, 12.35 Neuropathic foot ulcer and occult spina bifida. This young man presented with a painless ulcer on his foot (12.34). There was loss of sensation on the sole of his foot. Examination of his back revealed the faun tail, an indicator of occult spina bifida (12.35). Neuropathic ulcers on the foot occur on the ball of the big and little toes and the heels. A callosity forms which ulcerates, and the inactive ulcer has a noticeable rim of surrounding hyperkeratotic skin (*photo courtesy of Dr Adrian Ive and Dr Russell Hills*)

usually due to group A streptococci of M1 or M3 serotype). This results in an extremely painful, red, cellulitis-like swelling, which continues to spread despite appropriate antibiotics. Skin necrosis develops within hours or days, and patients may die unless the distinction with cellulitis is made and surgical debridement carried out. Streptococcal toxic shock (p 191) is an important complication with a poor prognosis. Similar acute necrotic or bullous changes can occur with other organisms such as *Vibrio* spp.

Necrotising infections—These are most common after surgical procedures, especially in elderly, diabetic or immunosuppressed patients. Most are due to a mixed aerobic and anaerobic infection. Meleney's synergistic gangrene usually occurs after abdominal operations and is due to a synergistic infection with *Staphylococcus aureus* and micro-aerophilic streptococcus. The wound becomes inflamed 2–3 weeks after the operation and then turns a dusky purple colour; subsequent necrosis causes extensive but superficial ulceration. Fournier's gangrene is a more aggressive disorder, with significant mortality; it affects the perineal region initially and is due to enterococci, *Bacteroides* spp. and others.

Gas gangrene—This may be either clostridial or non-clostridial. This results in extensive swelling, skin necrosis and little pain and has the potential for involvement of fat, muscle and bone. Gas may only be detected on radiography, and surgical debridement is required. The clostridial type was historically most commonly due to contaminated traumatic wounds in which devitalised tissue allowed the growth of *Clostridium* species (usually *Clostridium perfringens*) to cause localised cellulitis, with potential to progress into healthy muscle and fascial planes. Non-traumatic clostridial gas gangrene due to *Clostridium septicum* is becoming numerically more important in many countries, as a rapidly progressive infection associated with abdominal surgery or immune suppression. Necrotic ulcers and acute cellulitic legs should always be felt for crepitus, especially if bullae are present, and the patient is unwell and pyrexial.

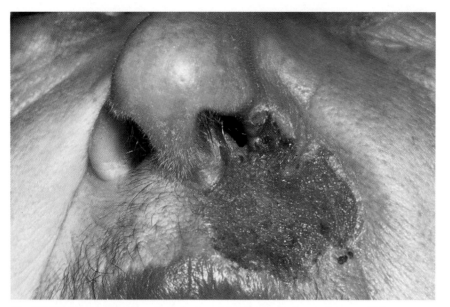

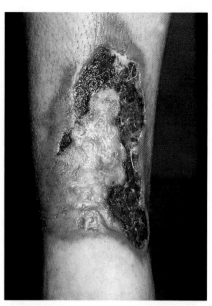

Fig 12.36 Neurotrophic ulcer in trophic trigeminal syndrome. This woman developed an ulcer on her upper lip and the side of her nose, due to constant picking and scratching at these sites, after destruction of her trigeminal ganglion for chronic facial pain (*see also* 2.46)

Fig 12.37 Ulcerated necrobiosis lipoidica. The ulcer is arising within a plaque of atrophic yellowish skin characteristic of necrobiosis lipoidica (*see also* 11.10)

Diabetes

Leg ulcers in diabetics arise from a combination of neuropathy, infection and ischaemia. Necrobiosis lipoidica occurs in approximately 0.3% of diabetics, but the likelihood of a patient with necrobiosis lipoidica having diabetes varies considerably between studies. Taking into account those with later development of diabetes, the correct figure is probably between 25% and 50%. Necrobiosis is caused by degeneration of the dermal collagen, although this is probably the consequence of a diabetic microangiopathy. The consequences for the skin are that the involved area of skin may ulcerate (**Fig 12.37**), and the ulcer develops within an area of abnormal skin, with the characteristic atrophy and yellow change due to subcutaneous fat becoming visible through the damaged collagen (*see* Fig 11.10).

13 Blisters and vesicles

INTRODUCTION

Blisters and vesicles are circumscribed, elevated swellings that contain free fluid. Blisters (**Fig 13.1**) are larger than vesicles (**Fig. 13.2**), although there is no general agreement about when a large vesicle becomes a blister. Arbitrarily, different authors define blisters as those greater than 5 or 10 mm in diameter. In practice, vesicles are generally only a few millimetres in diameter.

The shape and site distribution of blisters may provide a clue to the cause. Linear blisters (**Fig 13.3**) are usually due to contact-allergic reactions to plants, when the patient has brushed against the causative leaf or stem. In the

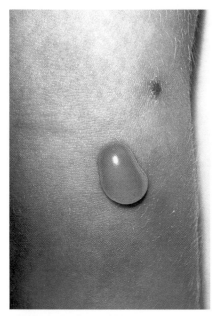

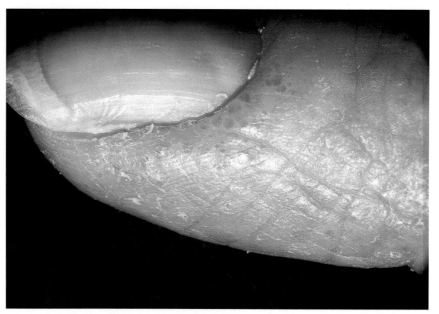

Fig 13.1 Bullous insect bite reaction. There is an adjacent erythematous papule caused by an earlier bite. Blistering reactions are common on the lower leg in children, especially after mosquito and horsefly bites

Fig 13.2 Small vesicles in the periungual skin. Acute eczema at any site may produce tiny intra-epidermal blisters due to intra-epidermal oedema or spongiosis. These blisters are fragile and rupture easily, surviving only on sites where the stratum corneum is thick, e.g. the palm or sole

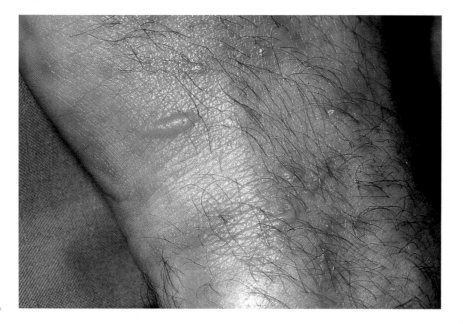

Fig 13.3 Linear blister. Contact-allergic reactions to plants, here to ivy, produce typical linear lesions, which may blister where the leaves brush against the skin

DIAGNOSTIC TIPS
AND PITFALLS

- Blisters or bullae are essentially the same as vesicles but larger

USA, poison ivy dermatitis is a common cause. In the UK, other ivys and the flowering indoor plant *Primula obconica* are possible causes. Giant hogweed causes a reaction on sun-exposed parts of the body; this may have a streaky pattern on the arms due to handling the hogweed or a more 'buckshot' pattern on the trunk in patients (usually young men) who have used a strimmer to clear rough pasture while stripped to the waist on a hot sunny day.

Blisters arise from a split within the epidermis or at the junction of the epidermis and dermis (**Fig 13.4**). The level of the split varies with different blistering disease (*see* below) and also largely determines the appearance of the blisters produced. Determining the level of the split on the basis of the physical signs is often a helpful indicator of the likely differential diagnosis.

DIAGNOSTIC TIPS
AND PITFALLS

- Blisters develop either from within the epidermis (intra-epidermal) or at the junction of the epidermis and dermis (subepidermal); these two main blister types can usually be distinguished clinically

234

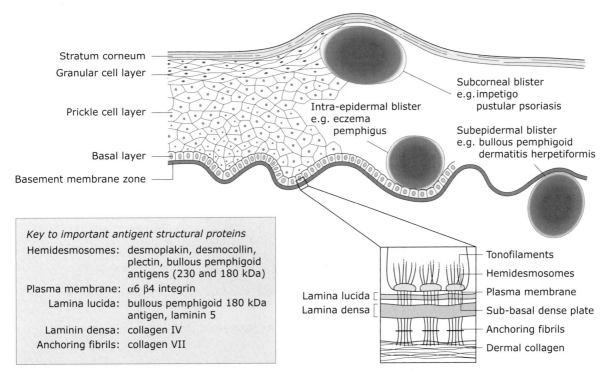

Fig 13.4 Subcorneal, intra-epidermal and subepidermal blister position in the skin. Subcorneal blisters are covered by the stratum corneum and thus are very fragile, surviving as blisters only in areas with a thick stratum corneum. Intra-epidermal or deeper epidermal blisters arise because of keratinocyte death (e.g. herpes simplex), oedema (e.g. eczema) or loss of intercellular adhesion (e.g. pemphigus); they may be multilocular and again usually only survive at sites with a thick stratum corneum. Subepidermal blisters occur following loss of adhesion between the epidermis and dermis (e.g. bullous pemphigoid) or dermal inflammation (e.g. dermatitis herpetiformis); because they have the thickest roof, they are the most robust

Table 13.1 Comparison of intra-epidermal and subepidermal blister clinical features

Presentation	Intra-epidermal	Subepidermal
Fragility	Thin roof, therefore fragile and may present as erosions with crusting, except on areas with thick stratum corneum, e.g. palm and sole	Tense robust blisters, but may present as erosions on areas of trauma, e.g. subepidermal blisters on the dorsum of the hands in porphyria cutanea tarda (13.39).
Blood content	Usually not haemorrhagic, but this may occur on dependent sites, e.g. legs, especially if there is noticeable upper dermal inflammation or oedema, e.g. eczema	Haemorrhage more likely to occur (13.5)
Blister spreading	Blistering, or more properly splitting of the epidermis, may be produced on apparently normal surrounding skin by gentle rubbing —a positive Nikolsky's sign (13.6–13.8)	Nikolsky's sign is negative. In bullous pemphigoid blisters, and most other blistering disorders, the blister may be extended into surrounding tissue by gently pressing on the blister roof (13.9, 13.10)
Morphology	Multilocular blisters in eczema (1.7), herpes zoster (13.16) and herpes simplex (2.26)	Generally unilocular, but occasionally multilocular blisters on the palms in bullous pemphigoid

There are no pathognomonic physical signs that enable a firm distinction to be made between subepidermal and intra-epidermal blisters, although the observer will be able to make a reasonably confident diagnosis based on the features described in **Table 13.1**. In general, a subepidermal blister is robust, fluid-filled and, possibly, blood-stained (**Fig 13.5**). An intra-epidermal blister by contrast has a thin roof and is therefore fragile and may not present as an intact blister (**Figs 13.6–13.8**) but as either shallow erosions or crusting. Since

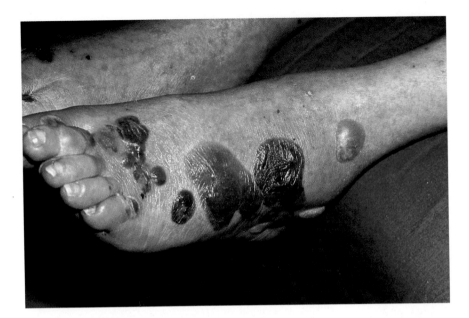

Fig 13.5 Blood-filled pemphigoid blister. Subepidermal blisters characteristically become blood-stained because they are formed at the junction with the dermis adjacent to dermal blood vessels. Bleeding into intra-epidermal blisters is often seen on the lower limbs

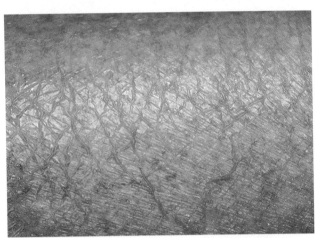

Fig 13.6

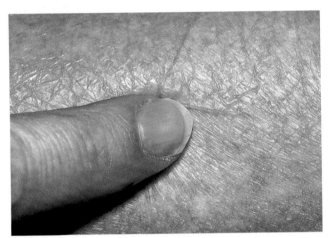

Fig 13.7

Figs 13.6–13.8 Nikolsky's sign. Shearing force from a fingertip applied to intact skin has produced separation of the epidermis from the underlying dermis. This sign can be seen in pemphigus, staphylococcal scalded skin syndrome or toxic epidermal necrolysis. Ruptured blisters in these conditions have a fragile 'rolled-up' appearance of the epidermal remnant at the edge of erosions (*see also* 13.14, 13.20, 13.43)

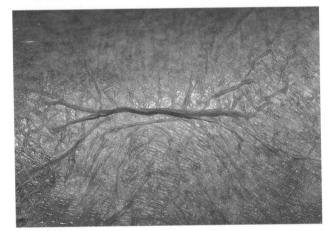

Fig 13.8

intra-epidermal blisters have the dermo-epidermal junction basement membrane between the blister and the dermal blood vessels, they are not usually haemorrhagic. These features are most noticeable when the split is very superficial, as in a subcorneal blister, compared with deeper levels of splitting within the epidermis, as occurs in pemphigus vulgaris.

Unfortunately, there are exceptions; intra-epidermal blisters on the palms and soles can be thick enough to withstand trauma, and bleeding may occur into eczematous (intra-epidermal) blisters, particularly on the lower limbs. A further complication is that the causative process also influences the signs; for example, infection also produces inflammation, which contributes physical signs that are not directly related to the pattern of blistering.

The colour of a blister may vary according to the cause, depth in the skin and duration. Blisters that contain neutrophils (pus) may be slightly greyish and cloudy or opaque initially, later turning yellow or green (*see* Chapter 14). However, a cloudy greyish colour of a blister may also occur due to epidermal cell death in the roof of the blister. This can be distinguished by puncturing the blister to see the fluid content. For example, blisters in vasculitis or erythema multiforme are often cloudy at an early stage, but this is due to epidermal damage, and the fluid content may be translucent.

Blisters can be divided according to the level of the split and in this chapter will be grouped as subcorneal, deeper intra-epidermal and subepidermal. Within each category of blister depth, there are several mechanisms for splitting. For example, intra-epidermal splits may occur due to faulty desmosomal connections between keratinocytes (in turn due to inherited defects or immunological damage), cellular damage (from drugs, bacterial toxins or physical damage), loss of nutrients (various causes of vascular obstruction) and others.

SUBCORNEAL BLISTERS

Subcorneal blisters are superficial blisters below the stratum corneum. Pemphigus variants that cause this level of split are discussed on p. 251–252.

Miliaria

Eccrine sweat ducts may become blocked, usually due to maceration induced by increased humidity; if increased sweating occurs, then multiple tiny fragile blisters containing the retained sweat are produced (**Fig 13.11**). These burst when touched with a finger and may be itchy (*see Fig* 14.16). Tiny clear miliaria (miliaria crystallina) are due to blockage in the acrosyringium

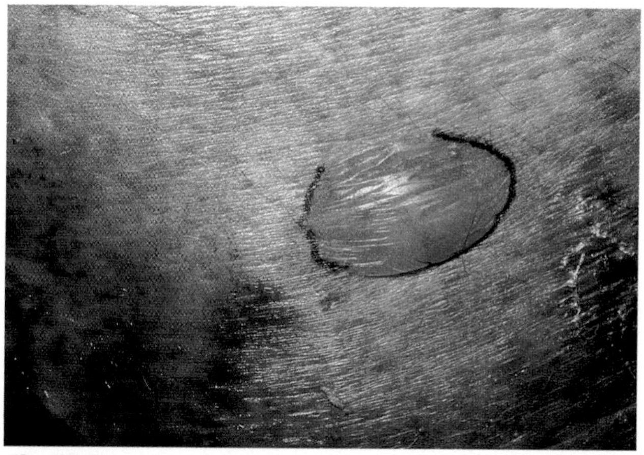

DIAGNOSTIC TIPS AND PITFALLS
• A cloudy greyish-coloured blister either may have a cloudy fluid content (early development of pus) or may be this colour due to epidermal death in the blister roof—these two can be distinguished by puncturing the blister

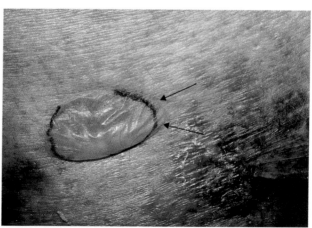

Fig 13.9

Fig 13.10

Figs 13.9, 13.10 Blister spreading by pressure in bullous pemphigoid. This can be shown with blisters at any level, in this case a subepidermal blister in bullous pemphigoid. After gentle pressure on the surface of an initially tense blister (13.9), the margin of the blister has spread laterally (arrows), and the increased space available for its fluid means that the blister is less tense (13.10). This occurs in virtually all blistering conditions and is not equivalent to Nikolsky's sign

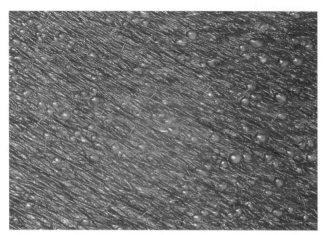

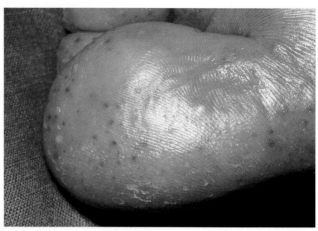

Fig 13.11 Miliaria. Widespread multiple tiny clear sweat filled miliaria appeared on the recently suntanned skin of this man after strenuous exercise

Fig 13.12 Early lesions of pustular psoriasis. In pustular psoriasis of the palms and soles, the early lesions may appear as tiny brownish vesicles, as shown here on the great toe. Small pustules are also visible

(the intra-epidermal portion of the sweat duct). Deeper obstruction may cause more inflamed lesions (miliaria rubra, 'prickly heat') or even pustules (*see* Fig 6.10).

Pustular psoriasis

Pustular psoriasis, as its name suggests, usually presents as a pustular eruption (see p. 237) rather than as blisters. However, pompholyx-type vesicles (**Fig 13.12**) can be seen in early lesions, especially in the localised variant that affects thicker skin areas of palms and soles.

Subcorneal pustular dermatosis

Subcorneal pustular dermatosis characteristically causes large pus-filled blisters, usually arranged in a complete or partial ring shape. Individual blisters may contain a pus level (**Fig 13.13**). This sign is also occasionally seen in bullous impetigo and bullous pemphigoid (**Fig 13.23**).

Staphylococcal scalded skin syndrome

In staphylococcal scalded skin syndrome (**Fig 13.14**), extensive blistering occurs with loss of sheets of skin. The phage type II staphylococcus is not found in the blisters but at some distant site (*see* p. 250). The subcorneal level of split in this disorder is important as it is clinically similar to toxic epidermal necrolysis (**Fig 13.43**), but the latter has an epidermal split due to necrosis of keratinocytes at all levels of the epidermis. Distinguishing between these two disorders has important therapeutic indications. A similar pattern of epidermal splitting occurs in toxic shock syndrome.

Impetigo

In impetigo, the blister roof is composed of stratum corneum only, so that it is extremely fragile and ruptures easily, producing a golden yellow–brown crust (*see* Fig 7.4). When present, the blisters are clear initially (*see* Fig 14.8) but later become turbid. The blister fluid oozes out from damaged blisters as a honey-coloured exudate (**Fig 13.15**). Other infections such as candidiasis may also cause subcorneal splitting.

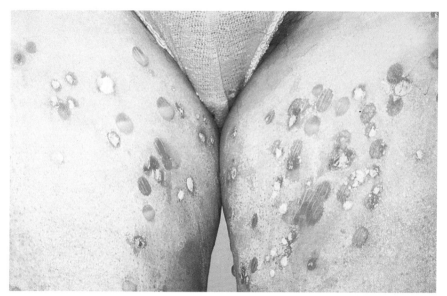

Fig 13.13 Subcorneal pustular dermatosis. This causes multiple large blisters with a well-defined pus level. Neutrophils sink to the bottom of the blister fluid with gravity. Pus levels may also occur in bullous pemphigoid (13.23), pemphigus and impetigo but are much less striking in these conditions

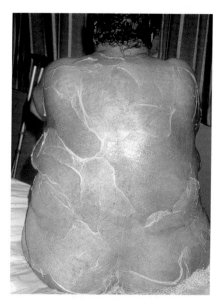

Fig 13.14 Staphylococcal scalded skin syndrome. This is an unusual event in a non-immunosuppressed adult. This was related to an infected wound, and the distinction from toxic epidermal necrolysis (a type of drug reaction, *see* 13.43) was crucial as the patient was taking antibiotics

DEEPER INTRA-EPIDERMAL BLISTERS

Deeper intra-epidermal blisters may arise owing to several mechanisms. Some, such as the acantholytic disorders and epidermolysis bullosa simplex, are discussed later (p. 253–255).

Friction blisters

Friction blisters may occur on the hands, for example after playing squash for the first time, and are caused by necrosis of epidermal keratinocytes.

Insect bites

Insect bites usually occur with surrounding inflammation and are arranged in groups (*see* Figs 2.25 and 15.8).

Eczema

With the exception of seborrhoeic eczema, all types of acute eczema may produce blisters (**Fig 13.2** and **13.41**, *see also* Fig 1.7).

Herpes simplex and herpes zoster

Herpesviruses infect and damage keratinocytes, which become enlarged ('ballooned') and separated from each other ('acantholysis'). Herpes simplex (*see* Fig 2.26) and herpes zoster blisters are multilocular initially (**Fig 13.16**) and usually pustular (*see* Fig 14.15). The remaining fragile epidermal strands break resulting in a unilocular blister. Umbilication is the result of skin necrosis caused by central vascular occlusion.

A further useful sign in evaluating herpes zoster is Hutchinson's sign. Involvement of the dorsum and sidewall of the nose in facial zoster signifies nasociliary nerve involvement, which is associated with ocular

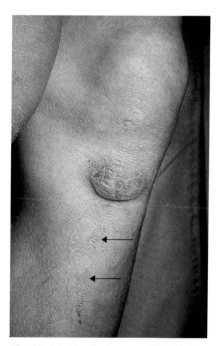

Fig 13.15 Staphylococcal impetigo blister. The blister roof is only as thick as the stratum corneum, so blisters are rarely seen. The blister has burst, and the characteristic honey-coloured exudate can be seen trickling down the leg (arrows)

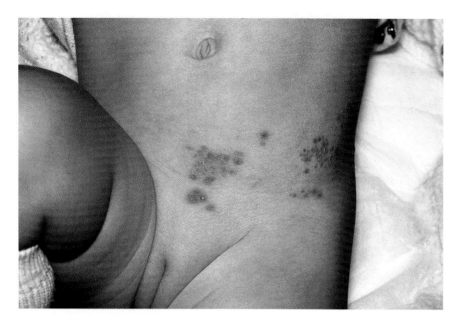

**Fig 13.16 Herpes zoster
(shingles) in an 11-month-old
child.** Babies may develop shingles
without evidence of preceding
chicken-pox; in these circumstances,
it is assumed that infection has taken
place *in utero* after the first trimester.
Here, the mother's other daughter
had chicken-pox 1 week before
delivery of this child

lesions. (Note also the sign described by Hutchinson in relation to longitudinal melanonychia, Chapter 19.)

Chicken-pox may present with scattered solitary blisters arising on an erythematous patch of skin; these rapidly become cloudy and umbilicated, and then the blister roof becomes necrotic (**Figs 13.17** and **13.18**).

Hand-foot-and-mouth disease

Hand-foot-and-mouth disease (coxsackie A) causes painful white vesicles with surrounding erythema on the fingers and toes (**Fig 13.19**) and associated small multiple painful mouth ulcers. The blisters are not multiocular, and the Tzanck test (*see* p. 74) gives negative results.

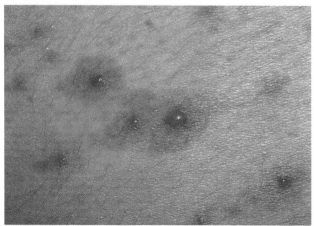

Fig 13.17

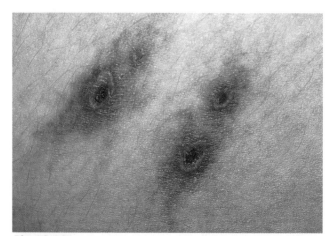

Fig 13.18

Figs 13.17, 13.18 Evolution of chicken-pox blisters in a pregnant woman. The initial blisters show the characteristic 'raindrop on a rose petal' appearance (13.17), followed 6 days later by blister necrosis (13.18). In the first trimester, chicken-pox infections may cause severe fetal abnormalities. Infection during the second trimester leads to undetected fetal chicken-pox, and these babies may develop herpes zoster without apparently having had chicken-pox (*see* 13.16). Maternal chicken-pox occurring a few days before delivery, when infection can present without the baby deriving benefit from maternal immunity, is associated with 20% mortality

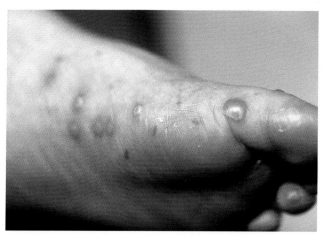

Fig 13.19 Hand-foot-and-mouth skin and oral lesions. Tiny painful cloudy blisters appear on the fingers, toes and mucous membranes of the mouth

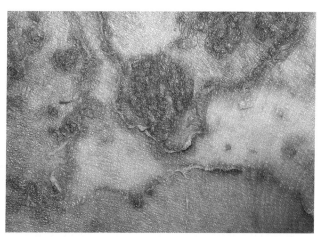

Fig 13.20 Pemphigus vulgaris. There are extensive erosions, crusts and white areas of dead blister roof on the side of this man's trunk. Owing to the fragility of the thin and damaged epidermal roof, intact blisters are relatively uncommon in this condition

Table 13.2 Comparison of pemphigoid and pemphigus

Bullous pemphigoid	Pemphigus vulgaris
Approximately 10 times more common than pemphigus vulgaris	Rare
Subepidermal blisters	Intra-epidermal blisters
70–90-year age group	60–70-year age group
Mucous membrane involvement 30%	Mucous membrane involvement 80%, and may occur several months before skin changes develop
Tense blister (13.24), blood filled (13.5)	Fragile blisters, erosions common (13.20)
Arise on urticated skin (13.26–13.27)	Arise on normal skin
Skin immunofluorescence: basement membrane zone linear IgG and C3	Immunofluorescence: intercellular IgG and C3
Nikolsky's sign negative. Blisters may be spread by gently pressing on the blister roof (13.9, 13.10)	Nikolsky's sign positive (13.6–13.8)

Pemphigus vulgaris

Pemphigus vulgaris causes widespread fragile blisters with erosions (**Fig 13.20**) and oral involvement (**Table 13.2** and **Fig 13.48**).

SUBEPIDERMAL BLISTERS

Burn blisters

In first-degree burns, the upper layers of the epidermis are destroyed. In second-degree burns, subepidermal blisters occur, and the upper layers of the dermis show heat-induced dermal necrosis. Blisters in coma or after prolonged pressure are similar.

DIAGNOSTIC TIPS AND PITFALLS

- A subepidermal blister is robust, fluid-filled and, possibly, blood-stained
- An intra-epidermal blister has a fragile thin roof and therefore bursts easily leaving either shallow erosions or crusting

241

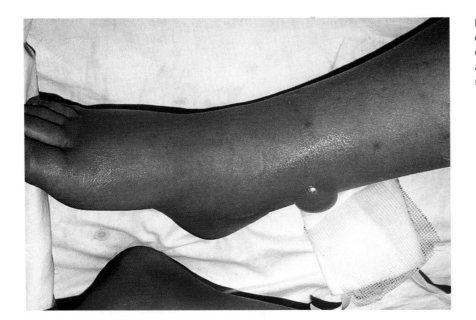

Oedema blisters

Oedema blisters occur in severe dependent oedema of the leg and are usually seen in people with right-sided heart failure and mild venous insufficiency. Rapid development of oedema, rather than the degree of swelling, seems to be the relevant factor. Large clear unilocular water-filled blisters appear on the oedematous lower limbs (**Fig 13.21**).

Dermatitis herpetiformis

Dermatitis herpetiformis (**Fig 13.22**) is an intensely itchy condition in which subepidermal blisters are occasionally seen if the patient can be prevented from scratching them (*see* Fig 15.3). When present, they are usually small, but occasionally, large tense blisters are seen, and these may be arranged in an annular pattern. Characteristic sites of lesions of dermatitis herpetiformis include the elbows, knees, buttocks and scalp. Skin immunofluorescence shows diagnostic granular IgA. The symptoms respond within days to oral dapsone in virtually all cases and in months to years to rigid adherence to a gluten-free diet in approximately 60% of patients.

Bullous pemphigoid

The main features of this disorder are listed in **Table 13.2** (*see also* p. 251).

Pemphigoid ('herpes') gestationis

Pemphigoid ('herpes') gestationis is a rare blistering disease similar to bullous pemphigoid in appearance, which occurs in pregnancy (**Fig. 13.28**). Although previously called herpes gestationis, it is not due to a viral infection.

Linear IgA disease

The name linear IgA disease relates to the appearance seen on direct immunofluorescence of clinically normal skin. It occurs in adults and children, approximately 50% of whom have associated mucous membrane lesions. In children, in whom the condition is also termed chronic bullous

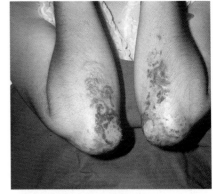

Fig 13.22 Dermatitis herpetiformis blisters. Typical distribution of multiple tiny blisters, most of which—being intensely itchy—have been destroyed by scratching. Haemorrhage into blisters is not uncommon in dermatitis herpetiformis (*see* 15.3), but these lesions are more inflamed and haemorrhagic than usual

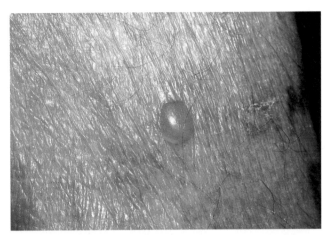

Fig 13.23 Bullous pemphigoid blister with pus level.
The leucocytes in a blister may settle, forming a collection
of pus at the bottom. Similar features are seen in other
leucocyte-containing blistering diseases (13.12, *see also*
14.15 and 14.16)

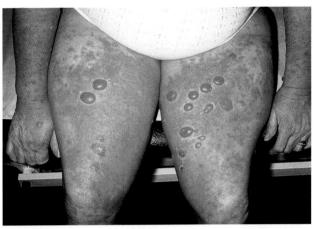

Fig 13.24 Bullous pemphigoid. Typical appearance of
multiple tense unilocular blisters, usually up to about 20
mm in diameter and arising on an inflammatory
background. The fluid content is a clear straw colour, but
haemorrhagic blisters are often present (*see* 13.5)

dermatosis of childhood, blisters are commonly present on the genitalia (**Fig
13.29**). There is no associated gluten enteropathy. Several drugs, notably
vancomycin, may cause linear IgA disease. Characteristically, blisters appear
in a ring shape, producing rosettes or clusters of blisters at the margin of a
lesion (**Fig 13.30**).

Erythema multiforme

Blisters may be due to both subepidermal oedema and epidermal necrosis and
thus may show various features. There may be large unilocular blisters or just
small blisters within a target-shaped lesion (**Fig 13.31**). Target-shaped lesions
are not unique to erythema multiforme (*see* p. 16). Blisters occur as a result
of epidermal death, so the blister roof may appear whitish and opaque. Oral,
genital and ocular mucous membranes may be affected, and if these features
predominate, the term Stevens–Johnson syndrome is used to describe this
variant of erythema multiforme (**Figs 13.32** and **13.33**). Toxic epidermal

DIAGNOSTIC TIPS AND PITFALLS

- Palmar blisters, other than
  those due to frictional injury
  or in early childhood, should
  suggest the possibility of
  erythema multiforme

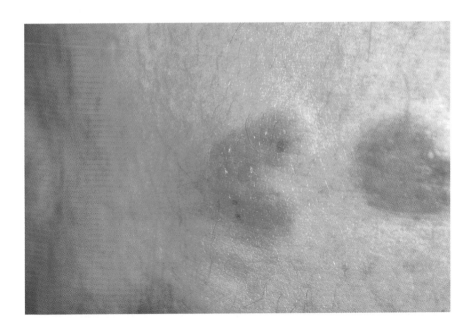

**Fig 13.25 Bullous pemphigoid
urticated plaques.** In bullous
pemphigoid, blisters arise on plaques
of urticated skin

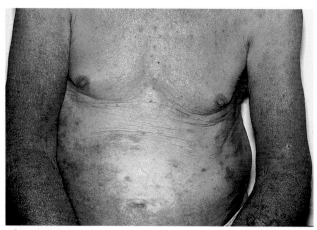

Fig 13.26

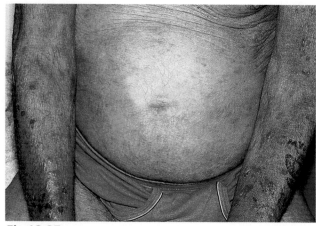

Fig 13.27

Figs 13.26, 13.27 Bullous pemphigoid in evolution. At the urticarial stage (13.26), the patient has widespread itchy red urticated areas on his arms and abdomen. Thirteen days later (13.27), blisters have appeared in these urticated plaques on his arms, but lesions on his abdomen have responded to potent topical steroids

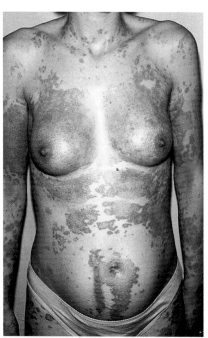

Fig 13.28 Pemphigoid ('herpes') gestationis. Six months into this woman's first pregnancy, she developed an extensive itchy blistering eruption. Blisters can just be seen on her lower arms and legs. Her rash was controlled by oral steroids, and she delivered a healthy normal child at term

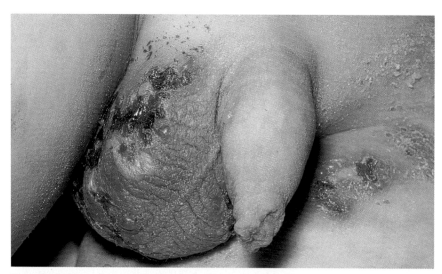

Fig 13.29 Chronic bullous dematosis of childhood. Genital and public lesions are typical. This child had been treated for several months for herpes simplex and impetigo. The child responded to sulfopyndine, with no recurrences after 12 months

necrolysis is another variant of erythema multiforme in which generalised erythema is associated with widespread skin peeling with or without mucous membrane involvement (**Fig 13.43**). Causes are listed in **Table 13.3**. Fixed drug eruptions have a similar histology in the acute phase.

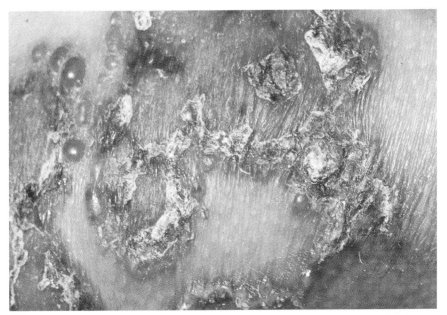

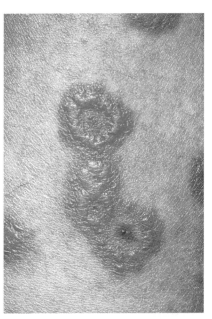

Fig 13.30 Adult linear IgA disease. Blisters appearing in a ring around the central crusted lesion, producing the 'cluster of jewels' appearance. Similar appearances are seen in dermatitis herpetiformis and pemphigoid (herpes) gestationis (*photo courtesy of Dr S Natarajan*)

Fig 13.31 Erythema multiforme. Typical target or iris lesions comprise a flat purpuric centre, a surrounding blister and a rim of erythema

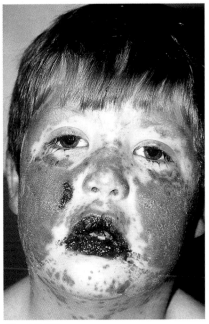

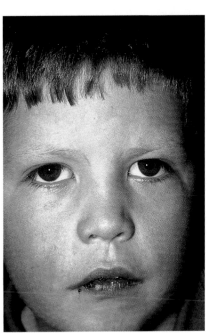

Fig 13.32

Fig 13.33

Figs 13.32, 13.33 Stevens–Johnson syndrome. This 8-year-old boy developed a severe mucous membrane type erythema multiforme reaction to cotrimoxazole (13.32). Sixteen days later, after the drug was stopped and with symptomatic therapy only, the rash had cleared (13.33)

DIAGNOSTIC TIPS AND PITFALLS

- Grouped blisters with an annular arrangement occur particularly in linear IgA disease and bullous pemphigoid

Others

Subepidermal blisters may occur in other conditions, such as porphyria and pseudoporphyria (*see* p. 253).

Table 13.3 Causes of erythema multiforme

Infections
Viral—herpes simplex (30%), hepatitis A and B, orf, others
Bacterial—streptococcal, tuberculosis, yersinia
Other—mycoplasma

Drugs (30%)
Antibiotics—sulphonamides, penicillin, tetracyclines, cephalosporins, isonicotinic acid hydrazide
Central nervous system—anticonvulsants, barbiturates
Other—non-steroidal anti-inflammatory agents, chlorpropamide, quinine, thiouracil, oestrogens

Other
Lupus erythematosus, neoplasia including leukaemia, pelvic tumours, after X-irradiation of tumours, inflammatory bowel
    disease, sarcoid

Idiopathic
Approximately 30% of cases are never associated with any particular cause, but many of these are probably related to occult
    herpes simplex

SKIN ABNORMALITIES THAT MAY BE CONFUSED WITH BLISTERS

Urticaria and weals

Patients often refer to weals (*see* Fig 1.5) as blisters, and it is important to establish that the supposed blisters actually contain clear fluid.

Lymphangioma

Lymphangioma presents as dilated lymphatic vessels, which appear on the skin as multilocular and intermittently blood-filled 'frogspawn'-like lesions (*see* Fig 9.70). Unlike blisters, they are fixed in position.

Myxoid cyst

Myxoid cysts are soft, dome-shaped lesions, usually on the finger or toe (**Fig 13.34**), which exude gelatinous material when punctured. They are unlikely to be confused with blisters because of their fixed position.

Cutaneous mucinosis

In focal cutaneous mucinosis, there are soft mucinous deposits; similar areas occasionally occur in pretibial myxoedema. Pressure on the surface of the lesion makes it compress like a semi-tense blister due to the semi-fluid mucin content (the 'waterbag sign,' **Fig 13.35**).

CONSEQUENCES OF BLISTER FORMATION

Erosions

As blisters burst, the underlying dermis or deeper layers of the epidermis are exposed as superficial erosions. Disorders of superficial blistering usually heal without scarring. Re-epithelialisation may occur from follicular remnants (**Fig 13.36**).

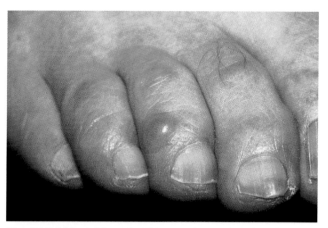

Fig 13.34 Myxoid cyst. This may be confused with a blister. If punctured, gelatinous clear fluid will drain from it. A connection between this cyst and the adjacent interphalangeal joint can be shown by the appearance of dye in the cyst after injecting dye into the joint space

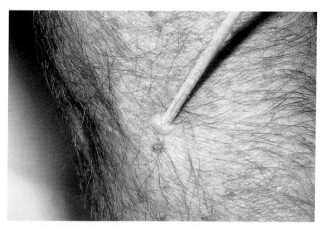

Fig 13.35 The 'waterbag sign'. The waterbag sign in focal cutaneous mucinosis, mimicking a blister. Pressure on the lesion makes it compress like a semi-tense blister (*photo courtesy of Dr GM White*)

Scarring

Scarring after blister formation is seen in cicatricial pemphigoid, porphyria, lichen planus, discoid lupus erythematosus, some types of epidermolysis bullosa and in secondarily infected blisters. These are described below.

Cicatricial pemphigoid

Cicatricial pemphigoid leaves areas of scarring alopecia on the scalp (**Fig 13.37**, *see also* Fig 18.26). Mucous membrane involvement produces oesophageal strictures, vulval and penile adhesions and adhesions between the conjunctiva and lower eyelid known as symblepharon (**Fig 13.38**).

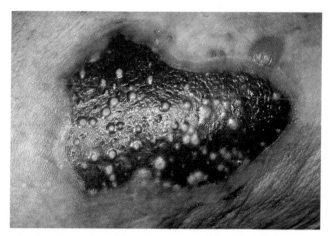

Fig 13.36 Healing in bullous pemphigoid erosion. Islands of regenerating skin are visible within the erosion as epidermal cells migrate upwards from follicles to colonise the eroded area

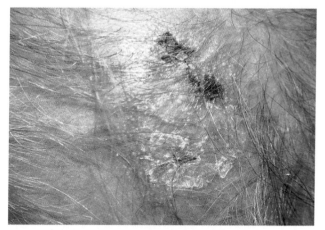

Fig 13.37 Cicatricial pemphigoid of the scalp showing scarring alopecia and milia. Scarring following blistering is a feature of the Brunsting–Perry type of bullous pemphigoid. Blisters may never be noticed by the patient. Such lesions are characteristically limited to the scalp or forehead and are not associated with mucous membrane scarring. This lesion has healed with milia formation (*see also* 18.26)

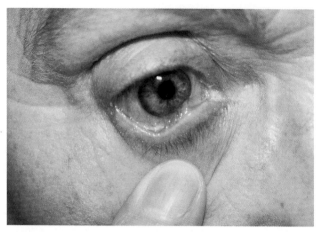

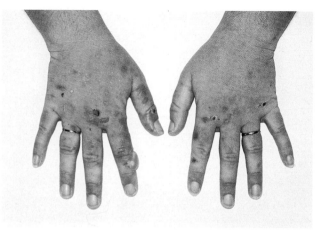

Fig 13.38 Cicatricial pemphigoid symblepharon. In cicatricial or scarring mucous membrane pemphigoid, lesions may be restricted to the eyes, genitalia and upper digestive tract. This woman has adhesions between the lower lid and conjunctiva of the eye

Fig 13.39 Porphyria cutanea tarda blisters. There are several large tense blisters, some of which are blood-stained, on the dorsum of this woman's hands. Areas of scaring and milia formation can also be seen. The provoking factor was excessive alcohol consumption (*photo courtesy of Dr Peter Farr*)

Porphyria

In porphyria, scarring occurs at sites of blister formation (**Fig 13.39**). These are usually seen on the back of the hand and are associated with skin fragility in the case of porphyria cutanea tarda. Scarring also occurs in some porphyrias in which blisters do not develop (**Fig 13.52**).

Inflammatory disorders of the basement membrane zone

Scarring is seen in discoid lupus erythematosus (*see* Fig 12.1), lichen planus (especially scalp or nailfolds) and dermatomyositis (*see* Fig 18.17).

Scarring epidermolysis bullosa

Epidermolysis bullosa (*see also* p 253) is the term applied to a group of disorders that (with the exception of epidermolysis bullosa acquisita, p 255) are all due to a variety of inherited structural defects of the skin in the region of the hemidesmosomes and basement membrane zone (**Fig 13.4**). The types that produce scarring are those with splitting at or below the level of the lamina lucida. The most scarring is seen in the 'dystrophic EB' types, which are due to defects in the anchoring fibrils (made of collagen VII) of the sublamina densa. This may be very disabling, producing a scarred mitten over the hands (**Fig 13.40**).

Secondarily infected blisters

Excoriation and infection of an erosion can lead to scarring in any condition if it is left untreated.

Milia

Milia are tiny white intradermal epidermal-lined cysts of keratin. Formed from sweat ducts and gradually extruded through the skin, they are commonly encountered in the healing phase of porphyria (**Fig 13.51**),

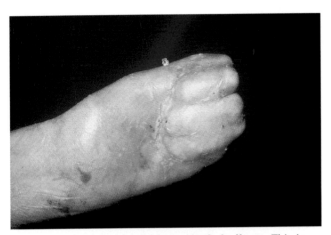

Fig 13.40 Dystrophic epidermolysis bullosa. This is the typical scarred mitten of this condition. Finger separation has been lost completely in this patient's left hand. The fingers, here, are clenched in a fist with the palm side towards the camera and the thumb uppermost. The finger bones can be identified only on radiography (*photo courtesy of Dr Colin Munro*)

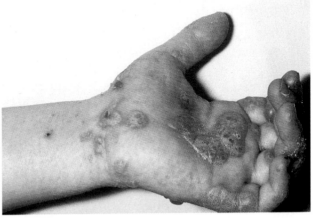

Fig 13.41 Pompholyx of the palms. Large fluid-filled blisters occur on the palms and soles. This pattern of eczema is usually endogenous. Occasionally, acute contact allergic reactions may present in this way

pemphigoid (**Fig 13.37**) and epidermolysis bullosa aquisita (**Fig 13.56**). They are also common in normal skin (*see* Fig 6.48).

MECHANISMS OF BLISTER FORMATION

Oedema of the epidermis

In eczema, multiple areas of spongiosis or intra-epidermal oedema join up to become small vesicles (**Fig 13.2**) but may become very large, for example on the palms in pompholyx eczema (**Fig 13.41** *see also* Fig 1.7).

Epidermal cell necrosis and epidermal cell damage

In viral infections of the epidermis, such as herpes simplex and herpes zoster, viral growth occurs within the epidermal cell, with subsequent cell death. Cells infected in this way swell (balloon degeneration) and burst (reticular degeneration), resulting in the coalescence of groups of cells. Multinucleate giant cells are created and can be identified with the Tzanck test (*see* p. 74).

Balloon and reticular degeneration also occur in hand-foot-and-mouth disease, although multinucleate giant cells are not seen.

Staphylococcal bullous impetigo

Staphylococcal bullous impetigo usually occurs in children as initially clear flaccid blisters, which rupture easily because the blister roof is made up of the stratum corneum only (**Fig 13.15**). Phage group II *Staphylococcus aureus* can be identified in all the skin lesions, and affected areas can be extensive (**Fig 13.42**). Disseminated bullous impetigo presents with widespread bullous lesions and scanty positive bacterial cultures and is associated with depressed immunity. *Staphylococcus aureus* is now recognised as the principal cause of all types of impetigo. *Streptococcus pyogenes* is found with *Staphylococcus aureus* in approximately 2% of patients and *Streptococcus pyogenes* alone in less than 2%.

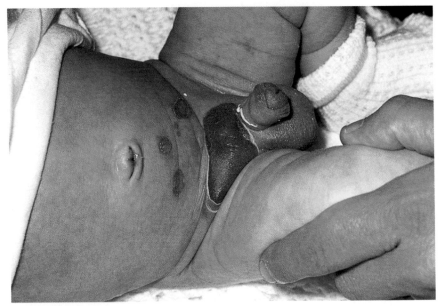

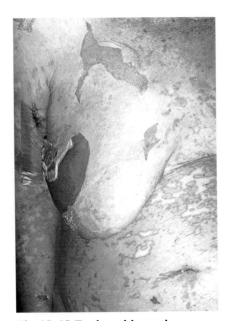

Fig 13.42 Widespread impetigo with skin shedding. There are wide areas of stratum corneum shedding in this baby's skin, with remnants visible at the periphery of the erythematous areas. Cultures from the skin grew *Staphylococcus aureus*. This condition is essentially the same as staphylococcal scalded skin syndrome but occurs as a localised response to staphylococcal infection

Fig 13.43 Toxic epidermal necrolysis. This example occurred as a result of hypersensitivity to allopurinol. Sheets of blister roof can be seen and can be produced by shearing stress even on clinically normal skin (Nikolsky's sign). Although the eroded areas and sheets of blistering are similar to staphylococcal scalded skin syndrome, the blister roof includes the full thickness of the epidermis. If in doubt as to the correct diagnosis, the differences can be shown rapidly on frozen sections. The confluent grey areas produced by the full-thickness epidermal death are similar to those of a more localised toxic urticated eruption (see 10.13); both toxic epidermal necrolysis and toxic urticated eruptions may be variants of erythema multiforme

Staphylococcal scalded skin syndrome

Staphylococcal scalded skin syndrome is caused by the same organism as bullous impetigo, but the large flaccid bullae do not contain staphylococci since the infection is based at a distant site, usually in the eye, nose or pharynx (**Fig 13.14**). The bullae are created by the release of a staphylococcal toxin called exfoliatin from the organisms at these sites; the toxin is cleared by the kidney. Since adult equivalent renal function is not achieved by healthy babies until approximately 2 years of age, very young children and adults with renal impairment are at risk. Another factor limiting the condition to very young children may be the presence of antibodies to the epidermolytic toxin, which can be identified in 75% of people over 10 years of age.

Toxic epidermal necrolysis

An important differential diagnosis for staphylococcal scalded skin syndrome is toxic epidermal necrolysis. This potentially life-threatening form of erythema multiforme occurs principally in adults, due to a drug reaction. The patient develops widespread hot, red skin. Within hours, the skin becomes painful and starts to peel off in large sheets (**Fig 13.43**). At this stage, the adjacent, apparently normal skin can be made to shear off or separate from the deeper layers by gentle rubbing. This is called a positive Nikolsky's sign (**Fig 13.6–13.8**).

In contrast to staphylococcal scalded skin syndrome, where the split is at the level of the stratum corneum, in toxic epidermal necrolysis, the split occurs at the subepidermal junction. These differences can be easily and rapidly distinguished in frozen-section histological examination of a skin biopsy sample or the blister roof.

Other causes of epidermal death

Epidermal death secondary to dermal ischaemia occurs in erythema multiforme (**Fig 13.31**), vasculitis (**Fig 13.45**, *see also* Fig 12.7), vascular occlusion,

> ## DIAGNOSTIC TIPS AND PITFALLS
>
> - Toxic epidermal necrolysis and staphylococcal scalded skin syndrome may be clinically very difficult to distinguish, but the epidermal histology and level of blister split are different

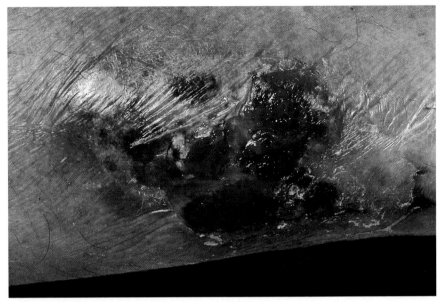

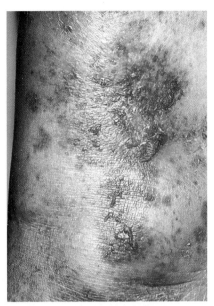

Fig 13.44 Pyoderma gangrenosum with blisters. Typical, rapidly enlarging, bluish or purple, inflammatory plaque leading to ulceration

Fig 13.45 Blistered vasculitis. Epidermal death and subsequent blistering are seen in areas of palpable purpura

necrolytic migratory erythema (annular blistering lesions, due to zinc deficiency or glucagonoma) and pyoderma gangrenosum. The latter may present with a large solitary blister with a necrotic roof (**Fig 13.44**, *see also* Figs 12.17, 12.18), which rapidly sloughs off to reveal the undermined ulcer. In vasculitis, the blisters (**Fig 13.45**) are usually blood-filled, easily burst and may be pustular (*see also* Fig 14.22).

Immune-mediated damage to intra-epidermal or subepidermal adhesion

Bullous pemphigoid

The main features of bullous pemphigoid are listed in **Table 13.2**. The subepidermal blistering is due to antibodies against the bullous pemphigoid antigens in the lamina lucida.

Bullous pemphigoid variants

Cicatricial pemphigoid may present with scarring of the mucous membranes (*see above*). The Brunsting–Perry variant presents as multiple small blisters on the head and neck (**Fig 13.46** and **13.47**) or scarred lesions on the scalp (**Fig 13.37**, *see also* Fig 18.26).

Pemphigus vulgaris and other pemphigus variants

The main features of this disorder are listed in **Table 13.2**. Blistering occurs due to immunological damage to desmosomal proteins (desmogleins 1 or 3 depending on the pemphigus variant), which normally provide 'spot-welding' between keratinocytes. Loss of these adhesion points causes the epidermal cells to separate from each other ('acantholysis'), which in turn causes blisters. The prototype is pemphigus vulgaris in which blistering is suprabasal, but in pemphigus foliaceous (*see* Figs 7.43 and 7.44) and pemphigus erythematosus, the blistering is subcorneal. There is also an endemic form of pemphigus found in South America and a paraneoplastic version of pemphigus that causes a rather lichenoid rash and severe cheilitis (**Fig 13.48**).

251

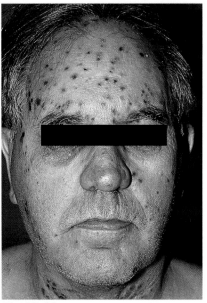

Fig 13.46

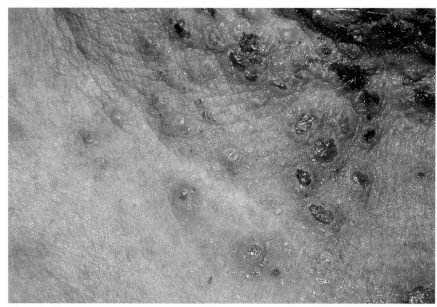

Fig 13.47

Figs 13.46, 13.47 Brunsting–Perry disease. Multiple small blisters and some associated erosions are visible on the face (13.46) and neck (13.47) in this variant of bullous pemphigoid

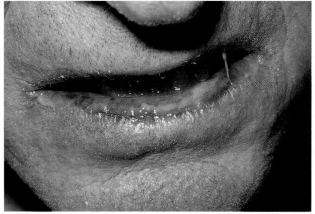

Fig 13.48 Paraneoplastic pemphigus. In this disorder, which is disproportionately associated with lymphoma, thymoma and Castleman's tumour, severe and therapeutically resistant cheilitis is a prominent feature. Bronchiolitis obliterans is a severe complication

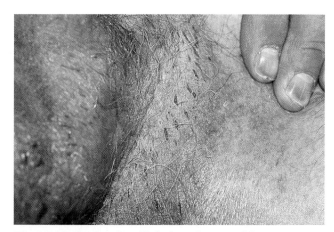

Fig 13.49 Benign familial chronic pemphigus (Hailey–Hailey disease) in the groin. Affected areas show crusting and little irregular splits or rents of the skin rather than overt blister formation

Acantholytic disorders

Benign familial chronic pemphigus, also called Hailey–Hailey disease (**Fig 13.49**) has an acantholytic histology similar to pemphigus vulgaris but is due to an inherited defect in desmosomes and is usually manifest as eroded plaques in the flexures. It is especially troublesome in hot humid weather. Other disorders in which acantholysis is a feature include Darier's disease (*see* Figs 7.29 and 7.30), Grover's disease (transient acantholytic dermatosis) and various isolated lesions (e.g. warty dyskeratoma). None of these present as blistering diseases.

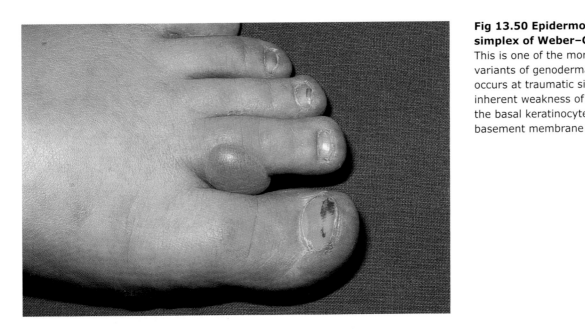

Fig 13.50 Epidermolysis bullosa simplex of Weber–Cockayne type.
This is one of the more common variants of genodermatosis. Blistering occurs at traumatic sites due to the inherent weakness of attatchment of the basal keratinocyte to the basement membrane

Blistering due to basal cell damage

Epidermolysis bullosa simplex

The commonest type of epidermolysis bullosa is epidermolysis bullosa simplex in which there is a defect in the hemidesmosomes attaching the basal keratinocytes to the basement membrane, which leads to splitting at the deep part of the basal cells of the epidermis. The feet are typically affected (**Figs 13.40, 13.50, 13.54 and 13.55**).

Acquired disorders causing basal cell damage

Inflammation at the junction between the epidermis and dermis, as seen in lichen planus and systemic lupus erythematosus, may result in the separation of the epidermis and the development of a subepidermal-type blister. This is a relatively rare event given the prevalence of these conditions, and blisters are not usually the presenting feature.

Dermal damage

Porphyria and pseudoporphyria

The skin manifestations of blistering and increased skin fragility followed by milia, scarring and hirsutes are seen in the cutaneous porphyrias. Porphyrin concentrations are abnormally high in blood and tissues. Visible light reacts with the tissue porphyrin, producing highly reactive active oxygen species. These cause lipid peroxidation, resulting in destruction of lipid-containing cell membranes. The porphyrias that produce skin signs include porphyria cutanea tarda, variegate porphyria, erythropoietic protoporphyria, congenital erythropoietic porphyria and hereditary coproporphyria. The last two are very rare and will not be discussed.

Porphyria cutanea tarda is the most common. Common provoking factors are excessive alcohol consumption, contraceptive pill and hepatitis C. The changes are best seen on hands that are both exposed to the sun and prone to minor trauma. Features include skin fragility, small blisters (**Fig 13.39**), i.e. 5–10 mm in diameter, which heal with milia formation (**Fig 13.51**), hypertrichosis, scarring and sclerodermatous changes in the damaged skin.

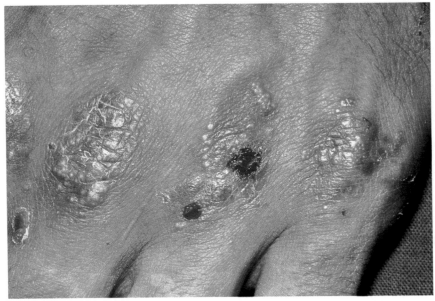

Fig 13.51 Milia in porphyria cutanea tarda. Milia are present as tiny white papules grouped together over the knuckles and dorsum of the hand in this man with porphyria cutanea tarda (*see also* 13.56)

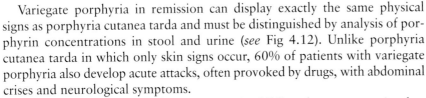

Fig 13.52 Erythropoietic protoporphyria scarring on the face in a child. There are several linear scars with well defined edges on the cheeks in this child with erythropoietic protoporphyria. Patients present with acute oedema, itching and pain in the skin after sun exposure

Variegate porphyria in remission can display exactly the same physical signs as porphyria cutanea tarda and must be distinguished by analysis of porphyrin concentrations in stool and urine (*see* Fig 4.12). Unlike porphyria cutanea tarda in which only skin signs occur, 60% of patients with variegate porphyria also develop acute attacks, often provoked by drugs, with abdominal crises and neurological symptoms.

Erythropoietic protoporphyria presents in childhood as acute sun intolerance, usually with acute oedema of the sun-exposed areas. Flat scars on the nose and cheeks are a very useful pointer to the diagnosis in the inactive state (**Fig 13.52**).

Pseudoporphyria, with similar signs but without demonstrable abnormalities of porphyrin metabolism, occurs in association with haemodialysis, drug-induced (furosemide, nalidixic acid, tetracyclines, naproxen), diabetes, and repeated sub-bed use in poorly tanning individuals (**Fig 13.53**).

BLISTERING AT SITES OF TRAUMA

Blisters commonly form in normal individuals after repeated and unaccustomed repeated friction, usually on the palms and heels. By contrast, in some bullous diseases, blisters form after relatively minor injuries and are usually apparent on the dorsum of the hands and feet and in the mouth.

In porphyria and pseudoporphyria, blisters and erosions occur at sun-exposed, trauma sites. The mechanism seems to be that sun exposure causes skin damage, and the damaged skin is then vulnerable to blister formation when traumatised.

In epidermolysis bullosa, blisters appear on non-sun-protected sites after trauma, and signs may develop in the first few days of life (**Figs 13.54** and **13.55**). This group of rare inherited diseases presents as blisters or erosions in children, usually at trauma sites such as the mouth, fingers, toes, knees. Healing with scarring occurs in some types of epidermolysis bullosa, and milia formation is common.

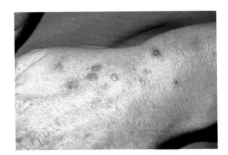

Fig 13.53 Sun-bed induced blisters in pseudoporphyria. In patients who tan poorly and regularly use UVA sun beds, blisters may appear on sun-exposed skin (*photo courtesy of Dr Peter Farr*)

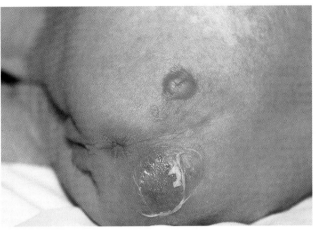

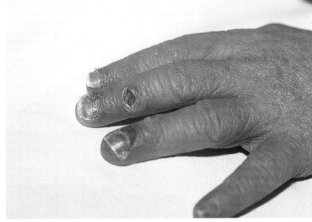

Fig 13.54

Fig 13.55

Figs 13.54, 13.55 Epidermolysis bullosa. Blistered buttock (13.54) and affected fingers (13.55) in a 2-day-old child with junctional epidermolysis bullosa. The child survived for 3 months

Acquired epidermolysis bullosa can develop in adults in association with a variety of systemic diseases, including multiple myeloma, diabetes, inflammatory bowel disease, amyloid, thyroiditis and pulmonary tuberculosis. Patients have increased skin fragility and trauma-induced blisters that heal with scarring (**Fig 13.56**). Unlike pseudoporphyria and porphyria, blisters also occur in the mouth, and nail changes are common. Immunofluorescence of the uninvolved skin shows linear IgG and C_3, i.e. similar to that seen in bullous pemphigoid.

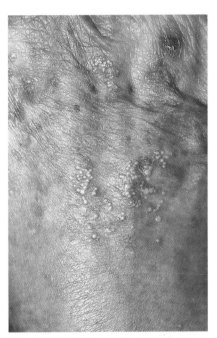

Fig 13.56 Epidermolysis bullosa acquisita on the dorsum of the hands. No blisters are present in these healing areas, but milia and a residual erosion are prominent; clinically, this eruption resembles porphyria cutanea tarda

14 Pustules

INTRODUCTION

A pustule is a localized collection of yellow–green fluid containing polymorphonuclear leucocytes and their breakdown products (**Fig 14.1**). Pustules may appear *de novo* following neutrophil-mediated inflammation, for example in a bacterial folliculitis. They may also be caused by gradual polymorph accumulation in a pre-existing clear vesicle, as occurs in herpesvirus infections. In this case, an initially clear vesicle becomes cloudy (a transitional stage sometimes called a vesicopustule), and subsequently, the more typical yellow–green colour develops. The distinction between these two methods of formation is useful in differential diagnosis, but is not always easy to determine unless lesions at different stages are present concurrently or unless individual lesions are observed at intervals. It can also be difficult to distinguish between an early vesicopustule with slightly turbid fluid content due to inflammatory cells and a vesicle with clear fluid content but a damaged overlying epidermis (*see* Fig 13.19), as both can be grey in colour. It is therefore simplest to reserve the term pustule for established lesions with the typical yellow or green colour.

Healing pustules may form a scab or crust in some disorders, notably palmoplantar pustulosis (**Fig 14.2**) where a brown scale develops as the pustule resolves. Pustules of the same duration tend to be relatively monomorphic, so the presence of resolving lesions at the same time as fresh pustules implies an ongoing process. Where pustules appear as crops, they are typical of vari-

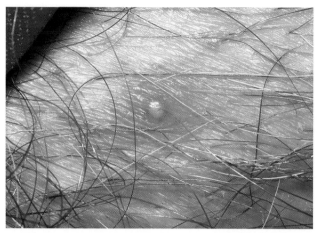

Fig 14.1 Follicular pustule (lesion in pubic area). The central hair clearly identifies this lesion as a follicular pustule (most likely to be infective in origin in this region of the body)

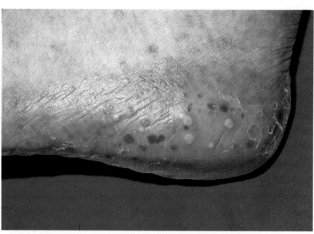

Fig 14.2 Palmoplantar pustulosis. The precise relationship of this disorder to psoriasis remains debatable, but the physical signs are typical. The pustules are fairly large (often 5 mm in diameter) and of several colours (yellow, green, and 'dried up' brown), on a well-defined erythematous scaly background

cella, in which new vesicles coexist with pustules and with necrotic old lesions; pustules at several stages of evolution are also typical of chronic disorders, such as palmoplantar pustulosis. The converse is not necessarily true, for example, the lesions of pityrosporum folliculitis tend to be fairly monomorphic irrespective of duration (**Fig 14.3**).

COMPARISON OF FOLLICULAR AND NON-FOLLICULAR PUSTULES

For clinical purposes, it is useful to determine whether the pustules are related to hair follicles, as infective causes of folliculitis are common. As well as having a central hair within the pustule, other features of follicular pustules, such as their size, discrete nature and density, are determined by the characteristics and density of the adjacent hair follicles (**Table 14.1**).

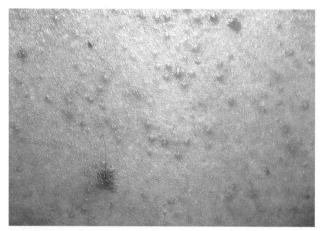

Fig 14.3 Pityrosporum folliculitis. This presents as fairly uniform scattered papules and small pustules, usually on the back

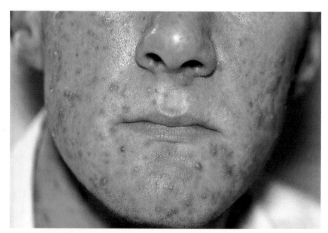

Fig 14.4 Gram-negative folliculitis. This boy developed widespread pustules after long-term antibiotic therapy for acne. Cultures grew a Gram-negative bacillus, and he responded to oral isotretinoin

Table 14.1 Comparison of follicular and non-follicular pustules

Follicular	Non-follicular	Comments
Limited to hair-bearing skin (14.1)	May affect any body site (14.2)	—
Central hair (14.1), e.g. facial acne (14.6)	No central hair (14.2)	May be difficult to identify small hairs,
Lesions are discrete (14.3)	Lesions may coalesce (14.7)	Non-follicular pustules may be discrete, especially in early stages Follicular pustules may coalesce at the deep aspect (14.9)
Density is related to normal follicles (14.3)	Density is not related to hair follicles (14.2)	Follicular pustules cannot be closer together than the local interfollicular distance. Some grouped non-follicular pustules (e.g. herpes simplex) may be approximately this density
Lesions are fairly uniform in size (14.3)	Lesions are often variable in size (14.2)	A less useful sign, as it is influenced by duration of lesions (any crop of pustules, follicular or not, tends to be fairly uniform in size)

A typical example of a follicular pustule, with a central hair emerging from the lesion, is an acute follicular infection, such as staphylococcal folliculitis (**Fig 14.1**). Hair may be less obvious in other examples, such as acne (**Fig 14.6**), where the sebaceous gland inflammation may be much more prominent than the fine hair of the associated hair follicle. By comparison, typical non-follicular pustules, such as those of generalised pustular psoriasis (**Fig 14.7**), have neither a central hair nor a regular pattern corresponding to follicular openings.

It is therefore often possible to reach a short list of differential diagnoses by determining whether a pustular eruption is follicular and whether there has been a discrete episode or an ongoing process. Other factors that may be

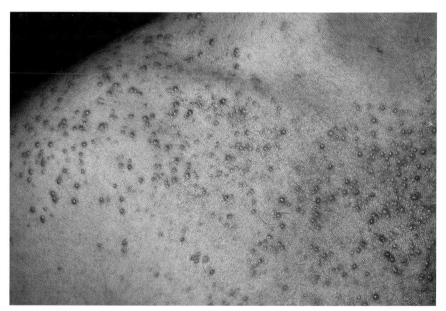

Fig 14.5 Steroid acne. Drug-induced acneiform eruptions tend to be more prominent on the trunk and the individual lesions more monomorphic in appearance than is the case in typical acne

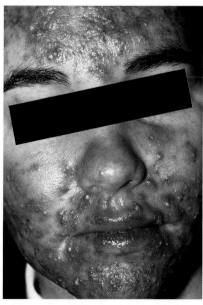

Fig 14.6 Pustules in acne. These arise from follicles, but the hairs are much less obvious.

259

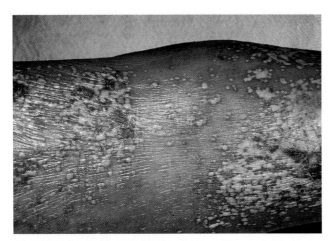

Fig 14.7 Pustular psoriasis. This eruption is non-follicular because it consists of superficial pustules that are variable in size, often closer to each other than the normal follicular density and have confluent areas. Note: any samples for identification of infection in a pustule or vesicopustular lesion must be taken from the inside of the lesion; remove the roof with a sterile blade or needle and swab the base of the pustule

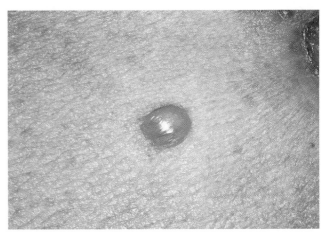

Fig 14.8 Impetigo. This generally causes larger blisters or crusting (*see* 1.13 and 7.4). Smaller pustules can occur, especially in the disseminated type of impetigo. This lesion shows a 'pus level' where the pus cells have settled by influence of gravity from the clearer fluid component; this feature is not specific but is seen in other superficial types of pustule such as subcorneal pustular dermatosis (Sneddon–Wilkinson disease) (*see* 13.13)

helpful include symptoms and previous history, body site (e.g. herpes simplex often occurs around lips and nose), distribution (e.g. zosteriform pattern) and clinical features of an associated dermatosis. Note, however, that some infective agents can cause both follicular and non-follicular pustules. For example, staphylococcal infection can cause simple folliculitis (*see* Fig 14.1) as well as larger, very superficial, subcorneal pustules in impetigo (**Fig 14.8**). When taking microbiology swabs from a pustule, the sample should be taken from the pustule base or undersurface of the removed pustule roof and not from the external surface.

CLASSIFICATION OF PUSTULES

In **Table 14.2** we have divided pustules according to their site (follicular or non-follicular) and the presence of other skin signs.

FOLLICULAR PUSTULES WITH FEW OTHER SKIN SIGNS

Staphylococcal pustules

Staphylococcal pustules are a classic example of the follicular pustule discussed above (*see* Fig 14.1). Occasional pustules of this type are a common finding, especially on a hairy chest or legs in men. In flexural regions, they may indicate that the patient is a chronic carrier of staphylococci. Diabetes mellitus should be excluded in patients with frequent or severe episodes of folliculitis, especially in cases with the deeper variants (furuncle or carbuncle, *see* below).

Lesions that are related to pustules include:

- Furuncle or boil—a deep inflammation of a hair follicle.
- Carbuncle—a deep inflammation of several contiguous follicles (**Fig 14.9**).

DIAGNOSTIC TIPS AND PITFALLS

- Follicular pustules have a central hair emerging from the discrete lesions and a distribution and density similar to the adjacent hair follicles

- Non-follicular pustules have neither a central hair nor a regular pattern corresponding to follicular openings

- Staphylococcal infection can cause both types of pustule. Simple folliculitis and non-follicular, very superficial, subcorneal pustules occur in impetigo

- Viral and bacterial swabs should be taken from the base or roof undersurface of a deroofed pustule and not from the external surface

- Abscess—a large deep collection of pus in any organ; in the skin, it may develop from a deep folliculitis but can also arise by direct penetrating infection around foreign bodies or from deeper infections. It can 'point' to the skin, with an obvious collection of pus, but generally presents as a nodule.

Pityrosporum folliculitis

This relatively common infection of follicles occurs in areas of high sebum production on the back (*see* Fig 14.3) and is caused by the same yeast that causes pityriasis versicolor. Tiny papules and pustules occur, sometimes with a faint brown peripheral pigmentation, as seen in seborrhoeic dermatitis.

> ### DIAGNOSTIC TIPS AND PITFALLS
>
> - Recurrent staphylococcal pustules in flexural regions may indicate that the patient is a chronic carrier of staphylococci or is diabetic

Table 14.2 Classification of causes of pustules

Follicular pustules (folliculitis)	
Few other skin signs	**With associated skin signs**
Infection Staphylococci (14.1), Gram-negative folliculitis (14.4) and others (*see also* non-follicular causes of infection) Pityrosporum folliculitis (14.3)	**Inflammation** Acne (14.6), rosacea (14.13) Perioral dermatitis (14.14) Chronic superficial folliculitis of the scalp Rare causes of folliculitis, e.g. perforating folliculitis, eosinophilic pustular folliculitis
Pseudofollicular Ingrowing hairs in beard area (pseudofolliculitis barbae) (14.10–14.12)	**Systemic disease with pustules** e.g. Behçet's disease (non-follicular pustules may also occur in Behçet's disease due to pathergy)
Drugs/chemical Steroids (14.5), halides, chlorinated hydrocarbons (chloracne), comedogenic agents	
Irritant Oils, tar	
Non-follicular pustules	
Few other skin signs	**With associated skin signs**
Pustules arising in other appendages Sweat ducts: miliaria pustulosa (14.16)	**Inflammation** *Psoriasis* Generalised pustular (14.7) Palmoplantar pustulosis (14.2, 14.20) Acropustulosis of Hallopeau (14.21) *Vasculitis* Various causes, e.g. Behçet's disease, gonococcal, bowel-associated reactive dermatitis–arthritis syndrome, pathergy (lesions at sites of needle injury in Behçet's disease, pyoderma gangrenosum) *Bullous disease* Subcorneal pustular dermatosis (13.13)
Infections (may be follicular) *Primary* Staphylococci (14.1) Candida (14.26) Dermatophyte (ringworm) fungi (14.25) Herpes simplex (14.15) Exanthematic pustulosis Rare—cytomegalovirus, listeria, syphilis *Secondary* Eczema, psoriasis, others	
	Drugs (including generalised pustular eruption, 'acute generalised eruptive pustulosis' (14.18, 14.19)) Sulphonamides, others
	Infestation Scabies (14.17)
	Other dermatoses Sweet's syndrome, transient pustular melanosis Erosive pustular dermatosis of the scalp (18.28)

Pseudofolliculitis barbae

These pustules present as papules and pustules at hair-bearing sites and thus are initially usually considered to be follicular in origin. However, as the name suggests, this common disorder is not actually follicular but is due to hairs growing back into the skin and thereby superficially traumatising the skin. These ingrowing hairs can be readily identified by lifting the non-follicular end of the hair out of the skin with a needle (**Figs 14.10–14.12**). Although follicular pustules in the beard area can be due to infection by staphylococci, herpes simplex and others, pseudofolliculitis barbae is more common and can be distinguished from a true folliculitis by careful inspection.

Oil and irritant folliculitis

Oil and irritant folliculitis have no specific features to distinguish them from staphylococcal follicular pustules, except for their history, distribution (which is related to the areas of contact) and sterility on culture.

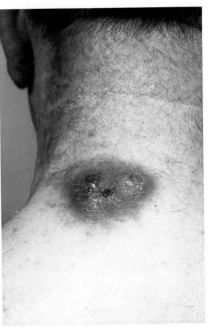

Fig 14.9 Carbuncle in a diabetic man. These lesions are due to deep infection of several adjacent hair follicles and often present as a nodule rather than a pustule initially

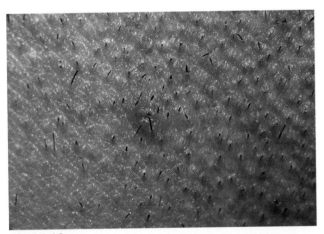

Fig 14.10

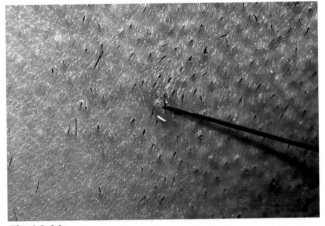

Fig 14.11

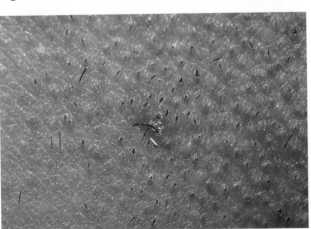

Fig 14.12

Figs 14.10–14.12 Pseudofolliculitis barbae. This is a common condition. The pustules are actually adjacent to the follicles in the beard area (14.10), as shown by lifting the ingrowing hair out of the pustule (14.11). This is a worthwhile manœuvre; not only does exploring the hair confirm the diagnosis (14.12), but it also relieves pain

FOLLICULAR PUSTULES WITH OTHER SKIN SIGNS

Acne

Acne causes a range of changes, including folliculitis. However, purely pustular acne is unusual, and typically, there are a variety of lesions at different stages of evolution (**Fig 14.6**). These are all primarily follicular and include papules, pustules, whiteheads, blackheads, nodules and cysts. The face is virtually always involved; in males, larger lesions and more persistent changes may be present on the upper back. A purely pustular eruption in a person with acne suggests the diagnosis of Gram-negative folliculitis (**Fig 14.4**).

Acneiform eruptions may occur through the use of chemicals such as chlorinated hydrocarbons, which cause chloracne, and of drugs including corticosteroids (**Fig 14.5**), halides, isoniazid and phenytoin. Drug-induced acneiform eruptions tend to be more prominent on the trunk and the individual lesions more monomorphic in appearance than is the case in typical acne. The variability of acne lesions is therefore a potentially useful physical sign.

Rosacea

In rosacea, follicular pustules are common but not always present. The most consistent abnormality is erythema and easy flushing, which leads to fixed telangiectasia that often persists when the pustules have resolved (**Fig 14.13**). Typical lesions are papules and pustules on cheeks, nose, chin and central forehead. Other features include rhinophyma—a thickening of the skin of the nose with dilated follicular openings and very prominent sebaceous glands. Ocular changes of blepharitis, conjunctivitis and scleritis may occur.

Perioral dermatitis

Perioral dermatitis is of uncertain cause but clinically has many similarities to rosacea, consisting of papules, pustules and a noticeable erythematous background. The distribution is more limited, and the classic site is a vague ring around the mouth, but with a few millimetres of sparing beyond the vermilion border (**Fig 14.14**).

Behçet's disease

A sterile folliculitis can occur in this multisystem disorder, although only very rarely as the presenting feature. Orogenital ulcers and cutaneous vasculitis are more common skin findings, and many other organ systems are affected. Patients may also develop pustules due to the presence of pustular vasculitis (*see* below) or at sites of needle injuries (e.g. venepuncture), a process termed pathergy.

NON-FOLLICULAR PUSTULES AND VESICOPUSTULES WITH FEW OTHER SKIN SIGNS

The classic vesicopustular disorders are herpesvirus infections, although several other disorders are also characterised by the progression from vesicles to pustules. Diagnosis is made by the history, associated skin and/or systemic

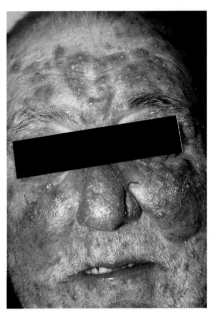

Fig 14.13 Rosacea. Papules and pustules are associated with diffuse erythema and prominent telangiectasia

DIAGNOSTIC TIPS AND PITFALLS

- Beard pustules may be due to pseudofolliculitis barbae, caused by hairs growing back into the skin and thereby superficially traumatising the skin. The end of these ingrowing hairs can be uncoiled or pulled out of the skin using a needle

DIAGNOSTIC TIPS AND PITFALLS

- Simple acne includes a range of lesions including papules, pustules, whiteheads, blackheads, nodules and cysts. A purely pustular eruption in a person with acne suggests the diagnosis of Gram-negative folliculitis or drug-induced acneiform rash

263

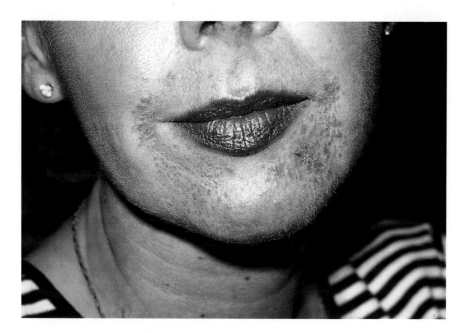

Fig 14.14 Perioral dermatitis. This patient has multiple erythematous papules appearing around her mouth but sparing the area immediately around the lips. This is often a consequence of mistaken topical steroid therapy of rosacea. The rash responds to oral tetracyclines

features, progression and specific tests. The last may include virology, microbiology, serology and histopathology. Rapid identification of virally infected vesicles can be made in some cases by electron microscopic or fluorescent antibody identification (e.g. herpesviruses), and a Tzanck smear test can be useful (*see* p. 74).

Herpes simplex

Herpes simplex is one of the commonest vesicopustular eruptions (**Fig 14.15**). Primary infection may occur on skin or mucous membranes (often a gingivo-stomatitis) and can be sexually acquired. The classic area for recrudescence to present is around the lips in the form of the typical cold sore. Lesions occur in a grouped ('herpetiform') pattern, often on a slightly red or oedematous base. Initially, they consist of monomorphic clear vesicles, which become yellow and somewhat umbilicated before crusting as the infection settles.

Herpes varicella-zoster

The herpes varicella-zoster virus causes two patterns of eruption (*see* p. 239).

Chicken-pox (varicella) generally occurs in the young age group; mild prodromal illness of short duration is followed by crops of vesicles that appear over a period of a week or so. The early lesions may have a pink halo of inflammation, which is said to resemble a raindrop on a rose petal (*see* Figs 13.17 and 13.18). Although occurring mainly on the trunk and face, the lesions are scattered and discrete. They become pustular, then necrotic and scabbed, often healing with some degree of scarring. Lesions at different stages are present after the first couple of days.

Herpes zoster or shingles is a recrudescence of infection in the posterior nerve roots, and the eruption has a dermatomal distribution (*see* Fig 2.21). The vesicles are preceded by pain in the affected dermatome, which is usually patchily covered by vesicles. These are often grouped together on an erythematous plaque, although less closely than in herpes simplex, but less scattered than in chicken-pox. The vesicles are generally larger than those occurring in chicken-pox or herpes simplex, and they may dry up with a less obvious

DIAGNOSTIC TIPS AND PITFALLS

- In some cases of herpes zoster, there may be just a few cold sore-like lesions, but the distribution of these is within a single dermatome, and there is usually dermatomal pain— misdiagnosis as herpes simplex is a pitfall, that leads to inadequate treatment

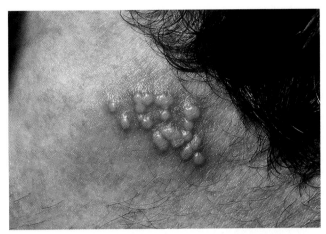

Fig 14.15 Herpes simplex infection. This case was acquired by direct inoculation from an infected lip while playing rugby ('scrumpox'). The individual lesions are all of the same duration and monomorphic in terms of size, shape and colour (*see also* 2.26)

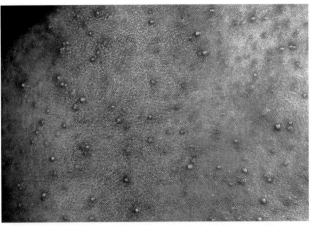

Fig 14.16 Miliaria. These deep miliaria are clinically pustular with associated erythema and swelling because of the degree of associated inflammation (*photo courtesy of Dr Adrian Ive*)

pustular stage but larger areas of crusting. There are many variations; zoster may present as pain without rash or occasionally as rash without pain. Shingles may also be seen in small children with no preceding history of chicken-pox, and it is assumed that the primary infection must have occurred *in utero* in such cases (*see* Fig 13.16). Note that in some cases, there may be just a few cold sore-like lesions in herpes zoster, but the distribution of these is within a single dermatome and is usually associated with dermatomal pain—misdiagnosis as herpes simplex is a pitfall that leads to inadequate treatment.

Neonatal toxic erythema

Neonatal toxic erythema is a common eruption occurring in over 50% of full-term neonates (*see* Figs 6.5 and 6.6). Individual lesions are red macules with a central pale white/yellow papule or pustule. The pustules are superficial and present around pilosebaceous follicles. They are not specific in appearance but are diagnosed by their timing, lack of associated illness, eosinophil content and sterility on culture.

Miliaria

Superficial miliaria are tiny clear vesicles (*see* Fig 13.11), but deeper inflammation of the eccrine duct (miliaria rubra, prickly heat, **Fig 14.16**) is a common cause of pustules and has the same association with hot humid conditions and exercise. This condition is common in babies (*see* Fig 6.10).

Toxic pustuloderma (acute generalised exanthematous pustulosis)

Acute onset toxic pustuloderma is short-lived. The condition occurs following a viral illness or as a reaction to a particular drug—usually to a sulphonamide, β lactam antibiotic or anticonvulsant. The drug-induced pattern is termed 'acute generalised exanthematous pustulosis' or 'AGEP.' Patients have widespread non-follicular pustules with an erythematous halo

DIAGNOSTIC TIPS AND PITFALLS

- In adults with acute onset of widespread skin pustules, consider pustular psoriasis, viral infections and a drug eruption

- In children with a pustular eruption, infection is the first consideration—neonatal toxic erythema can usually be diagnosed rapidly by staining a smear from the pustules and evaluating the eosinophil content

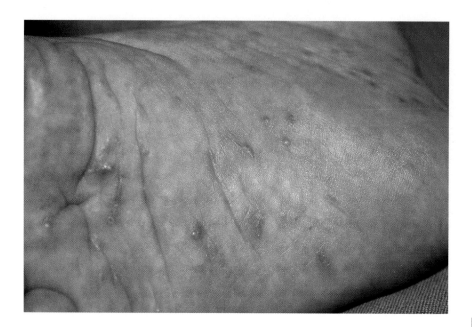

Fig 14.17 Scabies. This condition can cause prominent pustule formation, particularly on the feet in infants

(**Figs 14.18** and **14.19**). Although originally considered to be an exanthematic variant of pustular psoriasis, it can be distinguished by the lack of severe systemic upset, rapid spontaneous resolution and the absence of any history of psoriasis.

Differential diagnosis

Eruptive xanthoma is an uncommon but easily misdiagnosed disorder, which causes small yellow spots with a surrounding inflammatory halo (*see* Fig 3.35). This may simulate a non-follicular pustular disorder, but pus cannot be expressed from the interior of a pricked lesion.

> ### DIAGNOSTIC TIPS AND PITFALLS
>
> • Eruptive xanthoma produces small, transient yellow spots with a surrounding inflammatory halo. They may be confused with a non-follicular pustular disorder, but pus cannot be expressed from a pricked lesion

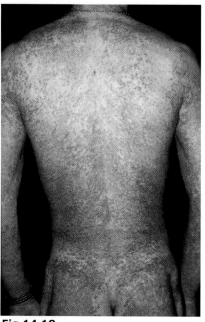

Fig 14.18

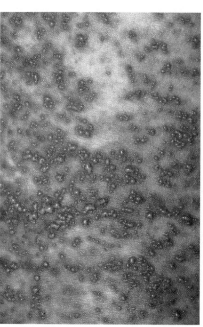

Fig 14.19

Figs 14.18, 14.19 Toxic pustuloderma. This man presented with widespread tiny pustules following a viral illness (14.18); he was not systemically unwell, and the rash cleared spontaneously in 7 days. There are multiple small pustules, some of which contain a fluid level (14.19) resembling that of generalised pustular psoriasis but without the same tendency to confluence of lesions (*see* 14.7)

NON-FOLLICULAR PUSTULES WITH OTHER SKIN SIGNS

Many pustules present with some degree of surrounding inflammation. In conditions where pustules are not due to primary infections, the rash of the underlying disorder is usually predominant. The number of pustules can vary considerably, for example, an extensive rash with a few pustules can occur in some infective processes such as ringworm (**Fig 14.25**) or candidiasis, but, conversely, pustule formation may be subtle, for example in infantile or partially treated scabies (**Fig 14.17**). Rashes in which pustules are a common feature at presentation are described below, whereas pustules that occur in primarily bullous disorders are discussed in Chapter 13.

Psoriasis

Various forms of pustular psoriasis are recognised. Generalised pustular psoriasis (**Figs 14.7** and **14.20**) is uncommon but potentially serious as it occurs in patients with widespread and rapidly increasing psoriasis and is associated with symptomatic systemic toxaemia. The individual psoriatic plaques are usually thin, very vascular, not very scaly and extensive (often confluent). The pustules are superficial and non-follicular; they appear in crops, are a whitish-yellow colour and often become confluent. They sometimes tend to be most prominent at the periphery of the plaques, and resolution leaves a thin rim of 'peeling' crust and stratum corneum.

Palmoplantar pustulosis (**Fig 14.2**) is a variant of psoriasis. It has a characteristic appearance of fairly large pustules at different stages (yellow, green and 'dried-up' brown) on an erythematous and scaling well-defined base. It affects the soles (often the side of the heel) more often than the palms. It can be asymmetrical, in which case, fungal infection should be excluded.

Acropustulosis (of Hallopeau) is a rare disorder that affects the distal part of the digits, usually the fingers, and which is morphologically similar to palmoplantar pustulosis. Pustules may occur under the nails, and the nail is often lost from affected digits (**Fig 14.21**).

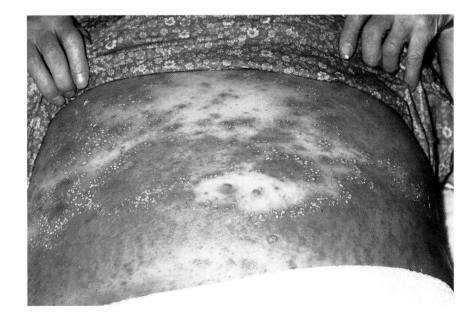

Fig 14.20 Generalised pustular psoriasis. There are multiple pustules at the margins of the erythematous areas

Scabies

Scabies is a common cause of vesicopustular eruption with intense itch (p. 276). Although there are always some other lesions, including linear burrows, papules, nodules, urticated lesions and eczematous lesions (*see* Figs 15.10–15.16), scabies is mentioned here because the pustular component may be the most obvious feature, particularly on the extremities in infants (**Fig 14.17**).

Eczema

Secondary infection of eczema is common, although identifiable pustules may not be present. Follicular papules and pustules are frequent when eczema involves hairy legs. Although staphylococci, and sometimes streptococci, are the usual cause, it is important to consider herpes simplex infections if there is a sudden worsening of eczema, with development of widespread pustular or crusted areas (eczema herpeticum, *see* Fig 15.25).

Vasculitis and related disorders

Pustules can develop as a result of several forms of injury to the skin where there is a polymorph infiltrate. Some arise internally in various forms of vasculitis, especially those where there is major vessel wall damage and fragmentation of polymorphs in a leucocytoclastic vasculitis. There are no specific features of the pustules that lead to a clear diagnosis in these disorders, but in general terms, it is reasonable to associate small pustules with disease of the smaller superficial vessels and larger pustules with a vasculitis of larger deeper vessels. Thus, the pustules that can occur in association with palpable purpura in Henoch–Schönlein disease (*see also* Chapter 17) are generally small (**Fig 14.22**), whereas those that present in pyoderma gangrenosum (*see* Figs 12.17, 12.18, 13.44) are larger (**Fig 14.23**).

Pustules are also a feature of acute febrile neutrophilic dermatosis (Sweet's disease, *see* 17.42), although this does not have any noticeable vessel wall damage, and both folliculitis and vasculitic pustules occur in Behçet's disease.

Fungal infection (ringworm and candida)

Dermatophytes that primarily affect humans or domestic pets do not usually cause obvious pustules in humans, although this can occur on hairy skin especially and particularly if the infection has been inappropriately treated with topical steroids, i.e. tinea incognito (**Fig 14.24**). By contrast, the more inflammatory response to infection with cattle ringworm often causes pustule formation at any site (**Fig 14.25**, *see also* Fig 15.20). In the scalp and beard area, this can cause a boggy inflammatory nodule (kerion) that may be studded with pustules, and in which the hairs become loose, causing subsequent alopecia.

Pustules often develop in candida infections in humans. Occasionally, external infection of a wide skin area can cause scattered monomorphic pustules (**Fig 14.26**), but the more common clinical picture is of a spreading infection from a flexural area. In this situation, the flexure is diffusely red and glazed or shiny in appearance, with satellite papules and pustules outside the confluent area of involvement (*see* Fig 5.26). By comparison, staphylococcal pustules in the flexures are discrete lesions.

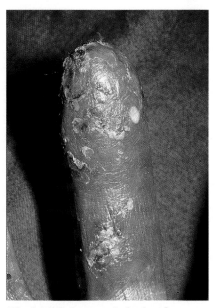

Fig 14.21 Acropustulosis of Hallopeau. Pustules are on the digits, with loss of nails. There is a background of erythema and scaling

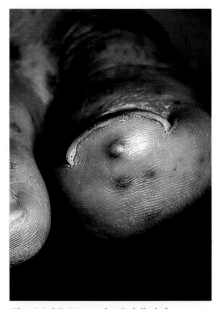

Fig 14.22 Henoch–Schönlein purpura. Pustule formation due to small-vessel leucocytoclastic vasculitis occurs on a background of scattered palpable purpuric lesions

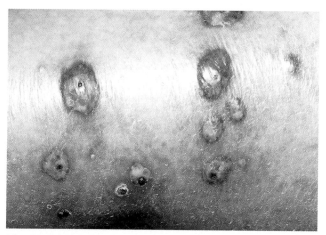

Fig 14.23 Pyoderma gangrenosum. This condition can cause large pustular lesions, which rapidly progress to form deep ulcers

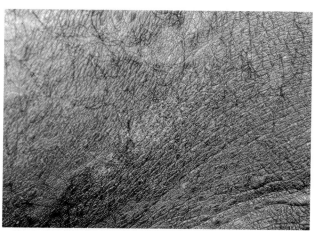

Fig 14.24 A fungal infection may result in pustules, and these are more likely to appear in mistaken steroid treatment of a dermatophyte skin infection. They should not be confused with a bacterial infection

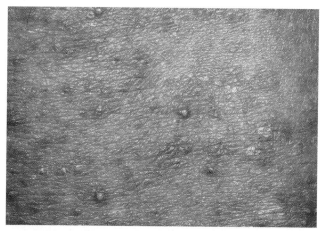

Fig 14.25 Cattle ringworm in a farm worker. This is generally more inflammatory than infection with human or cat/dog ringworm; pustules are a common feature and occur on a background of erythema and fine scaling

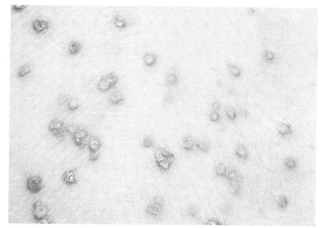

Fig 14.26 Candidiasis. This widespread infection affected most of the back and was apparent shortly after a prolonged surgical operation. The widespread scatter and monomorphic lesions without an obvious area of more prolonged infection suggest that this infection was acquired from a contaminated surface. Compare with the more typical appearance of napkin candidasis shown in 5.26

Excoriation, itch and eczema

INTRODUCTION

Excoriation (**Figs 15.1** and **15.2**) is a term used for the various patterns of skin damage inflicted by the patient as a result of picking or scratching. This usually occurs owing to the sensation of itch, and although itch is strictly a symptom rather than a physical sign, it is discussed in this chapter because it is such a common dermatological presentation. Itching may be due to cutaneous (**Table 15.1**) or systemic (**Table 15.2**) disease.

In itchy dermatoses (**Table 15.1**), other features of the skin disease are usually present, although in patients with dermatitis herpetiformis (**Fig 15.3**, *see also* Fig 13.22) or scabies, the specific lesions may be scanty and obscured

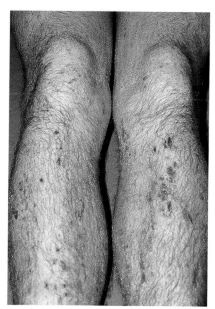

Fig 15.1

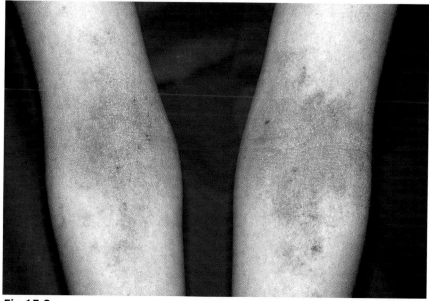

Fig 15.2

Figs 15.1, 15.2 Atopic eczema. Excoriated lesions (15.1) on this man's legs are due to scratching itchy atopic eczema. The excoriations obscure the extent and nature of the underlying problem. Compare with 15.2, where excoriation is localised to the elbow flexure in this girl with atopic eczema

Table 15.1 Common itchy skin conditions

Skin changes	Examples
Multiple separate lesions	Lichen planus, insect bites, urticaria
Diffuse rash	Scabies, eczema (particularly atopic), fungal infections, pityrosporum folliculitis, pityriasis rosea
Itchy blistering eruption	Dermatitis herpetiformis, pre-bullous pemphigoid, miliaria, pregnancy dermatoses

Table 15.2 Systemic causes of generalised pruritus

Renal
Chronic renal failure

Hepatic cholestasis
Intra-hepatic—primary biliary cirrhosis, drug-induced cholestasis
Extra-hepatic—obstructive jaundice

Blood
Polycythemia rubra vera
Iron deficiency
Chronic lymphatic leukaemia

Pregnancy

Endocrine
Thyrotoxicosis
Myxoedema

Neoplasia
Hodgkin's disease
Lymphomas and other solid tumours

Drugs
Opiates, aspirin hypersensitivity, hydroxyethylstarch infusions, ACE inhibitors

Parasitic infestation
Trichinosis, onchocerciasis
Threadworms—these cause only perianal itching

Psychogenic

Idiopathic
Approximately 50% of most series

by the secondary effects of scratching. In asteatotic eczema in elderly patients, physical signs of the underlying disorder may also be subtle; itch may be generalised, although the characteristic features are only prominent on the shins (**Fig 15.4**). Some disorders may have their most characteristic lesions in scratch marks, e.g. lichen planus (*see* Fig 8.22) and Henoch–Schönlein purpura (*see* Fig 17.23).

The term generalised pruritus is normally used for patients with itch but with no detectable primary disorder of the skin. Some patients have marked secondary features of excoriation that affect all sites, except for the mid-back, which the patient is unable to reach. This typically leads to an area over the lower scapulae and mid-back with a bilobed shape, known as the 'butterfly sign' (**Fig 15.5**). The extent of the spared area depends on the agility of the patient (compare **Figs 15.5** and **15.6**). Many patients with so-called idiopathic pruritus seem to have generally rather fine scaly skin, especially elderly patients, and the itching commonly responds to emollients and topical steroids. Other patients who have generalised pruritus 'without a rash' may

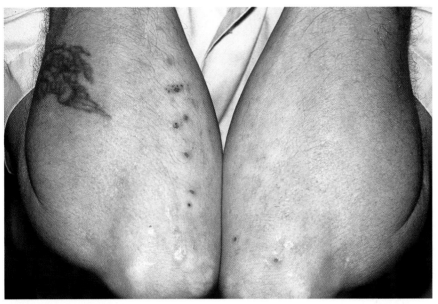

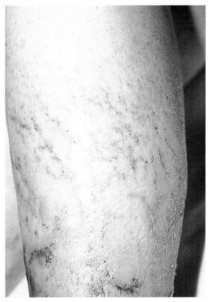

Fig 15.3 Excoriations in dermatitis herpetiformis. Itching occurs at the sites of blister formation, i.e. the elbows, knees, scalp and buttocks. Scratching bursts the blisters, and usually only grouped excoriations are visible at affected sites (*see* 13.22)

Fig 15.4 Asteatotic eczema. The red fissured cracks or 'crazy paving'-like appearance of the skin are shown on this woman's leg. Asteatotic eczema may be associated with widespread itchy dry skin, although this cracking of the skin may be clearly seen only on the shins

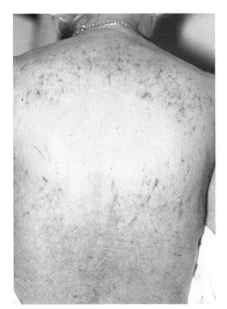

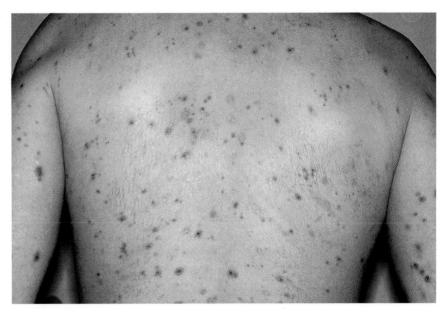

Fig 15.5   **Fig 15.6**

Figs 15.5, 15.6 Generalised pruritus. Excoriations on the back showing difference in extent of spared area. Sparing of the mid-back in an elderly woman (15.5) with idiopathic pruritus and in a young man with Hodgkin's disease (15.6). In the latter, there is just an arc-shaped area of sparing at the level of the shoulder blades

actually have subtle rash due to disorders such as urticaria or scabies or other early signs of a primary skin disorder. Some have an underlying systemic disease (Table 15.2), but approximately 50% have no obvious underlying abnormality. Diabetes mellitus is often cited as a cause of generalised pruritus, but recent evidence does not support this conclusion, although perineal itch (generally due to candidiasis) may occur in patients with glycosuria. Iron deficiency, even with normal haemoglobin concentrations, is an underestimated cause of generalised pruritus.

Various patterns of damage are produced by patients who pick, scratch and gouge their skin. Oval gouges are produced by picking, linear gouges by dragging the nail across the skin and fine linear abrasions by scratching sideways with the nails (**Fig 15.7**). Repeated rubbing results in polished and occasionally bevelled nails (*see* Fig 19.5).

Prurigo is a loosely applied term used to describe a range of unconnected itchy skin diseases. It is generally employed when excoriations, thickening or nodules develop as a result of scratching (*see* p. 285).

ITCH DUE TO DISCRETE FIXED LESIONS

Many papules may be transiently itchy, including seborrhoeic warts (*see* Figs 9.79–9.81) and naevi (*see* Figs 9.23–9.25). In most cases, this is an unhelpful feature, although in urticaria pigmentosa, the development of an itchy weal after scratching a tan-coloured macule (Darier's sign) is characteristic (*see* Figs 4.28–4.30).

ITCH DUE TO A RASH

Multiple solitary itchy lesions occur in lichen planus (*see* Figs 8.22 and 8.23), insect bites (*see* Figs 2.25 and **Fig 15.8**) and urticaria (*see* Fig 1.5).

More diffuse itchy rashes include eczema (particularly atopic eczema), fungal infections (**Figs 15.19–15.21**), pityrosporum folliculitis (**Fig 15.3**), scabies (**Figs 15.10–15.18**) and many exanthemata (*see* Chapter 10).

DIAGNOSTIC TIPS AND PITFALLS

- In cases of generalised pruritus, complete sparing of areas that are not accessible by the patient's hands (such as the 'butterfly sign' on the back) suggests that any rash is secondary to scratching rather than a primary dermatosis

DIAGNOSTIC TIPS AND PITFALLS

- In patients who have generalised pruritus without a rash, always examine carefully for skin dryness, dermographism or subtle signs of scabies before investigating possible systemic causes

- Most widespread pruritus is due to a dermatosis rather than to systemic causes

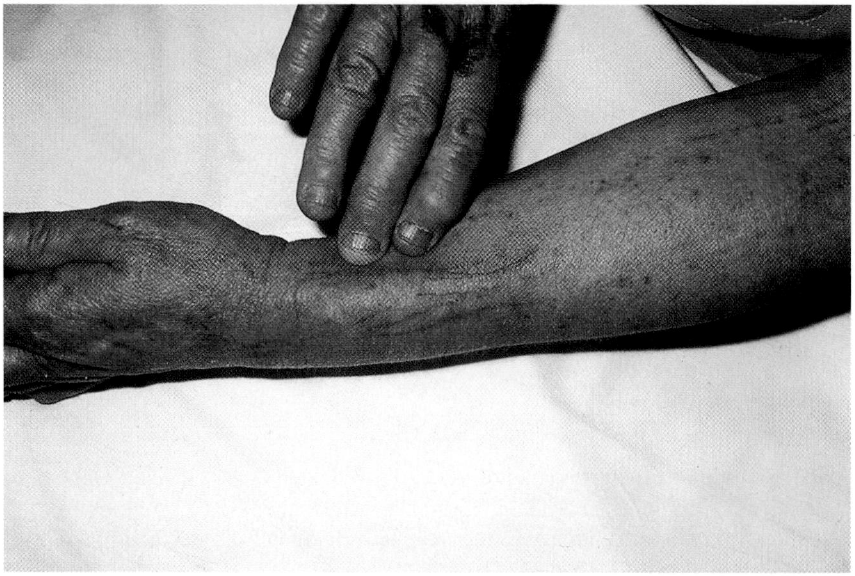

Fig 15.7 Fine scratch marks in mild eczema. Rubbing the nails sideways across the skin has resulted in localisation of the purpura in the scratch marks

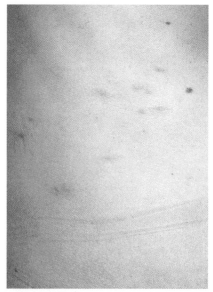

Fig 15.8 Papular urticaria. Cat flea bites have produced a group of itchy papules on this child's trunk. Cat fleas usually cause problems on the lower legs as they live in carpets. If pets are allowed to sleep in the beds or children lie on the carpets, bites appear at any site

Psoriasis (*see* Figs 8.8–8.15) may be itchy, especially during actively increasing involvement. The frequency of itch in psoriasis is probably underestimated because it is usually not as severe as in other common dermatoses such as eczemas.

In the blistering eruption of dermatitis herpetiformis (*see* Figs 13.22 and **Fig 15.3**), localised itching at sites of predilection is a constant and overwhelming symptom. Other conditions such as bullous pemphigoid are itchy in the pre-bullous urticarial phase (*see* Fig 13.25).

Insect bites (papular urticaria)

Bites from flying insects generally present no diagnostic difficulty and are obvious to the patient.

Cat and dog fleas usually cause papular urticaria (**Fig 15.8**) on the legs (*see* Fig 2.25). Papules and blisters present together with older excoriated and secondarily infected lesions. The fleas (**Fig 15.9**) hatch from eggs in the carpets of the house and will bite, but not live on, a passing human. Lesions may occur at any body site if the animal is allowed in the owner's bed.

Animal scabies mites will not live on humans but may bite and cause skin lesions. In dogs, scabies causes sarcoptic mange. In humans, lesions include itchy weals, papules and papulovesicles on the exposed sites, such as the abdomen, lower chest, thighs and forearms; facial lesions also occur in children. Other pet infestations such as that due to *Cheyletiella* (a mite of dogs, cats and rabbits that causes 'mobile dandruff') may be difficult to identify without the aid of an expert who can examine animal coat or litter brushings. If there are no pets in any house that the person visits, mites from rodents or birds (especially pigeons) should be considered as a cause of bite reactions. It may be necessary to discreetly examine clothing seams for body lice. Scalp and pubic lice can be easily spotted on hair, provided they are looked for. Scalp hair lice may affect the eyelashes. Pubic lice can spread to axillae, chest, thighs, beard and eyelashes (*see* Fig 18.49). Lice feed by piercing the skin with claws, injecting irritating saliva and sucking blood. They thus become engorged with blood and can be identified by the characteristic rust colour of their abdomen.

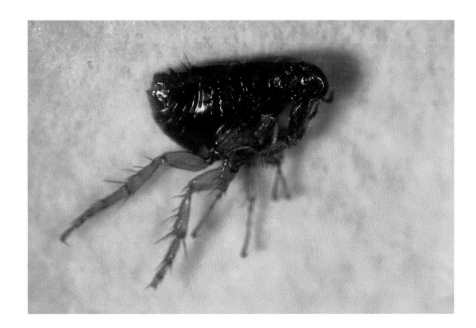

Fig 15.9 Microscopy of cat flea.
Cat fleas are commonly found in carpets and on coat brushings taken from domestic cats

Scabies

Infestation with the mite *Sarcoptes scabei* (**Fig 15.10**) produces an itchy eruption. The mite uses its powerful mandibles to dig a burrow in the stratum corneum, which it extends by 2 mm each day. The female lays 2–3 eggs a day at the end of the tunnel for around 30 days and then dies. The larvae hatch and migrate to a shallow pocket on the skin surface, where they can be transferred to a new host. Within 3 weeks of hatching, the larvae have moulted and are sexually mature mites. Copulation occurs on the skin surface. The male dies, and the female starts digging her burrow to lay her eggs (**Fig 15.11**). If it is assumed that infection takes place with one mite, then it will take a month or so before the mite population can reach a sufficient level and distribution to cause symptoms. Around 20 mites are required before the patient develops itching and rash. Initially, itching is mild, localised and relieved by scratching, as this may destroy mites. Itching starts to become most noticeable at night.

Patients usually have visible burrows (**Figs 15.12** and **15.13**). In adults, the best places to look are the side of the wrist, palms, fingers and finger webs; failing that, burrows can often be seen on the penis and around the nipples.

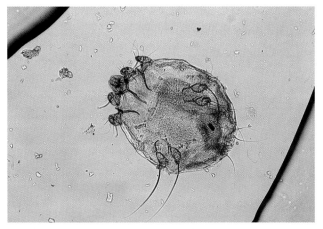

Fig 15.10 Microscopy of the scabies mite in potassium hydroxide preparations

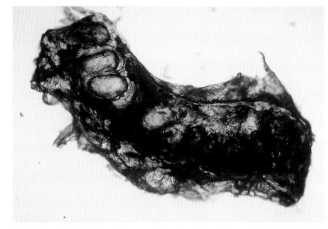

Fig 15.11 Scabies eggs. Burrow containing a row of scabies mite eggs

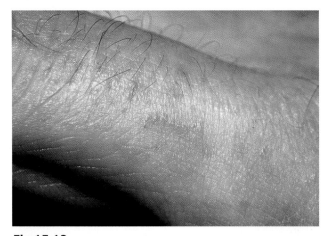

Fig 15.12

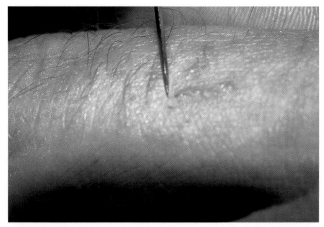

Fig 15.13

Figs 15.12, 15.13 Scabies burrow. This presents as scaly, slightly wavy ridges approximately 5–15 mm long. The mite is visible at the less scaly end, on the left side of the burrow, as a dark grey dot under the skin of the side of the finger (15.12). Mites can be retrieved using a triangular needle (15.13), to which the mites will stick once released from the burrow

Adult mites can be extracted from the burrow using a needle (**Fig 15.14**), preferably a triangular flat-sided needle, because the mite can be scooped on to the side of the needle without it disappearing down the hole, as may occur with a hollow needle. If burrows cannot be identified but there are excoriated lesions and papules, these can be scraped. The technique is painful and leaves a small erosion, so it must first be explained to the patient who must be able to cooperate; any residual potassium hydroxide left on the skin must be thoroughly washed off at the end of the procedure. The papule is scraped using a number 15 blade, after first applying one drop of 10% potassium hydroxide to the skin. The resulting mixture of skin and potassium hydroxide is then placed on a glass slide with a cover slip and examined under a microscope. Adult mites, eggs and scabies faeces may all be identified.

Burrows may be difficult to see in clean patients, and techniques such as enhancing burrows by applying ink or fluorescein may aid diagnosis (*see* Chapter 4).

In small children, burrows are best seen on the soles of the feet (**Fig 15.15**). Because small children are usually unable to cooperate, it is best to try to identify the mite in the parent rather than the child.

Secondary lesions result from scratching and infection. Infected pustules are common in small children (*see* Fig 14.17), and underlying scabies is a cause of (especially recurrent) impetigo. A 'buckshot' pattern of urticated or eczematous lesions is characteristic of scabies (**Fig 15.16**) and is due to the immunological response to mites rather than each lesion representing the site of a mite. This reaction takes some time to settle after treatment, as the immune system remains stimulated by dead mites in the skin. Eczematisation may also occur as a result of overzealous application of an irritant scabicide. Itchy nodules on the buttocks, genitalia (**Fig 15.17**) or axillae develop in approximately 5% of patients and persist for several months after the infection has been adequately treated.

It is also important to recognise more extensive variants of scabies. Crusted scabies (also historically known as Norwegian scabies because it was

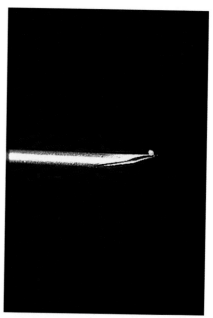

Fig 15.14 Mite on the tip of the needle. The mite is approximately 0.3 mm long. Females are larger than males

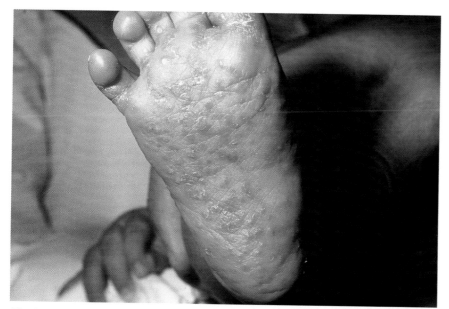

Fig 15.15 Scabies burrows on a child's foot. In infants, scabies burrows are usually best seen on the soles of the feet but also occur on the palms and face. Pustules may also be present (*see* 14.17)

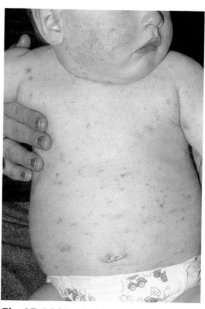

Fig 15.16 'Buckshot' pattern of scabies. Diffuse pruritic eczematous lesions on an infant are often confused with eczema.

277

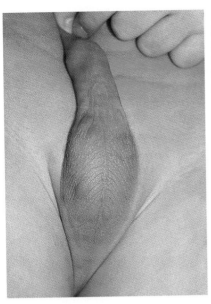

Fig 15.17 Scabies nodules on the genitalia of a child. Brownish-red itchy papules occur on the genitalia and axillae. These probably represent allergy to dead scabies mites but are not a sign of persistent infection

Fig 15.18 Chinese writing pattern of scabies. Hundreds of burrows may occur in some immunocompetent patients with prolonged scabies infestation. This differs from crusted (Norwegian) scabies in that each of the burrows is individually identifiable forming a pattern that has been likened to Chinese writing

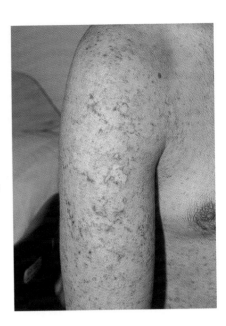

first desribed by two Norwegian dermatologists) consists of sheets of crusting, especially around the ears, eyelids and finger webs and usually occurs in immunosuppressed or demented subjects. The crusts contain hundreds of mites. Occasionally, non-immunosuppressed patients in whom the diagnosis has been missed or in whom treatment has been inadequate develop large numbers of burrows that may merge together in a pattern termed 'Chinese writing' scabies (**Fig 15.8**)

Fungal infections

Dermatophyte fungal infections produce scaling areas with a defined scaly advancing border. Itching is usually present but is not usually the most significant symptom. The diagnosis should be suggested by the asymmetrical or unilateral distribution and by the active scaly edge (*see* **Fig 15.19**). Note that fungal infection of the feet is usually symmetrical but on the palms it is usually unilateral, the two together being termed the 'one hand two feet' pattern (*see* Fig 7.18).

Mistaken steroid therapy of a dermatophyte infection alleviates the symptoms for the first 1 or 2 weeks as itching and scaling improve, but the fungus grows unchecked, and the risk of cross-infection is increased (**Figs 15.20 and 15.21**). The rash changes and becomes less scaly, diffusely red and possibly pustular and a clear advancing edge may be difficult to distinguish. When treatment is stopped the rash recurs, typically leading to further steroid application, increased diagnostic confusion, and, in time, steroid-induced skin atrophy.

Eczema

All eczemas are itchy, although this is minimal in truncal seborrhoeic eczema. In **Table 15.3**, the various types of eczema have been classified according to the frequency with which they are associated with itching.

Atopic eczema

Atopic eczema presents with itching, particularly in infancy when this may be the overwhelming symptom (**Fig 15.22**). This is in contrast to seborrhoeic

DIAGNOSTIC TIPS AND PITFALLS

- Recognition and treatment of scabies are usually possible from the physical signs, and it is a rewarding condition to diagnose and treat

- Most of the rash of scabies consists of non-specific lesions; a scattered 'buckshot' pattern and a mixture of urticarial and eczematised lesions are highly suspicious

- Multiple itchy nodules of the flexures or genitalia should be considered suspicious of scabies until proved otherwise

- Burrows are easiest to identify on hands, wrists and feet; pustules on the feet in babies are strongly suspicious of scabies

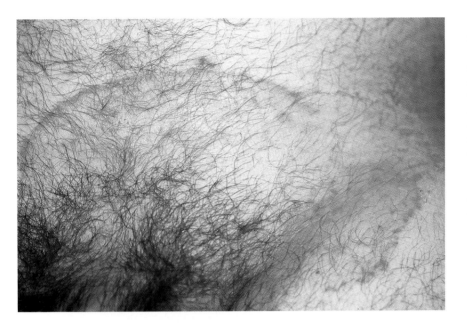

Fig 15.19 Fungal infection of the groin. This infection of the groin with *Trichophyton rubrum* has a red scaling border, and the central area is slightly pigmented. Fungal hyphae virtually disappear from the central area, being chiefly present in the scaly border. The previously infected skin seems to be relatively resistant to reinfection. Repeated infections producing concentric rings of annular scaling can occur in *Trichophyton concentricum* infections and steroid-treated fungal infections

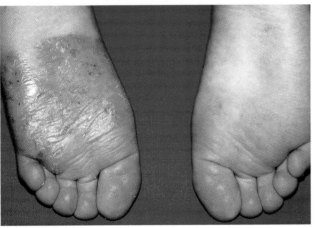

Fig 15.20

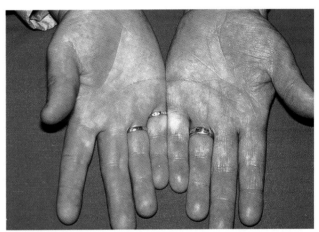

Fig 15.21

Figs 15.20, 15.21 Tinea incognito. This child has a steroid-treated fungal infection of her foot. The asymmetrical involvement indicates an exogenous cause. Steroid-treated fungal infections may not have an active edge, and are diffusely red and occasionally pustular. Because the fungus has grown unchecked, it is potentially more infectious. The child's mother developed tinea incognito of her left hand after applying a topical steroid to her daughter's foot for 2 months (15.21)

Table 15.3 Types of endogenous and exogenous eczema ranked according to itchiness

Endogenous	Exogenous
Atopic	Contact irritant
Lichen simplex	Contact allergy
Discoid	
Varicose	
Asteatotic	
Pompholyx	
Hyperkeratotic hand-and-foot	
Seborrhoeic	

DIAGNOSTIC TIPS AND PITFALLS

- Fungal infection should be considered in any asymmetrical itchy rash

- It is important to examine the feet if there is a unilateral red scaly eruption of the palm, as bilateral plantar or toe web fungal infection may be associated (one hand two feet syndrome)

eczema in infancy or infantile psoriasis, both of which upset the parent far more than the child. The distibution patterns vary with age—the characteristic pattern is involvement of the antecubital and politeal flexures, but in infants atopic eczema may be diffuse, and in older children the main involvement may be of the hands and feet. The closer morphology includes dryness, erythema, fissuring, lichenification (*see* below) and weeping (in acute phases or related to secondary infection, *see* Fig 4.25).

In atopic individuals, lichenification (**Figs 15.23** and **15.42**) occurs at sites of repeated rubbing or scratching, and these areas may become infected. Hair loss may occur at the outer borders of the eyebrows or on the temples (**Fig 15.23**) due to constant rubbing, and patients' bodies may be covered in excoriations (**Fig 15.1**). Affected individuals can be identified by their facies in which there is oedema and thickening of the infra-orbital skinfold—the Dennie–Morgan line (**Fig 15.24**). Patients often have co-existing dry skin or ichthyosis (*see* Fig 7.5). Children with atopic eczema are at risk from extensive and recurrent herpes simplex infections of the skin (**Fig 15.25**), warts and *Staphylococcus aureus* infections of the skin. Eczema may occur around mollusca contagiosa infections in normal and atopic individuals (**Fig 15.26**).

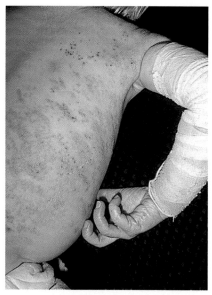

Fig 15.22 Scratching. This is a surrogate for describing itch in the younger child and is a cardinal physical sign for the diagnosis of infantile eczema. Note that the rash is diffuse on the trunk; the characteristic antecubital and popliteal involvement is a feature in older children

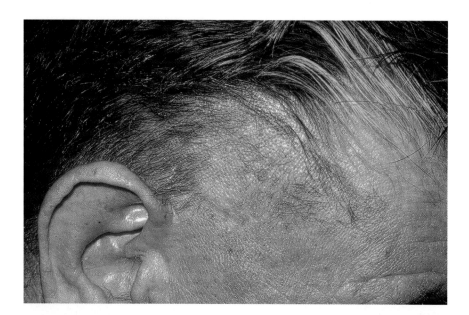

Fig 15.23 Rubbing. Alopecia, pigmentary disturbance and thickening of the skin (lichenification) due to chronic rubbing of the scalp margin in an adult with lifelong atopic dermatitis

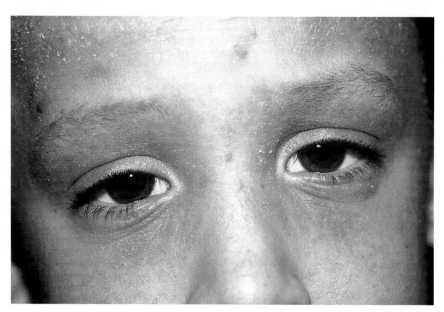

Fig 15.24 Atopic facies. Atopic eczema of the eyelids results in thickening and oedema of the infra-orbital skinfold—the Dennie–Morgan fold, producing the instantly recognisable atopic facies

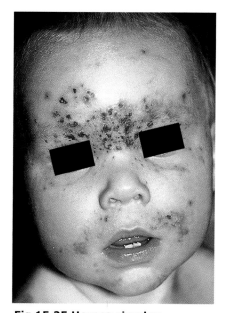

Fig 15.25 Herpes simplex infection in atopic eczema (eczema herpeticum). This 1-year-old has multiple well-circumscribed crusted and ulcerated herpes simplex lesions grouped together on his forehead. Earlier lesions are umbilicated vesicles. Children with atopic eczema are vulnerable to this complication, which is also called Kaposi's varicelliform eruption. Herpes simplex infections can also occur in the lesions of Darier's disease, pemphigus foliaceous and ichthyosiform erythroderma

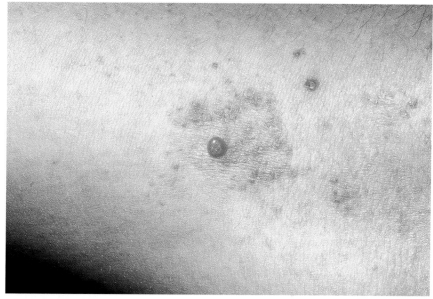

Fig 15.26 Molluscum contagiosum and surrounding eczema. Approximately 10% of children with mollusca contagiosa develop eczema around the lesions. If lesions are extensive, there may be broad areas of eczematisation. This disappears when the mollusca resolve. Children with atopic eczema are also more likely to develop warts, probably because of the combined effects of repeated scratching, the immune-suppressing effects of topical steroids or the altered cutaneous immunity that exists in atopic eczema

Lichen simplex

Constant rubbing results in linear lichenification. Common sites include the nape of the neck, proximal forearm of the non-dominant side, shin (**Fig 15.27**), palm, top of the foot, scrotum, labia majora and perianal skin. On the legs, lateralisation of lichen simplex is independent of handedness.

Discoid eczema

Discoid eczema most commonly affects the limbs of adults (**Fig 15.28**); the subacute oozy eczematous lesions often become infected.

Pompholyx eczema

Pompholyx eczema is characterised by multiple palmoplantar vesicles (**Fig 15.29**). This is usually an endogenous pattern of eczema, although acute allergic reactions may present in this way.

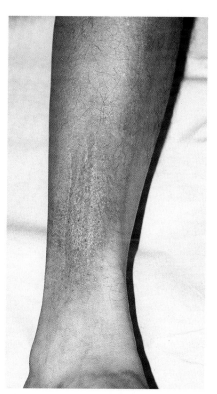

Fig 15.27 Lichen simplex. There is a linear area of lichenified and excoriated eczema on this man's shin

Chronic hyperkeratotic hand and foot eczema

Chronic hyperkeratotic hand and foot eczema may not be particularly itchy (**Fig 15.30**). Patients may have hyperkeratosis at other friction sites, e.g. elbows and knees. Most cases seem to involve some degree of physical damage, being either caused or perpetuated by friction, picking and rubbing at the palmar skin.

Contact eczema

Itching in contact allergic or irritant eczema (**Figs 15.31** and **15.32**) is generally proportional to the acuteness and severity of the eruption, which in turn depends on the type of agent causing the reaction, the degree and frequency of exposure and (in the case of allergic types) the degree of immunological reaction provoked. Thus, contact eczemas are by their very nature highly variable in extent and severity. With a few exceptions, such as the lichenoid appearance due to allergy to colour developers or depigmentation associated with allergy to some chemicals in rubber manufacture, the close-up morphology is not useful in suggesting either the diagnosis of contact, as opposed to any other dermatitis, or the cause. Some examples are shown in **Figs 15.31–15.40**.

By contrast, the body site distribution is much more important in suggesting both the diagnosis and the causative agent. For example, allergy to rubber gloves or footwear (**Figs 15.33–15.35**) is typically symmetrical and localised to sites of contact. Hand eruptions may be caused by contact allergic or irritant eczema, but endogenous eczema and other non-eczematous rashes occur on the hands. Asymmetrical hand 'dermatitis' should always raise concerns about fungal infection (*see* Fig 7.18), but true contact dermatitis may be asymmetrical if only one hand is in contact with the offending allergen (**Figs 15.36** and **15.37**). A summary of the main features of common hand rashes is given in **Table 15.4**.

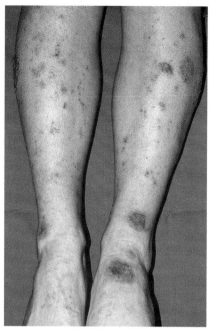

Fig 15.28 Discoid eczema.
Nummular or round patches of acute exudative eczema on the legs. Secondary infection is common

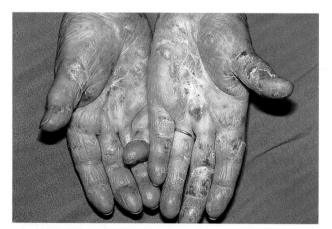

Fig 15.29 Pompholyx eczema. There are large tense multilocular blisters on this woman's palms. Similar changes were present on her feet

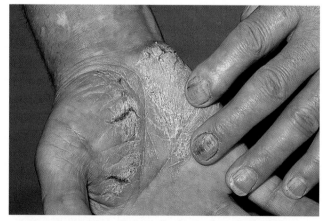

Fig 15.30 Hyperkeratotic dermatitis of the palms.
This is thought to be primarily frictional in origin and is more common in men. The typical picture is of a relatively well-circumscribed area of marked hyperkeratosis with a small inflammatory component. Note in this patient that there is also a habit tic nail dystrophy due to picking at the nail surface (*see also* 19.30)

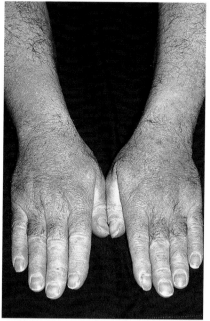
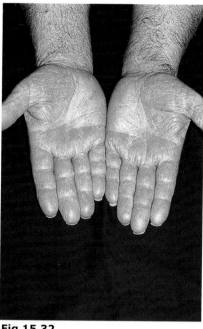

Fig 15.31

Fig 15.32

Figs 15.31, 15.32 Contact irritant eczema of the hands. The dorsum of the hands is covered in scaling and fissures (15.31), compared with the palms, which are relatively spared (15.32). Irritant eczema usually, but not invariably, involves the dorsum of the hands, the fingers and the sides of the fingers. Spread on the palms also occurs

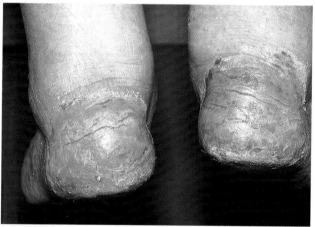
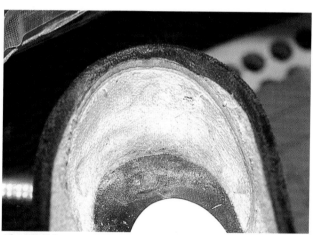

Fig 15.33

Fig 15.34

Figs 15.33, 15.34 Slipper heel rubber allergy. This patient (15.33) was allergic to the rubber supports in the heel of her slippers. Cutting away a small part of the cloth cover at the heel (15.34) revealed the rubber

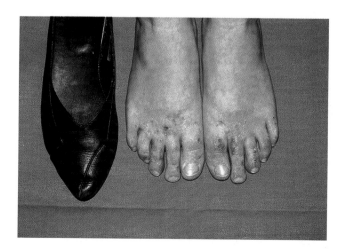

Fig 15.35 Shoe allergy. This young woman had a symmetrical rash on her feet caused by the rubber-based glue used to stick the various layers of her shoe leather together

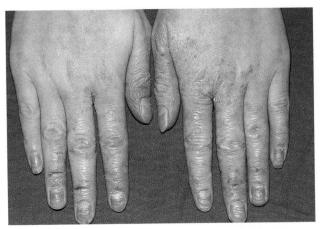

Fig 15.36 Asymmetrical chronic 'dermatitis'. This should always suggest the possibility of fungal infection. However, in this hairdresser, the reaction was eczematous, due to a black dye. The asymmetry is because implements such as scissors were held in the dominant right hand and wet hair between fingers of the more severely affected left hand

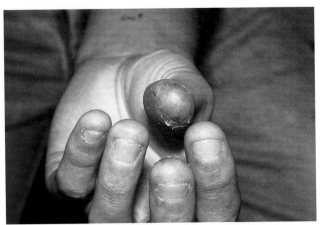

Fig 15.37 Epoxy resin allergy. The rash may be localised to the fingertips, and this seems to occur particularly in men who use epoxy resin glues to lay floors. Alternatively, the patient can be so sensitive that symptoms occur on the face from vapour contact alone. Unilateral fingertip eczema (mainly affecting the thumb, index and middle fingers) is common in cooks who handle garlic, and bilateral changes of this type occur in florists due to handling plants

Table 15.4 Guide to the differential diagnosis of hand eczema*

	Symmetrical	Feet similarly affected	Other sites involved	Vesicles present	Itch
Fungal infection	No	Sometimes	Toenails	Sometimes	Yes
Hyperkeratotic palm and sole eczema	Yes	Yes	No	No	Yes
Pompholyx eczema	Yes	Yes	No**	Yes	Yes
Hyperkeratotic and chronic pustular psoriasis	Yes	Yes	Yes	Sometimes (13.12)	Mild
Contact allergic	Yes	No	Yes	Yes	Yes
Contact irritant	Yes	No	No	Yes	Yes
Porphyria cutanea tarda (13.39)	Yes	No	Face	Blisters, scarring and milia	No

*Dogmatic diagnosis of the aetiology of hand eczema on the basis of physical signs alone is unreliable. In many cases, irritant eczema coexists with endogenous or allergic eczema.
**Acute pompholyx may be accompanied by a more widespread scattered eczema.

Urticaria

Urticarial weals are itchy red raised dermal swellings with surrounding erythema that last less than 24 hours. Oedema of the deeper structures can cause swelling of the face, particularly on the lips and tongue (*see* 16.2–16.4). Other examples of urticarial eruptions are shown in 1.5, 16.1, 16.8 and 16.10.

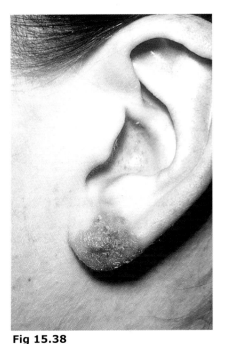

Fig 15.38

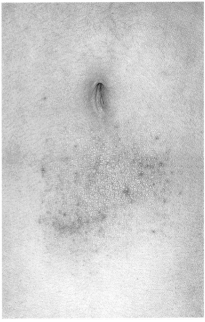

Fig 15.39

Figs 15.38, 15.39 Nickel allergy.
Allergy to nickel is common; approximately 10% of women and 5% of men patch tested give a positive result. Metal jewellery, especially pierced earrings (15.38), is the probable source. Nickel in jean stud buttons or buckles of a belt causes the localised patch of eczema on the central abdomen (15.39)

Nodular prurigo, lichenification and picker's nodule

The terms nodular prurigo, lichenification and picker's nodule describe changes that occur as a consequence of contact rubbing, scratching or picking.

Nodular prurigo

Nodular prurigo is a chronic idiopathic itchy condition usually seen in elderly men and women, who develop discrete nodules 5–30 mm in diameter, usually on the extensor aspects of the limbs, as a result of constant scratching (**Fig 15.41**). The original cause of the scratching is normally obscure, although many patients have a background of atopic diseases. In these circumstances, there is a possibility that emotional stress may play a part. Similar nodular lesions can be seen in patients with a longstanding systemic cause for their pruritus.

Picker's nodules

Picker's nodules are solitary nodules caused by constant scratching. They can occur at any site but are common on the scalp and hands. Tumours and foreign-body reactions may have to be distinguished by biopsy.

Lichenification

Lichenification is the development of thickened patches of skin with increased skin markings due to constant scratching in a predisposed atopic subject (**Fig 15.42**). This is discussed more fully on p. 138.

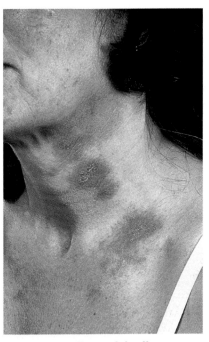

Fig 15.40 Nail-varnish allergy.
This results in allergic contact eczema on the eye lids and side of the neck rather than the fingertips (*photo courtesy of Dr Adrian Ive*)

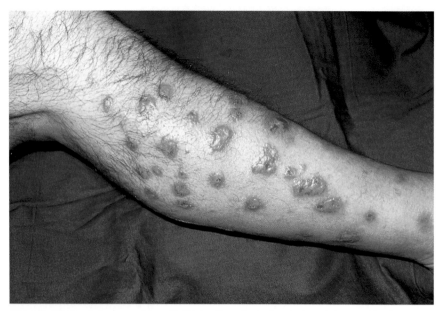

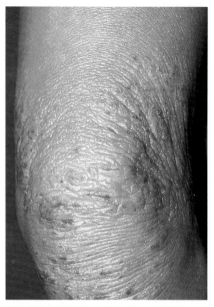

Fig 15.41 Nodular prurigo. Multiple discrete indurated nodules on the legs. Some have an excoriated surface. In this case, the only causative factor identified was iron deficiency due to previous gastrointestinal bleeding

Fig 15.42 Lichenification of the knees in a child with atopic eczema. In reverse-pattern atopic eczema, the extensor rather than the flexor surfaces are affected. This pattern is associated with a worse prognosis

EXCORIATIONS WITH A PSYCHOLOGICAL CAUSE

Various patterns of self-inflicted skin injury are recognised (**Fig 15.43–15.47**), and these are described below. In all such cases, there is usually no underlying pathological basis for the lesions, with the possible exception of mild acne in acne excoriee (**Fig 15.45**). Patients may freely admit that they are scratching or gouging at their skin, as in the case of 'tycoon's scalp' and parasitic delusions, or may be at pains to try to mislead or obscure the cause of their skin rash, as occurs in trichotillomania (*see* Fig 18.41) and dermatitis artefacta (**Fig 15.46** and **15.47**). In neurotic excoriations (**Fig 15.43**) and acne excoriee, patients will admit reluctantly to scratching or picking their skin.

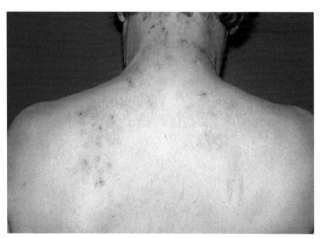

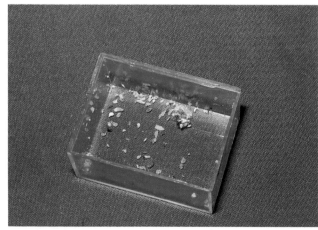

Fig 15.43 Neurotic excoriations. These are most prominent on the left upper back as this is the site that the patient can reach with the dominant right hand

Fig 15.44 The 'matchbox sign'. A collection of carpet fluff and small fragments of wood and skin scale produced by a patient with delusions of parasitosis

Widespread excoriations

Neurotic excoriations

With neurotic excoriations, the patient freely admits to rubbing, scratching or picking of the skin when asked. There is no attempt to confuse or obscure the origin of the lesions (**Fig 15.43**). Patients are often greatly distressed by their symptoms. There may be an associated psychiatric illness.

Delusions of parasitosis

With delusions of parasitosis, the patient has a monosymptomatic delusional psychosis that his or her skin is infested with insects. Often, the patient will show the collection of what he or she believes to be evidence of the infection, classically producing a collection of debris in a small carton (the 'matchbox sign', **Fig 15.44**). This usually turns out to be pieces of rolled-up skin or clothing threads but must be examined under the microscope to exclude genuine infestation. The skin shows scars and erosions on accessible sites, usually the arms and legs.

Excoriations localised to one area

Acne excoriee de jeune fille

Constant picking or scratching of minor acne lesions can result in the excoriated lesions being more severe than the underlying condition. It occurs to a minor degree in many people with mild acne, but becomes a major problem in a few individuals. Lesions are characteristically on the face (**Fig 15.45**), with superficial excoriations and erosions. Scarring due to secondary infection is a common associated feature.

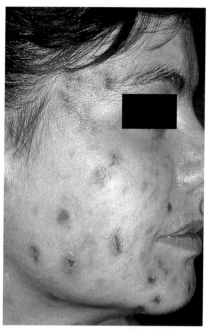

Fig 15.45 Acne excoriee. Multiple deep excoriations of the face in a patient with relatively mild acne initially. She had also been investigated for anorexia and weight loss

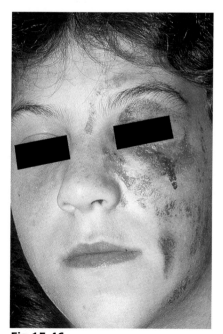

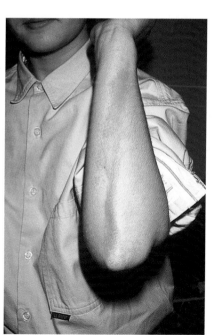

Figs 15.46, 15.47 Dermatitis artefacta. This young woman (15.46) has produced linear excoriations and crusted erosions on the left side of her face. The child (15.47) and her sister both had acute onset linear erythema of the extensor aspect of each forearm; friction, possibly with the side of a match box, was thought to be the cause (*see also* 2.49)

Fig 15.46

Fig 15.47

Dermatitis artefacta

Dermatitis artefacta—These self-induced skin lesions are easiest to diagnose and manage in teenagers in whom excoriations and superficial skin injury (**Figs 15.46** and **15.47**) are the most common pattern of artefact. Excoriations on the face and the breast (*see* Fig 12.10) are common, particularly in young women. The lesions themselves are of geometric shape and unnatural distribution, often being perfectly circular or having unusually linear morphology and a sharp demarcation from normal skin. By contrast, eczema, a common differential diagnosis, has an ill-defined edge. In elderly patients, the artefact can take on many different forms, including swollen limbs (*see* Fig 17.45), bruising, skin ulcers, etc., and can be diagnosed only by exclusion of other causes.

Scalp and hair manipulation

Tycoon's scalp—Constant rubbing and scratching of the scalp produces excoriations and finally hair loss. The patient will admit to rubbing, but wants an explanation as to why it is itchy. No primary scalp abnormality is present. Affected individuals are said to be intense and demanding, hence the flattering diagnostic label.

Trichotillomania—Damage to the hair produced deliberately by the patient results in patterned hair loss with broken hairs, but areas of complete baldness are not a feature (*see* Fig 18.41).

16 Weals

INTRODUCTION

A **weal** is a transient swelling of the skin due to the accumulation of tissue fluid in the dermis. Individual lesions may take the form of a plaque, papule or nodule, which lasts less than 24 hours. However, new areas may continue to appear, and the eruption as a whole may continue for weeks. The raised central lesion or weal is usually surrounded by a rim of erythema known as the **flare** (**Fig 16.1**, *see also* Fig 1.5). Characteristically, the weal resolves leaving no residual change on the skin, but after very severe urticaria, some bruising or purpuric change may be visible.

There are various types of **urticaria** (**Table 16.1**, *see also* Fig 1.5 and **Table 16.2**), and some of those with specific or useful physical signs are discussed below. Note that the term 'urticaria' describes a process and gives little indication of the cause. Weals can also be created by direct physical measures such as intradermal injection of saline or pharmacologically by intradermal injection of histamine or other vasoactive agents.

Localised extravasation of fluid also occurs in other conditions, in which additional physical signs develop, and the areas of swollen skin vary significantly from typical urticaria. These conditions include angio-oedema, urticarial vasculitis and the urticated lesions that occur in several inflammatory skin conditions. The term 'giant urticaria,' which has been loosely

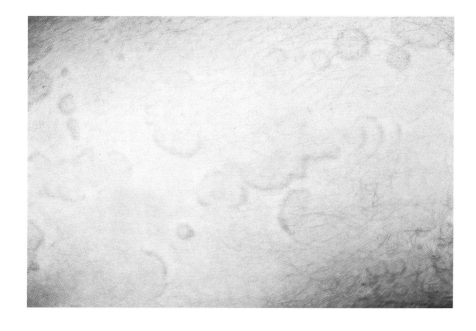

Fig 16.1 Typical urticarial weal.
The paler central area with a red border forms annular, arciform and polycyclic lesions

Table 16.1 Comparison of ordinary urticarial weals and angio-oedema

	Urticaria	Angio-oedema
Distribution	Any, but often trunk mainly	Hands, feet and face including tongue
Border	Sharply defined	Diffuse
Flare	Yes	No
Duration	Minutes to hours	May be 2 or 3 days
Symptoms	Itch	Tightness, pain

Table 16.2 Causes of urticaria

Idiopathic
Physical—cholinergic, dermographism, pressure, vibration, cold, heat, solar
Allergic—IgE-dependent mast cell degranulation—atopic, some foods (eggs, shellfish, strawberries, etc.; may be systemic reaction or direct contact urticaria), drugs, radiocontrast media, bee stings, helminth infestation
Non-allergic chemical-induced (histamine releasing agents)—salicylates, codeine, morphine, antibiotics (ciprofloxacin, rifampicin, vancomycin), plasma expanders, ACE inhibitors, curare and derivatives, azo dyes and benzoates (in foods)
Vasculitic and complement abnormalities—reactions to blood products, serum sickness, lupus erythematosus
Specific triggers, uncertain mechanism—infections (especially viral, occult bacterial), hormonal, exercise

applied to both angio-oedema and large lesions of ordinary urticaria, does not determine any particular cause of urticaria and is therefore of limited value.

URTICARIA

The clinical appearance of urticaria rarely identifies a specific cause, although some physical urticarias are distinctive. The diagnosis of urticaria is usually made from the patient's description of transient lesions. It is important to be aware of the possible confusion between the duration of the overall process and the duration of individual lesions when taking the history. Lesions that come and go or move around from day to day are essentially diagnostic of urticaria. If in doubt, it is helpful to draw around a lesion with a ballpoint pen and to ask the patient to note whether the lesion moves from the outlined area over the next 24 hours (*see* Figs 4.2 and 4.3). The speed of change is unhelpful in identifying a cause.

If a cause is identified (**Table 16.2**), this is also usually from the history rather than from the appearance of lesions or from laboratory tests. Even where there is a fairly characteristic pattern, such as the linear weals of dermographism (**Fig 16.7**) or the tiny papular weals with a prominent surrounding flare in cholinergic urticaria (**Fig 16.10** *see also* Figs 4.34 and 4.35), the clinical history may be just as useful as actually seeing a lesion. However, it is helpful to be able to actively elicit a physical sign to confirm a diagnosis, and this can often be achieved in the group of physical urticarias that are discussed below.

Dermographism (=dermatographism)

Anyone's skin will weal if lashed hard enough. People with dermographism have a much lower threshold, and stroking the skin firmly with a blunt, narrow object or simply scratching the skin will provoke a weal (**Fig 16.8**). This linear weal develops usually within minutes and lasts 5–30 minutes. Delayed dermographism describes the rare phenomenon of weals appearing up to 48 hours after provocation. Pens, keys, orange sticks and similar objects are usually available to elicit these weals, and 'pens' with adjustable pressures can be used for research purposes. If a patient is taking an antihistamine when examined, this will commonly block the weal response but not the flare, so that the history of linear weals after scratching may be adequate to make the diagnosis in this situation. Dermographism can occur as an isolated entity or in conjunction with either other physical urticarias or other causes of urticaria (**Fig 16.8**).

Terms that cause confusion are black dermographism and white dermographism. Black dermographism (*see* Fig 3.18) is neither a cutaneous physical sign nor a weal. It occurs under gold jewellery and is produced by metallic gold on the skin surface. White dermographism (**Fig 16.9**) is a cutaneous response but not a type of weal. It is a vasoconstrictive response, which is produced by a gentle stroking pressure, and it occurs non-specifically in many patients with confluent areas of erythema or erythroderma of any cause.

Cholinergic urticaria

Weals of cholinergic urticaria are typically only 4 or 5 millimetres in diameter but have a prominent and wide flare (**Fig 16.10**, *see also* 4.34 and 4.35). The weals are provoked by sweating caused by exertion or heat, and they can be experimentally produced by injection of cholinergic agents, exercising the patient or immersion of the patient in a bath of water at 42°C. The last test is more reliable and reproducible than exercise but rather more involved. Note that a clinical history of urticaria related to water needs careful evaluation to avoid confusion (**Table 16.3**); small lesions that might be confused with cholinergic urticaria include dermographism due to jets of water in a shower and the lesions of aquagenic urticaria.

Other physical urticarias

Provocation of lesions can be achieved in several other physical urticarias. These are considered together here as the lesions, which occur naturally, do

DIAGNOSTIC TIPS AND PITFALLS

- A weal is a transient swelling of the skin that lasts less than 24 hours and resolves leaving no visible change

- In idiopathic urticaria, very severe wealing on the legs may resolve leaving bruising or purpuric change

- The diagnosis and cause of urticaria (if there is one) are usually made from the patient's history

- Dermographism cannot be elicited if the patient is taking oral antihistamines

- Cholinergic urticaria has a distinctive clinical appearance, with typically small weals surrounded by a prominent and wide red flare

- Urticaria apparently provoked by water contact has a number of causes, including cholinergic urticaria, dermographism, aquagenic urticaria and idiopathic urticaria

Table 16.3 Causes of urticaria related to water

Type of urticaria	Cause
Cholinergic urticaria	Sweating
Dermographism	Jets of water, towelling after bathing
Heat urticaria	Heat
Cold urticaria	Cold
Aquagenic urticaria	Water (weals present)
Aquagenic pruritus	Water (itch not weals, occurs after bathing; exclude polycythaemia rubra vera)

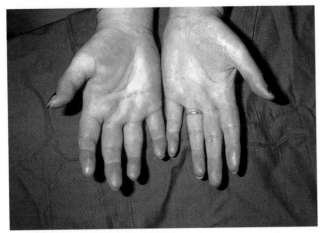

Fig 16.2 Angio-oedema. Deeper swelling is less sharply defined, not associated with a flare component and may last longer than the usual dermal weals of ordinary urticaria. When the hand is affected, as shown (right hand), the usual symptoms are tenderness, stiffness and functional impairment

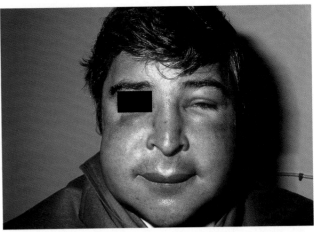

Fig 16.3 Facial swelling in angio-oedema. This is very apparent when lips or eyelids are involved, as shown here

not have a specific physical appearance (although the history may be diagnostic). Thus, cold urticaria can be produced by application of an ice cube to the skin (Fig 16.11) or localised immersion in cold water, heat urticaria by application of tubes of hot water or immersion, pressure urticaria by hanging weights from a focal point (this reaction is delayed several hours after the stimulus) and so forth. Oral antihistamines should be stopped before doing these tests, as wealing may be inhibited even though abnormal erythema can still occur. Immersion of large areas of skin in cold water can be dangerous in cold urticaria as it may cause systemic symptoms of histamine release.

ANGIO-OEDEMA

Angio-oedema is a deeper form of urticaria, caused by the same inflammatory process but producing tissue fluid accumulation at a deeper level in the deep dermis, fat and submucosa. It does not have the visible flare of a dermal weal, and the tissue fluid is less sharply defined. It therefore presents as a diffuse subcutaneous swelling (Figs 16.2–16.4). It typically affects the extremities (face, hands and feet), possibly because it is most apparent at these sites. Although angio-oedema can be quite transient, the fluid volume of any lesion is much greater than a simple dermal weal; this, and possibly the difference in body sites affected compared with 'ordinary' urticaria, causes angio-oedema lesions to be more persistent than simple weals. The other difference from ordinary urticaria (Table 16.1) is that urticarial weals are itchy, whereas angio-oedema is often described as tight or tender; this is probably due to the larger fluid volume of the lesions and the tendency for angio-oedema to occur in the more tightly tethered skin of the head and extremities.

Angio-oedema occurs in association with almost all types of urticaria and at specific sites of contact with a causative agent (e.g. contact urticaria, cold urticaria). The development of angio-oedema in a patient with urticaria therefore has no specific diagnostic significance.

Angio-oedema without urticaria is the typical lesion of a deficiency of the C1 esterase inhibitor. In this rare and potentially life-threatening condition, patients present with angio-oedema but not urticaria. They may experience a prodromal reticulate erythema on the chest wall but not simple urticaria. An

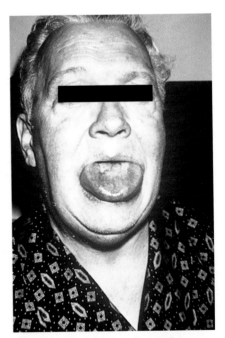

Fig 16.4 The tongue in angio-oedema. The tongue is a relatively common site in angio-oedema. If the mouth and lips are the only sites affected on a regular basis then it is worth considering contact urticaria due to foods

important differential in angio-oedema, in which facial and arm swelling is fixed, is superior vena cava obstruction (*see* Fig 17.44) in which additional features are present, notably venous distension on the chest.

URTICARIAL VASCULITIS

Urticarial vasculitis causes weals that may be indistinguishable from ordinary urticaria but which may have unusual features. These include long duration of individual lesions, purpura or residual bruising, pain rather than itch, minimal response to antihistamine drugs and unusually shaped lesions (**Fig 16.5**). The presence of purpura, especially on the lower legs, is a poor discriminator because this may occur after severe but otherwise histologically and clinically ordinary urticaria (**Fig 16.6**). Histological examination distinguishes severe urticaria and urticarial vasculitis. As the name suggests, lesions of urticarial vasculitis are caused by a small vessel vasculitis with immune complex deposition in vessel walls, and serum levels of complement components C3 and C4 may be reduced (hypocomplementaemic urticarial vasculitis). This may occur as an isolated entity or associated with disorders such as lupus erythematosus.

URTICATED LESIONS

Some eruptions clearly have an urticarial component, having both raised lesions due to extravasated fluid and an erythematous flare, but the lesions last for several days, and other features of the underlying disorder are present (**Table 16.4**). Such lesions are best described as 'urticated.' For example, urticaria itself does not have an epidermal component, but plaques of eczema may be both scaly and urticated. Similarly, urticaria does not consistently

DIAGNOSTIC TIPS AND PITFALLS

- Angio-oedema is a deeper form of urticaria, produced by tissue fluid accumulation in the deep dermis, fat and submucosa

- Angio-oedema is commonly associated with urticaria, and its development therefore has no specific diagnostic significance

- Deficiency of the C1 esterase inhibitor is a rare and potentially life-threatening condition that presents with angio-oedema without urticaria

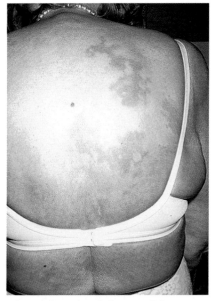

Fig 16.5 Urticarial vasculitis. An unusual stellate-shaped lesion, which lasted several days, with residual bruising and histological evidence of vasculitis, in a patient with hypocomplementaemia

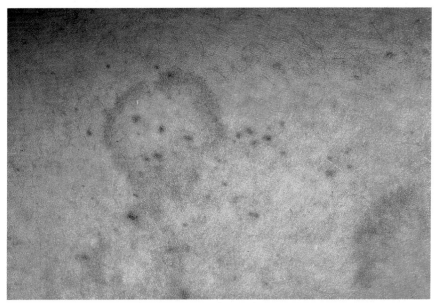

Fig 16.6 Purpura occurring in a banal lesion of urticaria with no evidence of vasculitis

Table 16.4 Features of urticated eruptions that differ from ordinary urticaria

Individual lesions persist for over 24 hours

Additional features are present:
 Scaling
 Blister formation
 Purpura or vasculitis
 Non-urticated skin lesions also present
 Systemic symptoms

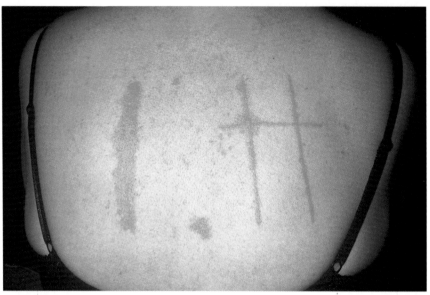

Fig 16.7 Dermographism. Typical linear weals produced by stroking the skin with the blunt end of a pen

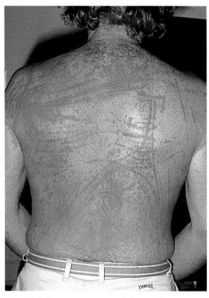

Fig 16.8 Dermographism due to scratching, on a background of a florid urticarial eruption caused by antibiotic treatment

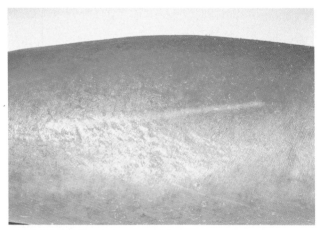

Fig 16.9 White dermographism. Vasoconstrictive response to gentle stroking of the skin in a patient with erythrodermic eczema

Fig 16.10 Cholinergic urticaria. Small papules with a prominent surrounding flare (*see also* 4.34 and 4.35).

Table 16.5 Disorders in which urticated lesions may be present

Eczemas

Papular urticaria (bite reactions), scabies, insect stings

Immunobullous diseases, especially bullous pemphigoid, dermatitis herpetiformis, pemphigoid gestationis

Toxic urticated erythema

Henoch–Schönlein purpura, other vasculitides

Others, e.g. familial Mediterranean fever, Well's syndrome, polymorphic eruption of pregnancy

Localised lesions, e.g. urticaria pigmentosa

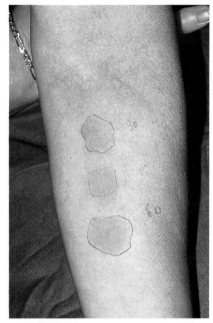

Fig 16.11 Ice-cube test in cold urticaria. The weal appears within a few minutes of removing the ice cube, which is usually applied for 5 minutes. This patient had a dose-related response, the smaller weal occurring after an application of only 15 seconds and progressively larger responses at 30 and 60 seconds

occur at the same site and have an association with a visible persistent lesion, but urticated lesions are a typical feature of urticaria pigmentosa (*see* Figs 4.28–4.30 and 9.53).

Toxic urticated erythema is a label rather than a diagnosis but is a useful term to describe an acute eruption that is usually predominant on the trunk, has an exanthematous pattern (*see* Fig 10.13) of urticated lesions and is a non-specific reaction pattern in some drug and viral reactions. Further examples of disorders in which urticated lesions are common are listed in **Table 16.5**.

17 Erythema and vascular disorders

ERYTHEMA

The interaction of different pigments in the skin is discussed in Chapter 3. Changes in redness are the predominant colour change in most skin disorders, although some pathological processes are purely related to other pigments, such as melanin. Furthermore, most changes in redness are due to changes in blood flow rather than to altered blood constituents, and changes in relative amounts of oxygenated haemoglobin are generally secondary to altered flow.

Erythema is an increase in redness due to increased visibility of intravascular blood and is therefore usually the result of vasodilatation (Table 17.1). In most cases, the individual vessels are not visible to the naked eye. Telangiectasia, which consists of individually identifiable vessels, may occur on a background of chronic vasodilatation (as in rosacea) but is not necessarily associated with diffuse redness.

It is important to recognise that redness is a normal colour component of all skin but may be difficult to see in sun-tanned, racially pigmented or very pale skin. Furthermore, vasodilatation is a labile process, subject to various controlling mechanisms. These factors affect erythema in both normal and pathological skin and are listed in Table 17.1.

Table 17.1 Some factors influencing erythema

External	Light source, observer's perception of erythema
Factors altering light reflection	Topical applications (e.g. oils) Thickness and quality of scale, epidermis, and dermis
Vascular anatomy	Density, depth, tortuosity, anastomoses and shunting, vessel type (arterial, venous, capillary), state of vessel wall
Blood	Erythrocyte count and haemoglobin level
	Proportions of oxyhaemoglobin and others (deoxyhaemoglobin, methaemoglobin, etc.)
Factors influencing vasodilatation	Body temperature (skin and core), posture, exercise (skin flow and competing muscle flow) Neurological (emotion, sympathetic nerves) Local effects (trauma, inflammation, pH, vasodilator metabolites) Tissue chemicals (histamine, catecholamines, prostaglandins, etc.) and drugs (pharmacological or idiosyncratic effects)
Other pigments	Melanin, haemosiderin, extravasated blood, etc.

Table 17.2 Shades of red

Shade of red	Examples
Bright 'scarlet' red	Campbell de Morgan spots (6.24) Pyogenic granuloma (9.65) Flexural rashes, especially candidiasis (5.26) Erysipelas (17.1)
'Ordinary' red	Psoriasis (8.9) Palmar erythema (17.11)
Brownish-red	Bowen's disease (8.17) Seborrhoeic eczema (17.2) Secondary syphilis
Pinkish-red	Pityriasis rosea (7.21)
Violaceous/purple	Dermatomyositis (17.8, 17.9) Lichen planus (8.22) Lupus pernio (5.3)
Dusky/blue	Cyanosis, methaemoglobinaemia Vascular insufficiency Some angiomas (17.3)

Important points in assessment of erythema

Shades of red

Various shades of red characteristically predominate in some disorders. (**Table 17.2**). Some of these are also discussed in **Table 3.1**. As an example, lichen planus is typically rather purple in colour. This is due to the combination of a red colour (due to vasodilation caused by inflammation) and a blue colour (due to disrupted brown melanin pigment lying in the upper dermis, which appears blue at this depth owing to the optical properties of the skin). This is also why resolving lichen planus lesions have a greyish or blue–brown shade—this is the residual colour after the red inflammatory contribution has subsided.

Blanching

The physical sign of 'blanching on pressure' is often ascribed undue importance by non-dermatologists but is actually not a very useful sign—failure to blanch on pressure, which usually (but not always) indicates extravasated blood, is much more relevant. Most common rashes have an erythematous component which, because it is caused by vasodilatation, will blanch on pressure. The presence of blanching therefore just confirms that erythema is produced completely or in part by flowing intravascular blood. Indeed, normal skin will also blanch on pressure (*see* Fig 3.20). Lack of blanching on pressure may indicate the presence of extravascular blood (*see* Purpura, p. 310–312), but some localised vascular lesions are also difficult to blanch. The limitations of this sign are therefore as follows:

- Blanching of erythema is a feature of virtually all skin eruptions, so the presence of blanching has limited diagnostic value.
- Some characteristically purpuric disorders also have a blanchable erythematous component. For example, the urticated lesions seen in Henoch–Schönlein purpura blanch on pressure, whereas the purpuric vasculitic component does not.
- Some angiomatous lesions with purely intravascular blood are difficult to blanch with pressure (**Fig 17.3**). This may be because they are very small, and adequate pressure cannot be applied to the relevant site without obscuring vision of the lesion. It may also occur because it is difficult to apply adequate pressure on soft areas such as the abdomen.
- In urticarial weals, extravasation of fluid into the dermis causes compression of dermal vessels leading to blanching of any associated vasodilatation. The weal may therefore not blanch further on external pressure despite being caused by increased blood flow.

Even when correctly performed, this sign may be misleading, as a mild degree of purpura is very common in inflamed skin, especially on the lower legs of elderly people, in dermatoses that are not primarily purpuric (*see* Fig 10.7).

Disorders characterized by erythema

Flushing

Flushing is a transient erythema usually of the face, upper trunk and upper arms. Frequent and prolonged flushing can be associated with fixed erythema or telangiectasia, for example in rosacea or in carcinoid syndrome. Physiological flushing occurs in everybody, at different thresholds, as a normal emotional response. Causes of flushing are listed in **Table 17.3**.

The cause of flushing is generally diagnosed from the history and associated features rather than by examination, as the physical signs of physiological and pathological flushing are identical, except in disorders with additional fixed telangiectasia, e.g. carcinoid syndrome. The patient should be asked about drugs, alcohol, chemical exposure and associated symptoms such as bronchospasm, gastrointestinal symptoms, headache and sweating.

Facial erythema

Facial rashes are discussed in more detail in Chapter 5. Red or erythematous lesions of the face may be transient (e.g. many febrile exanthemata), fixed (e.g. naevus flammeus) or variable (e.g. rosacea). Facial erythema is common in febrile illnesses in childhood but is also a characteristic feature of scarlet fever and erythema infectiosum (slapped cheek syndrome, *see* Fig 10.9). In scarlet fever, there is a typical circumoral pallor (*see* Fig 10.10); in erythema

---

Table 17.3 Causes of flushing

Generalised	Physiological	Emotional, thermal, menopausal, hot foods
	Drugs	Alcohol (*see* below)
		Nitrates and other vasodilators, theophyllines, nicotinates, histamine, bromocriptine, tamoxifen
	Chemicals	Radiographic contrast media, inhaled solvents (17.4)
	Food additives	Nitrites, sulphites, monosodium glutamate
	Alcohol	*Physiological*
		Racial variation (especially Oriental races)
		Interactions
		Drugs: chlorpropamide, disulfiram
		Chemical: inhaled solvents (e.g. dimethylformamide, trichlorethylene)
	Pathological	Mastocytosis, phaeochromocytoma, carcinoid syndrome, other peptide-producing tumours, hereditary angio-oedema
Localised	Physiological	Triple response to skin injury
	Facial	Fever, rosacea Neurological abnormalities
	Acral	Erythromelalgia, resolving episodes of Raynaud's phenomenon

infectiosum, there is a less prominent but more specific sign, which is reticulate erythema of the arms (**Fig 17.6**). Red lips are a feature of Kawasaki disease (*see* Figs 10.11 and 10.12), often with red swollen palms and soles.

'Butterfly rash'—This term describes a distribution of mid-facial erythema, which affects each cheek and may extend across the nose in a butterfly shape (**Fig 17.5**). It causes one of the most common problems of differential diagnosis in dermatology, mainly because one of the differential diagnoses, systemic lupus erythematosus, is potentially serious. In fact, most patients with this pattern of erythema have rosacea, seborrhoeic dermatitis, other eczemas, such as atopic or contact dermatitis, or transient erythema due to sunburn, cellulitis (**Fig 17.1**) or systemic viral infections.

Clinical differential diagnosis therefore needs to take other features into account. It is uncommon to have systemic lupus erythematosus with a butterfly rash on the face in the absence of other symptoms. Rosacea often affects the chin and forehead as well as the cheeks and has pustular lesions.

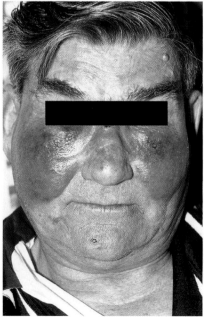

Fig 17.1

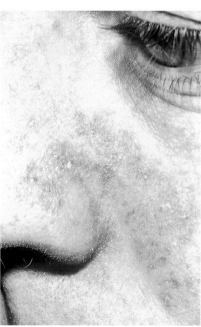

Fig 17.2

Figs 17.1, 17.2 Shades of red. Compare the beefy red colour of erysipelas (17.1) with the typically brownish-red colour of seborrhoeic dermatitis (17.2). Additional useful physical signs shown here are the sharp demarcation and oedema of erysipelas and the typical nasolabial fold distribution of seborrhoeic dermatitis (compare also with the more pink or violaceous red colour and mid-cheek distribution of lupus erythematosus, 17.5)

Seborrhoeic dermatitis affects the nasolabial area rather than the maxillary mid-cheek region, may be associated with dandruff, blepharitis or scaling of the eyebrows and is often at the browner end of the spectrum of red colours.

Reticulate erythema

Reticulate erythema describes a net-like pattern (*see* Fig 2.23). It may occur as a physiological variant (*see* Fig 6.22), in livedo (*see* p. 306), transiently in some infections or as a fixed pattern. Examples are given below.

Erythema infectiosum (fifth disease, slapped cheek syndrome, parvovirus B19 infection)—A bright red 'slapped cheek' appearance (*see* Fig 10.9) is very typical of this disease. However, apart from being rather persistent and often occurring in an apparently well child, the appearance of this part of the eruption may be similar to flushing of the cheeks in any febrile child. The more specific part of the eruption is a striking reticulate erythema on the arms (**Fig 17.6**).

Erythema ab igne—This condition is not uncommon. It is due to thermal damage to the skin and is usually found on the shins of elderly patients who sit close to a fire, although it can occur at other sites due to local application of heat, e.g. a hot water bottle (*see* Fig 6.23). Although initially red, there is a tendency to hyperpigmentation and hyperkeratosis, the latter having features similar to actinic keratosis. Development of pre-malignant or malignant tumours in affected skin is not uncommon. The pattern is basically that of the livedo distribution (*see* p. 306). Chronic heat damage causes epidermal dysplasia and extravascular leakage of blood cells. As the skin heats up, the radiant heat is conducted away into the systemic circulation by the cutaneous blood flow. Skin blood flow is less within the reticulate purple component because this follows the 'watershed' area of mixed blood flow between adjacent feeder vessels of the skin. These areas of relatively poor blood flow therefore reach a higher temperature than the central paler areas and thus experience the consequence of heat damage more profoundly.

Genodermatoses—A reticulate pattern of erythema is a feature of some genodermatoses. A photosensitive tendency is often also present—although the reticulate erythema is an early and fixed feature, e.g. in Rothmund–Thompson syndrome (**Fig 17.7**).

Fig 17.3 Superficial clustered angiomatous vessels. These can be difficult to blanch and may resemble purpura

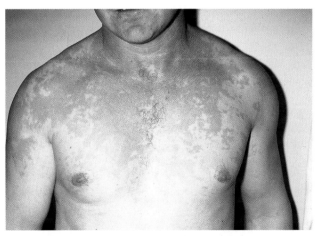

Fig 17.4 Flushing. In this case, flushing was an exaggerated reaction following solvent exposure and was most pronounced on the face and upper torso

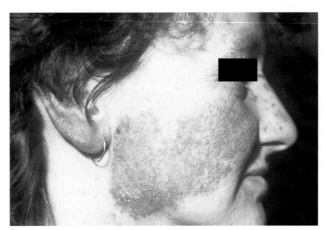

Fig 17.5 Butterfly facial rash of lupus erythematosus. This is much less common than other disorders, which may produce a similar pattern (seborrhoeic and atopic dermatitis, rosacea)

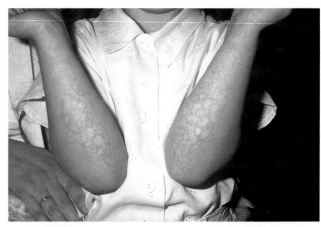

Fig 17.6 Reticulate erythema of the arms. The presence of this sign increases the diagnostic specificity of the 'slapped cheek' appearance of parvovirus B19 infection

Streaky erythema

Bleomycin therapy—Can cause a streaky or 'flagellate' pattern of truncal erythema, which becomes pigmented as the redness fades (*see* Fig 3.9). Streaky red whiplash-like marks with subsequent pigmentation also occur due to contact with photosensitising psoralen chemicals from *Umbelliferae* such as hogweed (especially if children have used the stems of such plants during play fights). The most common cause of a streaky erythema is dermatomyositis.

Dermatomyositis—A streaky pattern of violaceous coloured erythema on the trunk is virtually pathognomonic of dermatomyositis (**Fig 17.8**), although other signs are likely to be present and streaky erythema is not a requirement to make this diagnosis. The other prominent site of linear erythema, of the same violaceous colour, is along the dorsum of the fingers (**Fig 17.9**). The usual sign described on the fingers is smooth, purplish-coloured papular lesions over the dorsum of the joints (Gottron's papules, *see* Fig 5.21), although rather more extensive linear erythema is actually more common.

Acral and palmar erythema

Redness is a common feature of many dermatoses that affect the palms. Many of these affect other body sites, but only the palms may be affected in some patients with psoriasis, contact dermatitis (*see* pp. 284–285), lichen planus or dermatophyte infection (*see* Fig 7.18). Diffuse erythema of the weight-bearing plantar skin, especially of the forefoot, occurs in juvenile plantar dermatosis (*see* Fig 5.24), and the palms or fingertips are affected in a small proportion of patients with this disorder. In all of these situations, there are additional physical signs, notably scaling, although this may be subtle in dermatophyte infection.

Red palms and soles are an early feature of Kawasaki disease in children; swelling and peeling occur later (*see* Figs 10.11 and 10.12).

Various patterns of acral erythema occur due to chemotherapeutic drugs, some of which are characterised by damage to the sweat apparatus. One of the commonest is a sharply demarcated and 'glazed' erythema due to 5-fluorouracil (**Fig 17.10**).

Erythema and a 'burning' pain of the soles of the feet occur in erythromelalgia; some cases are due to myeloproliferative disease and respond to antiplatelet drugs such as aspirin.

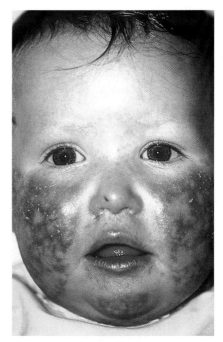

Fig 17.7 Reticulate erythema. This is a feature of some genodermatoses, including Rothmund–Thompson syndrome, where the face is typically affected (*photo courtesy of Dr F A Ive*)

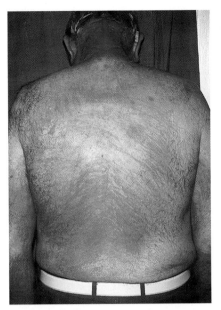

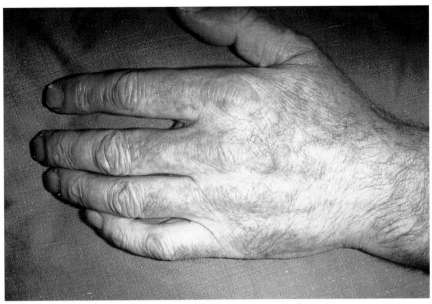

Fig 17.8 Dermatomyositis. This is characterised by a streaky pattern of violaceous erythema, which may resemble scratch marks

Fig 17.9 Dermatomyositis. Typical purple-coloured lesions on the dorsum of the fingers, which form linear streaks and are associated with prominent nailfold telangiectasia and giant capillary loops (*see* 19.43)

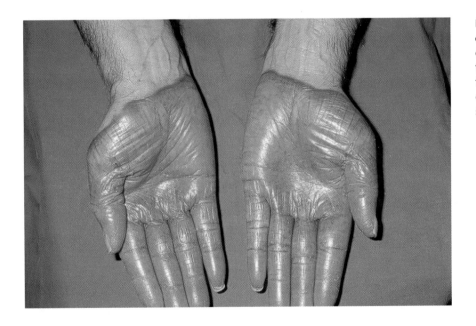

Fig 17.10 Erythema of the palms due to 5-fluorouracil. This reaction occurs in about 30% of patients treated with the drug and shows this typical sharp demarcation. Nail changes may also occur, but symptoms are usually mild

Erythema with purpura of the palms and soles extending to the wrists and ankles and with a sharp proximal cut-off point occurs in purpuric gloves and socks syndrome due to parvovirus infection.

Acral erythema with blistering, and histology showing epidermal necrolysis, is a recently described and rare pattern that seems to be specifically associated with hepatitis C infection.

Palmar erythema without scaling occurs in several conditions; it may be relatively diffuse but often most apparent on the hypothenar eminence (**Fig 17.11**). Gentle diascopy may reveal pulsatile flow.

Causes of palmar erythema without scaling include:

- Pregnancy and oral contraceptive drugs.
- Hepatic disease.
- Thyrotoxicosis.
- Rheumatoid arthritis.
- Hyperglobulinaemia in other chronic diseases: leukaemia, bacterial endocarditis, obstructive lung disease.

Other causes of erythema

Most rashes cause erythema to some extent. Maculopapular rashes are discussed in Chapter 10, and causes of erythroderma are described on p. 27. Extensive areas of erythema occur in pityriasis rubra pilaris (*see* Fig 2.43).

Sunburn can affect any body site and is noted specifically here because of the predictable time course of erythema. This develops about 6 hours after the exposure, peaks at 12–24 hours after a single insult and fades with fine peeling.

PALLOR AND VASOSPASTIC DISORDERS

Generalised pallor may be caused by anaemia, hypopituitarism, albinism or lack of sun exposure. The causes of white skin lesions are discussed in Chapter 3. This chapter discusses vascular causes of pallor (**Table 17.4.**).

Raynaud's phenomenon

Raynaud's phenomenon is a clinically characteristic sequence of vasospastic changes, usually in the fingers. Vasospasm causes fingers to turn white (**Fig 17.13**) or sometimes blue, followed by a period of dull purple (dusky) coloration then a reactive red or pink hyperaemic phase before returning to normal.

The important diagnostic features are:

- Variability: different digits are affected at different times and for different periods.
- Typical sequence of colour changes.
- The colour change shows a sharp cut-off point from normal skin proximally.

The main differential diagnosis is acrocyanosis, which is a fairly common problem, presenting as pale or dull (dark) 'dusky'-blue extremities in

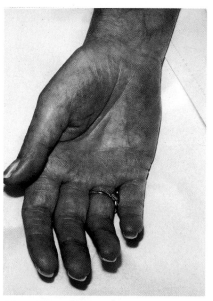

Fig 17.11 Palmar erythema. This is generally most prominent on hypothenar and thenar areas

Table 17.4 Vascular causes of pallor	
Physiological	'Vascular motting' (*see* 6.22) Cutis marmorata (*see* 6.21), including an exaggerated congenital form (cutis marmorata telangiectactica, 17.15)
Occlusive arterial disease	Atherosclerosis, other (*see* later) (17.43)
Vasospastic disorders	Raynaud's phenomenon (17.13) Steal effect and around many erythematous lesions (17.12); especially associated with angiomas and with psoriasis (Woronoff's ring)
Localised	Naevus anaemicus (*see* 3.19)
Neurological	Migraine, carpal tunnel syndrome (may cause early vasodilatation and later pallor or vasospasm)
Others	Weals (Chapter 16)

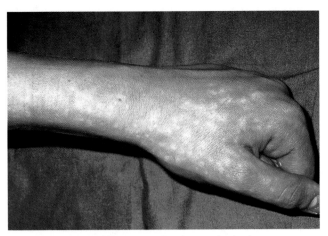

Fig 17.12 Steal effect. Localised vascular lesions, sometimes even quite tiny angiomas, often have a pale halo

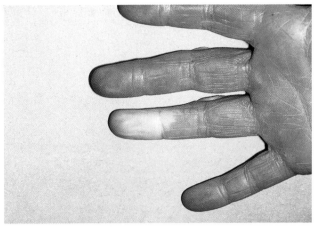

Fig 17.13 Raynaud's phenomenon. This is characterised by an extreme, sharply demarcated pallor

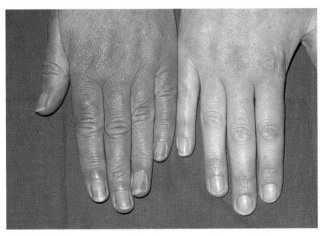

Fig 17.14 Acrocyanosis. There is a diffuse dusky purplish colour to the skin compared with a person with normal circulation

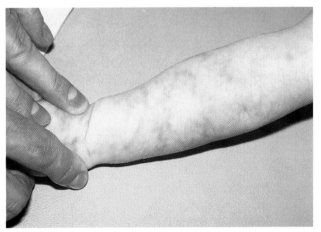

Fig 17.15 Cutis marmorata telangiectatica. A fixed livedo pattern with skin atrophy also, present at birth but often improving spontaneously during childhood. Compare with the 'broken' pattern of livedo in connective tissue disorders (*see* 17.16) (*photo courtesy of Dr F. A. Ive*)

cold conditions (**Fig 17.14**). By comparison with Raynaud's phenomenon, acrocyanosis is less well localised, usually symmetrical, affects all fingers, fades out towards the wrist, has a slower onset and is more closely related to duration of cold exposure. It does not cause trophic changes, sclerodactyly or cuticle or nail changes, although these can all occur as a long-term consequence of Raynaud's phenomenon. Blue staining of the hands from contact with wet denim jeans (e.g. sitting on the hands) has been termed 'acrocyanosis of Levi'. A frequently misdiagnosed and probably under-recognised differential diagnosis of Raynaud's phenomenon is Achenbach's syndrome—this is due to rupture of a small vein and causes sudden onset of a swollen blue finger that is usually tender and sometimes recurrent but without the vasospasm of Raynaud's phenomenon.

The causes of Raynaud's phenomenon are varied (**Table 17.5**). The cause cannot usually be diagnosed by examination of the hands alone. Clinical features at other body sites, such as rashes of connective tissue diseases, livedo associated with hyperviscosity, evaluation of peripheral pulses and associated neurological features, may help to establish a diagnosis.

Table 17.5 Causes of Raynaud's phenomenon

Idiopathic
(Raynaud's disease)

Arterial
Compression
  Thoracic outlet disorders, trauma/fractures
Occlusions
  Stenosis, thrombi, emboli, arteriosclerosis, Buerger's disease (thromboangiitis obliterans), small vessel occlusion in hyperviscosity disorders (*see* below)
Collagen-vascular disease and vasculitis
  Systemic sclerosis/scleroderma, polyarteritis nodosa, lupus erythematosus, dermatomyositis, rheumatoid disease, Sjögren's syndrome

Neurological
Cervical spondylosis, compression syndromes, reflex vasoconstriction, hemiplegia and other chronic neurological disorders with disuse

Haematological
Hyperviscosity disorders (polycythaemia, cryoglobulinaemia, dysproteinaemia, etc.)

Endocrine
Hypothroidism

Drugs/toxic
α-blockers, nicotine, vinyl chloride, ergot derivatives, methysergide, heavy metals, bleomycin

Trauma
Vibration white finger

Livedo

Livedo is a specific pattern of impaired blood flow, which is usefully considered at this point. The pattern is determined by the distribution of arterial blood supply to the skin and relates to the fact that there is a relative 'watershed' area of slower flow between each adjacent area of blood supply. Thus, any disorder that slows blood flow further may make this watershed distribution more prominent, as the blood at this region is deoxygenated and thus more blue in colour. The livedo distribution has a reticulate pattern with a chicken-wire appearance, often most noticeable on the lower legs. It may occur as a physiological response to cold, in association with abnormal vasospasm or with vascular inflammation. The last generally causes fixed patches of livedo separated by areas of normal skin, known as 'broken livedo'. Some causes are listed in **Table 17.6**.

TELANGIECTASIA

Telangiectasia is the term used to describe visible small blood vessels in the upper dermis. The causes are listed in **Table 17.7**. Some of the more useful patterns and important causes are discussed below.

Physical signs of telangiectatic disorders

The diagnosis of telangiectatic disorders is usually made clinically, and factors such as age of onset, sex and family history are important. Associated features such as diarrhoea and bronchospasm in carcinoid syndrome may provide clues to the underlying cause. However, the appearance of the telangiectasia

Table 17.6 Causes of livedo

Physiological
Especially infants (6.21)

Idiopathic
Cutis marmorata telangiectatica (17.15)

Inflammatory vascular disorders
Polyarteritis nodosa (17.16), livedo vasculitis, antiphospholipid syndrome,
Sneddon's syndrome, leucocytoclastic vasculitis, other collagen vascular diseases

Vascular obstruction
Protein: hyperviscosity syndromes such as cryoglobulinaemia (17.28),
cryofibrinogenaemia, macroglobulinaemia
Erythrocyte: polycythaemia, sickle cell disease
Crystals: oxalate, calcium
Emboli: Lipid—cholesterol or atheromatous emboli
  Other emboli—Subacute bacterial endocarditis, atrial myxoma

Erythema ab igne (6.23)

Drug-induced
Amantadine, catecholamines, quinine, quinidine

Table 17.7 Causes of telangiectasia

Hereditary and genodermatoses
Hereditary haemorrhagic telangiectasia
Angiokeratomas, including Fabry's disease
Ataxia telangiectasia
Rothmund–Thompson syndrome (17.7), Bloom's syndrome
Xeroderma pigmentosa

Primary/idiopathic
Angiomas (including Campbell de Morgan spots), angiokeratomas
Vascular naevi, spider naevi (17.17) (also occur secondary to liver disease)
Angioma serpiginosum (17.3)
Generalised essential telangiectasia (17.20), unilateral naevoid telangiectasia
Thread veins (6.27)

Secondary
Chronic vasodilatation
  Sun exposure, varicose veins, rosacea, chronic bronchitis ('costal fringe'),
  hepatic cirrhosis
Hormonal/metabolic
  Oestrogens, pregnancy, corticosteroids (exogenous or Cushing's syndrome),
  carcinoid syndrome, mastocytosis (telangiectasia macularis eruptiva perstans,
  (17.19)
Physical damage
  Erythema ab igne (6.23)
  Post-radiotherapy (11.9)
Atrophic disorders
  Poikiloderma (1.16), corticosteroid administration (11.3)
  Necrobiosis lipoidica, etc. (11.10)
Connective tissue diseases
  Dermatomyositis (17.8), scleroderma and related disorders (11.39),
  graft-versus-host disease
  Lupus erythematosus (11.1)
Drugs
  Nifedipine and other calcium channel antagonists (may be photo-distributed)
  Corticosteroids
Localised lesions
  Basal cell carcinoma, keratocanthoma (9.93)

is characteristic in several disorders, such as generalised essential telangiectasia, or may indicate a group of disorders, such as nailfold telangiectasia in the connective tissue diseases. There are also some useful general points:

- Telangiectasia will blanch with pressure. However, it can be difficult to blanch tiny angiomas, possibly because sufficient pressure cannot be applied.
- Many angiomas and vascular naevi are oestrogen-dependent so their apparent development during pregnancy is not an uncommon feature.
- The mucous membranes should be examined as well as the skin, e.g. lip and tongue lesions in hereditary haemorrhagic telangiectasia.

The main patterns of telangiectasia are listed below.

Radiating pattern (spider naevus)

A spider naevus is a recognisable pattern of telangiectasia in which a central bright red papule—an arteriole seen end-on—supplies blood to radiating telangiectases. The resulting appearance somewhat resembles the handle and spokes of an umbrella. The diagnostic sign is blanching of the radiating vessels when just the central, sometimes pulsatile and visibly raised, arteriole is compressed (**Figs 17.17** and **17.18**). The central pulsation may be made visible by partial compression using diascopy.

Spider naevi are seen commonly on the face in childhood and adolescence but can also occur in pregnancy, alcoholism, chronic liver disease (especially with portal hypertension), thyrotoxicosis and hereditary haemorrhagic telangiectasia (*see* Fig 5.9) and can also be related to oestrogen intake.

Focal grouped ectasias and matted pattern

Focal areas of telangiectasia occur in many conditions and are rarely clinically specific. The pattern is of multiple serpiginous vessels that appear to interweave; if enough vessels are visible, this gives rise to a matted (i.e. tangled) appearance. However, a single feeding blood vessel is not apparent, unlike in a spider naevus.

Small groups of vessels of this type are the most common type of telangiectasia in some naevoid vascular lesions, scleroderma and other connective tissue disorders. Similar, but smaller or less tightly grouped lesions, can occur

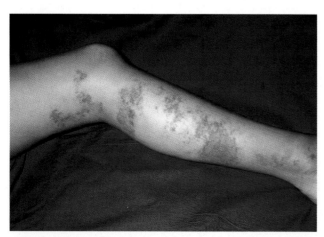

Fig 17.16 Polyarteritis nodosa with cutaneous livedo. The reticulate dusky discoloration is often patchy in intensity ('broken livedo')

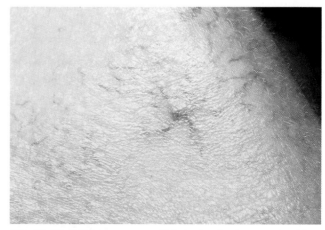

Fig 17.17 Spider naevus. This lesion is characterised by the central arteriole and radiating telangiectatic vessels; central pulsation may be visible

in radiation scars (*see* Fig 11.9), discoid lupus erythematosus (*see* Fig 11.1), rosacea and hereditary haemorrhagic telangiectasia (*see* Fig 5.9). Superficial small linear or serpiginous telangiectatic vessels are a feature of several discrete skin lesions, notably basal cell carcinoma (*see* Fig 9.73). Larger, more matted looking, lesions may be apparent in cutaneous mastocytosis (especially in the variant known as telangiectasia macularis eruptiva perstans, **Fig 17.19**), Cushing's syndrome and carcinoid syndrome.

Linear and arborising pattern

Tiny linear or wavy vessels, sometimes loosely grouped, are very common. They are relatively large diameter venous vessels, and more blue than red. Common sites include the upper back in young adults, the legs (especially in women, *see* Fig 6.27) around the costal margin of patients with chronic bronchitis and on the nose and cheeks in rosacea or chronic flushing.

More prominent lesions with a branching or arborising pattern are typical of generalised essential telangiectasia (**Fig 17.20**) and also occur in a more limited distribution on the lower legs as a common finding related to venous insufficiency ('venous flare').

Punctate and papular pattern

Punctate or papular telangiectasia is seen in a variety of disorders, and some small ectatic (dilated) vessels, or vessels viewed end-on, may appear as punctate lesions in many of the disorders already discussed. These are common in hereditary haemorrhagic telangiectasia and on the face in scleroderma.

More localised punctate telangiectasia is seen in radiation scars and in atrophie blanche (**Fig 17.21**).

Small or early lesions in some disorders that are usually classified as angiomatous rather than telangiectatic may actually have the appearance of telangiectasia when viewed carefully. This is the case in patients with cherry angiomas (Campbell de Morgan spots) (*see* Fig 6.24) and angioma serpiginosum (**Fig 17.3**).

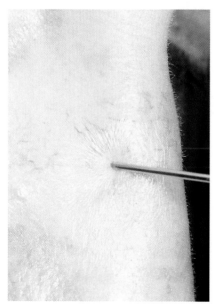

Fig 17.18 Spider naevus. The lesion can be blanched by point pressure on the central vessel (same lesion as in 17.17)

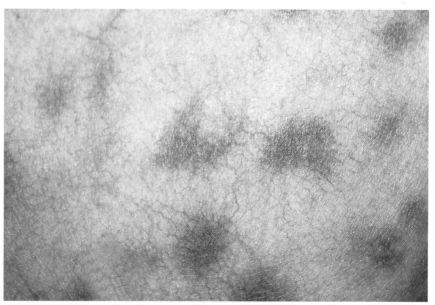

Fig 17.19 Telangiectasia macularis eruptiva perstans. This is a form of chronic cutaneous mastocytosis, in which a matted pattern of telangiectasia is observed

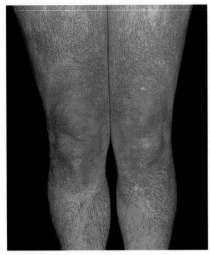

Fig 17.20 Arborising telangiectasia. This condition describes the linear tree-like branching pattern of vessels seen in essential telangiectasia. At a distance, this resembles a sheet of erythema on the leg

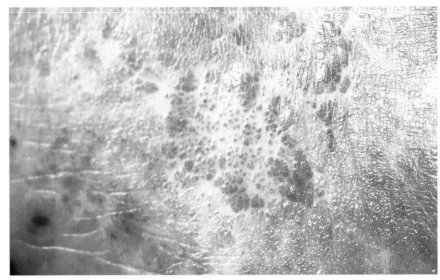

Fig 17.21 Atrophie blanche. This is a feature of venous disease in which punctate telangiectatic vessels with a scar-like appearance are visible in white areas

Angiokeratoma corporis diffusum (Fabry's disease) also falls into this category of small superficial ectatic vessels (i.e. telangiectasia) making up angiomas; this is an X-linked disorder, which is therefore found in males. Lesions occur around the buttocks and genital area but can be widespread, and internal involvement in this condition affects vessels of the heart, kidneys, eyes and nervous system. It is due to an enzyme defect (α-galactosidase deficiency), and it is interesting that cutaneous angiokeratomas with a similar appearance and distribution have been described in other disorders with rare enzyme deficiencies.

Nailfold telangiectasia

Nailfold telangiectasia is one of the hallmarks of connective tissue diseases discussed in Chapter 19, and it is most prominent in dermatomyositis (*see* 19.42–19.43).

PURPURA, VASCULITIS AND BRUISING

Extravasation of blood may present as bleeding, bruising (ecchymosis) and smaller purpuric lesions, which are the most important dermatological manifestations of intradermal bleeding (**Table 17.8**). Tiny pinpoint purpuric lesions are also known as petechiae. Most purpura is macular; palpable purpuric lesions suggest either a vasculitis or dysproteinaemia. Vasculitis is discussed in more detail on p. 317–322.

Ecchymosis or bruising is usually purple-coloured initially and then changes to appear blue, grey, green and yellow. Bruises are most likely to be the result of physical damage to vessels by external trauma but are occasionally due to clotting defects; they are less likely to have a dermatological cause than smaller purpuric spots. It is important to be aware that fixed bruise-like lesions may represent Kaposi's sarcoma in HIV infection.

Large sheets of brusing and necrotic lesions may occur in patients with thrombophilic disorders such as protein C deficiency or resistance and in purpura fulminans and disseminated intravascular coagulation (which may be

Table 17.8 Causes of purpura

Decreased platelet number or function	Hereditary/congenital Idiopathic thrombocytopenic purpura Other haematological disorders, e.g. leukaemias Increased consumption (large haemangiomas, hypersplenism, disseminated intravascular coagulopathy) Infections, uraemia, drugs and toxins
Vascular causes	Capillaritis and vasculitis (idiopathic, toxic/infective, drugs, systemic diseases) Altered connective tissue (age/actinic-related, corticosteroid, scurvy, lichen sclerosus, Ehlers–Danlos syndrome, amyloidosis) Non-specific (minor feature in many dermatoses, especially on the legs—prominent feature in stasis dermatitis, pigmented purpuric dermatoses (17.25, 17.26), clothing dye contact dermatitis, histiocytosis X) Traumatic (pinch and friction injuries, talon noir (9.47), splinter haemorrhages (19.51), suction purpura (artefactual, limb prostheses))
Other blood abnormalities	Dysproteinaemias Clotting disorders (usually cause bruising) Circulating anticoagulants Autoerythrocyte sensitisation

Table 17.9 Types of extravasation of blood related to underlying causes

Underlying cause	Petechiae	Larger bruises	Bleeding (e.g. gums, joints)	Inflammation (i.e. palpable purpura)**
Coagulation defect	+/–	++	++	–
Platelet defect	++	+	+	–
Collagen defect	Some, e.g. scurvy amyloid, EDS	++	Some, e.g. scurvy, EDS	–
Vessel wall abnormality	++	+/–	Some, e.g. HSP*	++

– Not a feature.
+/– Not characteristic.
+ Common (but depends on severity).
++ Typical.
EDS = Ehlers–Danlos syndrome.
*In Henoch–Schönlein purpura (HSP) bleeding from gut wall may occur, but bleeding from gums is not a feature.
**Vasculitis may only be evident on histological examination.

provoked by sepsis). Thrombophilic disorders also predispose to coumarin necrosis (*see* Fig 12.5).

Features that may help to determine the underlying defect causing extravasation of blood are given in **Table 17.9**.

Before discussing the main physical signs of the skin lesions themselves, it is worth noting a few additional points in the examination of patients with purpura:

- Always consider symptoms or signs in the mouth (**Fig 17.22**), joints, abdomen and eyes. For example, platelet disorders may cause bleeding from the gums, haemarthroses are a feature of some common clotting disorders, and Henoch–Schönlein purpura may be associated with joint pain or effusions and with colicky abdominal pain.
- Examine the eyes in all patients with purpura that might be due to thrombocytopenia. In particular, vitreous or fundal haemorrhages suggest a significant thrombocytopenic state and indicate a degree of urgency for

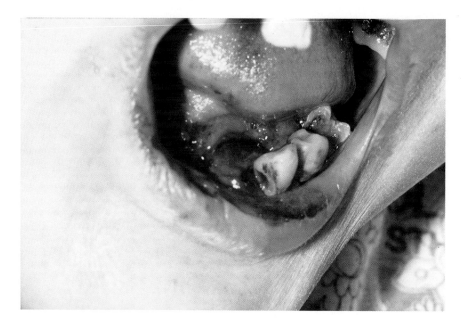

Fig 17.22 Haemorrhagic bulla of the gum in a patient with scurvy

diagnosis and treatment. Examination of the conjunctivae and fundi may also be rewarding in patients with purpuric skin lesions due to subacute bacterial endocarditis.

- Consider the importance of other skin findings, and assess whether the degree of purpura is out of proportion to the site and extent of associated skin disorder. This is discussed further on p. 316.
- Purpuric changes on the lower legs (*see* Fig 10.7) may occur in association with inflammatory dermatoses, especially in patients with oedema.

The main physical signs that are useful in the diagnosis of purpura are described below.

Blanching

Purpura will not blanch under pressure, as it is due to erythrocytes in tissue rather than within (compressible) vessels. As discussed above, this is not always a helpful physical sign. In purpuric disorders, it is important to remember the following points:

- An inflammatory component will blanch, so partial blanching may occur in vasculitic disorders or dermatoses of which purpura is a component.
- Lesions of capillaritis or resolving vasculitis may lose all their red colour when compressed but still retain visible reddish-brown haemosiderin staining as evidence of previous extravasation of blood.

Variability

Purpuric lesions are individually transient. They are bright red or purple initially but become darker purple and later brown as their haemoglobin content is degraded to haemosiderin. This feature distinguishes them from angiomas, which are fixed, and it is also helpful to determine if the process is ongoing. A good example is Henoch–Schönlein purpura, in which crops of lesions occur over a period of time, such that lesions of different age can be distinguished by their colour (**Fig 17.23**).

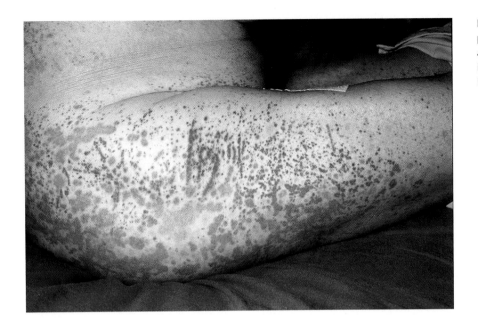

Fig 17.23 Henoch–Schönlein purpura. The lesions of different ages have colour varying between bright red recent purpura and brown haemosiderin of the earliest lesions

Inflammation

Palpable purpura implies an inflammatory component rather than simple extravasation, although sufficient leakage of blood in thrombocytopenia may cause palpable lesions. In most cases, therefore, the presence of palpable purpura suggests the diagnosis of vasculitis, including dysproteinaemias. However, deeper bruising (ecchymosis) alone may be palpable simply because of the volume of blood in the tissues. It is also important to distinguish angiomas that may be palpable but which are fixed and do not fade over a period of time (*see* above).

Absence of palpable lesions does not exclude vasculitis as a cause of purpura, although subtle elevation of the lesions is usually apparent on careful inspection.

Patterns

Different patterns of purpura may be diagnostically useful and are therefore described below.

Linear

Purpura that is provoked by minor injury can appear as lines made up of many individual purpuric spots. If thrombocytopenia is excluded, then the cause is likely to be either a dysproteinaemia (**Fig 17.28**) or an alteration to the supporting tissues of the dermal vessels (especially in amyloidosis, **Fig 17.24**).

Circular/annular

Vaguely circular purpuric lesions, often including the lower limbs, are a typical feature in a group of disorders known as pigmented purpuric dermatoses (**Fig 17.25**). These are due to low-grade chronic capillaritis and therefore exhibit petechiae at different stages. The background brownish-orange colour is largely due to haemosiderin, and a mild epidermal scaling component may also be present. Performing the Hess test (*see* p. 68) may cause increased purpura within the lesions. The dusting of pinprick-sized orange–red purpuric lesions in these disorders is known as a Cayenne pepper appearance (**Fig 17.26**).

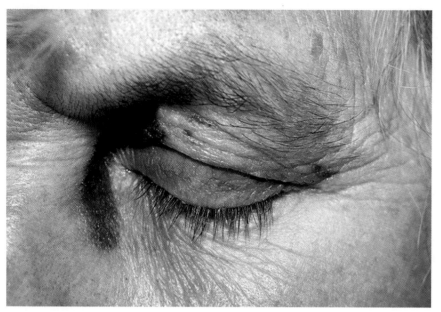

Fig 17.24 Panda sign. Amyloidosis with linear cutaneous purpura after minimal trauma on the fragile skin of the eyelid pressure from bedding. Diffuse bruising of the eyelids due to amyloidosis is known as the Panda sign

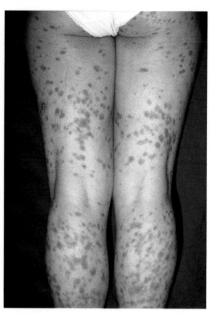

Fig 17.25 Pigmented purpuric dermatosis. The lower leg is the common body site for this group of disorders in which a low-grade capillaritis causes mildly scaling reddish-brown lesions with prominent haemosiderin content

Annular or 'cockade' (rosette-like) lesions of vasculitis on the face occur in young children with a disorder known as acute haemorrhagic oedema of infancy, Seidlmayer's syndrome or Finkelstein's disease. This is probably a variant of Henoch–Schönlein purpura.

More sharply demarcated circular lesions, especially on the face, and purpuric spots of a uniform colour, are strongly suggestive of artefactual disease.

Reticulate

A reticulate pattern of purpura within individual skin lesions has been described as specific for vasculitis due to deposition of IgA immune complexes (Henoch–Schönlein purpura). This is a relatively unusual sign (**Fig 17.27**).

Rashes with an overall reticulate pattern may have an element of purpura that is in the same reticulate distribution. This occurs to some extent in erythema ab igne on the lower legs (*see* Fig 6.23) but is most important in conditions that cause livedo (seen in dysproteinaemias, **Fig 17.28**), and vasculitic disorders such as polyarteritis nodosa or cholesterol embolisation (**Table 17.6**).

Overall distribution of purpura or bruising

Purpura confined to isolated urticated inflammatory lesions is discussed on p. 316.

Lower legs—Purpura localised to the lower legs is not very discriminatory, as purpura may appear within any inflammatory dermatosis at this site due to the increased hydrostatic pressure encouraging vessel walls to burst when inflamed. Furthermore, most small-vessel vasculitic disorders are most apparent on the lower legs. Note that the combination of lower leg and buttock involvement by palpable purpura is suggestive of Henoch–Schönlein purpura.

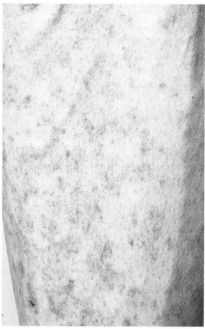

Fig 17.26 Pigmented purpuric dermatosis. Close examination reveals dusting of pinprick-sized haemorrhages, known as a Cayenne pepper appearance

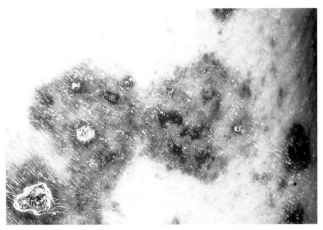

Fig 17.27 Henoch–Schönlein purpura. A reticulate pattern of purpura within lesions is said to be specific for vasculitis with IgA immune complex deposition

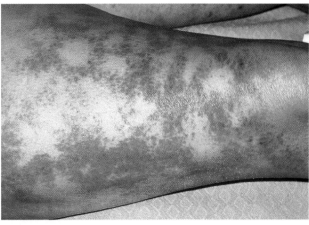

Fig 17.28 Reticulate purpura. This patient has cryoglobulinaemia (*see also* 17.39)

Erythema elevatum diutinum, a type of vasculitis that causes rather chronic fibrotic plaques, often affects the knees.

Palm and sole—A distinctive pattern of purpura on the hands and feet and adjacent distal limbs has been described as 'purpuric gloves and socks syndrome.' It is one of the skin eruptions that occurs owing to infection with parvovirus B19, which also causes the slapped cheek syndrome (fifth disease, *see* **Fig 17.6**). Oddly, purpuric lesions of the palms rarely occur in some bullous disorders in which purpura is not a feature generally, including dermatitis herpetiformis and toxic epidermal necrolysis.

Head and neck, periorbital—Fine petechial haemorrhages confined to the head and neck occur as a result of acutely raised intravascular pressure related to severe retching, coughing or the Valsalva manoeuvre. Because they all occur at the same time, the purpuric spots are all of the same colour (**Fig 17.29**).

This distribution of purpura is also common in amyloidosis (Panda sign), but in this, there are also grouped purpuric spots related to mild injury, and a more chronic course is apparent from the history and the presence of lesions of different colours.

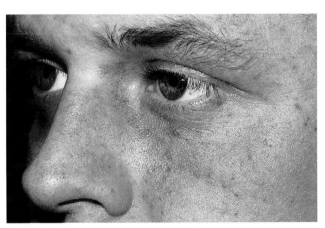

Fig 17.29 Purpura of the eyelids. This patient had a severe episode of vomiting

Periorbital—Ecchymosis may occur in children with neuroblastoma ('racoon sign').

Abdominal—In a patient with abdominal pain, bruising of the flanks (Grey–Turner sign) due to spread of haemorrhage to the retroperitoneal space or along or around the umbilicus (Cullen's sign) due to spread of haemorrhage along the falciform ligament is strongly suggestive of acute haemorrhagic pancreatitis. A periumbilical 'thumb-print' pattern of bruising occurs in immunosuppressed patients with *Strongyloides* infection.

Associated features

Connective tissue changes—Small sheets of purpura with irregular edges and often about 1–2 cm in diameter are a common feature in thinned skin due to chronic actinic damage (*see* Fig 6.14) or as a side–effect of long-term or high-dose oral or topical corticosteroid treatment (*see* Fig 11.3).

Lichen sclerosus is a further cause of purpura related to connective tissue changes (Fig 17.30). The small (usually about 2–5 mm in diameter) areas of purpura occur on a background of smooth, white atrophic skin. The degree of purpura may cause diagnostic problems (Fig 17.31). The main importance of this disorder is that it often involves genital skin in either sex and at any age, and the presence of genital purpura in children can give rise to concern about sexual abuse (Table 2.6).

Rashes—Purpura is a common component of many rashes. It may occur partly due to scratching, in which case it may have linear patterning and be associated with other signs of excoriation. However, it may also occur as a consequence of the high hydrostatic pressure in the lower legs (*see* Fig 10.7). In these situations, it is a matter of experience to decide whether the purpura is in proportion to the degree of inflammation and the general vascular status of the affected limb (Fig 17.32).

Urticated lesions—These are part of the spectrum of palpable purpura discussed above. They are especially common in Henoch–Schönlein purpura but also in other vasculitic disorders. Some reactions to insect bites may exhibit purpuric changes due to anticoagulants produced by the biting insect to prevent blood clotting during feeding—these include the central purpuric spot in lesions due to bedbug bites (purpura pulicosa) and the red–blue lesions caused by crab lice (maculae ceruleae). Purpura within urticarial lesions is also a feature of urticarial vasculitis (*see* Fig 16.5).

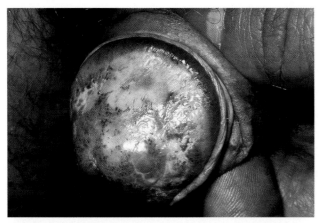

Fig 17.30 Lichen sclerosus. Altered upper dermal connective tissue alters the supporting matrix of blood vessels and is a cause of purpura

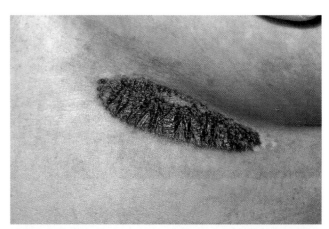

Fig 17.31 Lichen sclerosus with prominent purpura. The purpuric component may be the main clinical feature of this condition. This is most likely in lesions with major itch and scratch or, as in the inframammary region shown here, in flexural lesions where the skin is subject to shearing stress

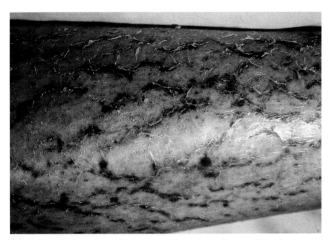

Fig 17.32 Purpura between ichthyotic scaling in a man with Hodgkin's disease. Purpura can occur in asteatotic eczema, which is quite similar, but the amount of purpura shown here is out of proportion to the degree of scaling

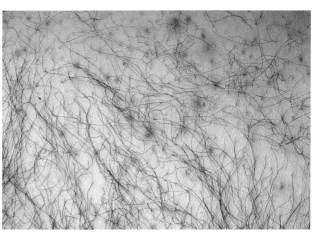

Fig 17.33 Follicular hyperkeratosis and purpura in scurvy

Follicular purpura—This is the hallmark of scurvy (**Fig 17.33**), although larger and deeper bleeding may occur and eventually cause 'woody' fibrosis. Other features that may be present include 'corkscrew' hairs (*see* Fig 4.44), which are actually multiply kinked rather than a spiral shape (*see* Fig 6.4), and bleeding from gums (**Fig 17.22**). Follicular eruptions, including purpura, are disproportionately frequent in HIV infection.

Splinter haemorrhages—These (*see* Figs 19.51 and 19.52) are purpuric lesions that develop a linear shape because of their site under the nail. The most common cause is trauma, but the most important causes are related to embolic and vasculitic disorders such as subacute bacterial endocarditis. Note that there may be evidence of vasculitis elsewhere, especially on the digital pulps (Osler's nodes) (*see* Fig 19.53) and other areas of the hands and feet (Janeway's lesions).

VASCULITIS

Several signs of vasculitis have already been discussed in relation to purpura. However, vasculitis can cause many other types of lesion, including pustules, necrosis, livedo and inflammation of fat (panniculitis). Problems that arise when considering vasculitis include:

- Clinically similar patterns are produced by many causes.
- Both clinical pattern and histological features may vary during the course of a vasculitic process and may be altered by non-specific factors such as localisation to areas of vascular stasis.
- Physical signs may be very variable, depending in part on the speed and degree of tissue anoxia. For example, temporal arteritis may cause extensive ulceration of the scalp (*see* Fig 12.26) but generally does not cause any obvious cutaneous abnormality.
- Some vasculitic disorders are characterised by lesions that do not overtly suggest a vascular aetiology, for example, the destructive vasculitis of Wegener's granulomatosis or the small scaling papules of pityriasis lichenoides (**Fig 17.36**).
- The type of blood vessels affected in the skin may not reflect the main pathological features of the disease; for example, Wegener's granulomatosis causes a granulomatous vasculitis of medium-sized arteries, but the skin lesions may be a small-vessel neutrophilic vasculitis.

- The situation is further confused by the wide range of different classifications of vasculitis, which may be based on clinical features, presumed aetiology or histological features such as size of vessels affected and types of inflammatory cells present. These are all useful in different ways:
  - Classification by clinical pattern is useful when faced with a patient with vasculitic lesions, but few patterns are 100% specific.
  - Classification by cause is especially useful as a memory jog for the tests that may need to be performed in patients with vasculitis but does not encourage a selective approach to investigation of individual cases.
  - Classification by immunological mechanism is useful from a scientific point of view but does not always translate easily into a clinically useful form.
  - Classification by histological features is useful and may help to predict outcome. For example, granulomatous vasculitis is generally more destructive than lymphocytic vasculitis, but the diagnosis is usually clinicopathological rather than pathological alone.

As none of these is the single best way to divide up vasculitic disorders, a classification based primarily on known causes of vasculitis is given for reference (Table 17.10). The main text describes the different clinical presentations, with a selected differential diagnosis for the various clinical presentations. Some lesions, in which there is vasculitis but which do not immediately suggest vasculitis on a clinical basis are mentioned in more appropriate chapters. For example, pyoderma gangrenosum (*see* Fig 12.17) usually presents because of ulceration and pityriasis lichenoides (**Figs 17.36–17.38**) as papules.

Clinical patterns

Clinical patterns of vasculitis may be quite varied. They are rarely specific, and a mixture of different patterns may occur in the same patient; for example, palpable purpura and cutaneous ulceration may be present simultaneously or sequentially. Additionally, some causes of vasculitis can give rise to a

Table 17.10 Causes of vasculitis

Drugs	Blood products, sulphonamides, other antibiotics, thiazides, allopurinol, phenytoin, non-steroidal anti-inflammatory drugs
Infections	Direct vascular damage e.g. syphilis, tuberculosis, infective ulcers/abscesses, etc. Septic emboli Immunological reactions e.g. meningococcus, gonococcus, viral
Arteritis and 'collagen vascular disease'	Wegener's granulomatosis, polyarteritis nodosa Churg–Strauss disease, giant cell arteritis Lupus erythematosus, rheumatoid disease Sjögren's syndrome, systemic sclerosis Behçet's disease Antiphospholipid syndrome
Other chronic disorders	Vasculitis associated with ulcerative colitis, cystic fibrosis, lymphomas and 'tuberculides'
Thermal	Perniosis (chilblains)
Uncertain or multiple causes	Henoch–Schönlein disease 'Hypersensitivity vasculitis' Nodular vasculitis Urticarial (hypocomplementaemic) vasculitis Hypergammaglobulinaemic purpura Erythema elevatum diutinum

variety of clinical patterns; for example, sulphonamides may cause serum sickness, typical leucocytoclastic vasculitis and erythema nodosum. Despite these limitations, it is useful to consider some typical patterns as they may help to narrow the search for a cause.

Palpable purpura

An eruption consisting of multiple palpable purpuric papules, most prominent on the lower legs, with each lesion generally about 5 mm in diameter, is one of the most common forms of vasculitis (**Fig 17.34**). It is the hallmark of a small-vessel leucocytoclastic vasculitis (leucocytoclasia is the histological identification of fragmented neutrophil polymorphonuclear leucocyte nuclei in and around the damaged vessels). This pattern is seen in:

- Some drug eruptions.
- Collagen vascular diseases.
- Antiphospholipid syndrome.
- Cryoglobulinaemia and other hyperglobulinaemic states.
- Henoch–Schönlein purpura.
- Association with systemic infections.
- Embolic vasculitis, e.g. cholesterol emboli, atrial myxoma.

Note:

- Urticated lesions can occur in any of these causes but are typical of Henoch–Schönlein purpura; it is probably best to reserve the label of true Henoch–Schönlein purpura for patients with IgA immune complex deposition in vessel walls.
- Physical factors such as gravity (lower legs most floridly involved), pressure (e.g. tops of socks, **Fig 17.35**) and exercise may all enhance the development of lesions.
- Pustules, necrosis, larger nodules and ulcers may all develop in any of the causes listed.
- Systemic malaise, arthritis, myalgia, nephritis and pyrexia may be a feature of any of the causes listed.
- Always suspect and exclude systemic infections and drug eruptions in patients with palpable purpura. Note that septicaemia can cause palpable purpura.

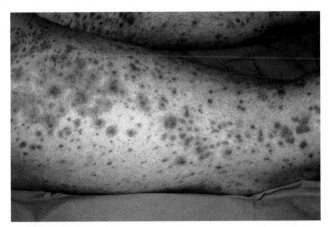

Fig 17.34 Palpable purpura. This is the hallmark of a small-vessel leucocytoclastic vasculitis

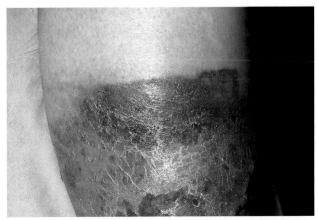

Fig 17.35 Leucocytoclastic vasculitis with lesions accentuated by pressure from elastic in socks (*see also* 2.39)

Other papular vasculitides

Papular lesions that are less obviously purpuric may occur in a form of lymphocytic vasculitis known as pityriasis lichenoides chronica (**Figs 17.36** and **17.37**). This disorder consists of multiple brown papular lesions, generally about 5 mm in diameter, which may exhibit a shiny scale ('mica scale') on the flat-topped surface. Except in those individuals in whom a more acute and necrotic version occurs initially (pityriasis lichenoides et varioliformis acuta, *see* below), it is more likely to be diagnosed as guttate psoriasis or a viral exanthem than as a vasculitis. Pityriasis lichenoides et varioliformis acuta (PLEVA) is an acute vasculitis seen mainly in children and young adults (**Fig 17.38**). Lesions are papular, haemorrhagic or necrotic and heal with scarring.

Pustular vasculitis

Pustules may develop in a leucocytoclastic vasculitis (*see* Fig 14.22). Consider also Behçet's disease (folliculitis-like pustules) or gonococcal vasculitis (relatively few, widely scattered, pustular vasculitic lesions with arthritis). *See also* Chapter 14.

Necrotic and destructive lesions

Necrosis may occur in many vasculitides but is generally preceded or accompanied by palpable purpura (**Fig 17.34**), inflammatory papules or other evidence of a vasculitic process, such as livedo. Haemorrhagic blisters may be a feature initially, followed by a hard black eschar of dead tissue (**Fig 17.39**). Similar haemorrhagic blisters may occur in some drug eruptions with a leucocytoclastic vasculitis, notably iododerma/bromoderma, and as part of the spectrum of pyoderma gangrenosum (*see* Fig 14.23). Infective pyoderma may be clinically similar.

In general terms, significant necrosis and destructive lesions are most likely to occur in granulomatous vasculitis, e.g. Wegener's granulomatosis or lymphomatoid granulomatosis, or in vasculitis affecting large or medium arterial vessels, e.g. polyarteritis nodosa. As usual, there are exceptions; pityriasis lichenoides et varioliformis acuta is a lymphocytic vasculitis of small vessels but may be quite destructive (**Fig 17.38**).

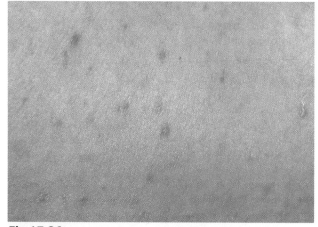

Fig 17.36

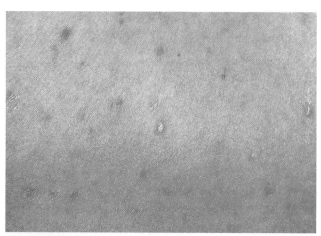

Fig 17.37

Figs 17.36, 17.37 Pityriasis lichenoides chronica. Small brown papular lesions, which are not overtly vasculitic. Gentle scraping of the central papule shown in 17.36 has made the typical 'mica' scale more apparent (17.37)

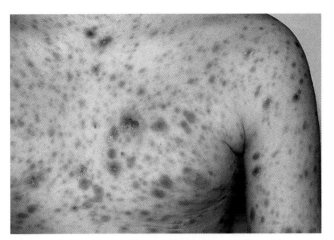

Fig 17.38 Pityriasis lichenoides et varioliformis acuta. The eruption is typically polymorphous and includes necrotic, papular and haemorrhagic lesions

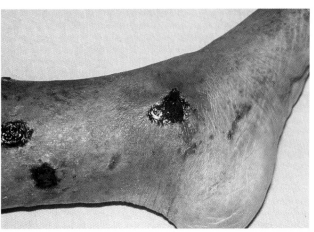

Fig 17.39 Necrosis in a patient with leucocytoclastic vasculitis. The dead tissue forms a hard black eschar. This was an exacerbation of disease in the patient with cryoglobulinaemia shown in 17.28

Nodular lesions and plaques

Nodular lesions and plaques may occur in conjunction with smaller palpable purpura lesions, but some specific patterns of nodular lesions with a vasculitic histology can be recognised.

Nodular vasculitis—This consists of purple nodules, often on the calf, which may ulcerate. This is really a descriptive label rather than a diagnosis; indeed, the term is often used for nodular vasculitic lesions where no other cause has been identified.

Erythema induratum (Bazin's disease)—This is a subset of nodular vasulitis that is associated with tuberculosis. Panniculitis is a deep inflammation of fat in which vasculitis may be either causative or a secondary feature. It generally presents as tender red inflamed nodules or plaques, often on the lower legs, and is generally less purple and less likely to ulcerate than a more superficial vasculitis. Causes of panniculitis in which vasculitis is an important feature include polyarteritis nodosa and thrombophlebitis. Lesions may produce deep tethering and a dimpled appearance as they resolve.

Erythema nodosum—This is an acute lymphocytic vasculitis that affects dermis and fat. It causes multiple tender red nodules that are usually most prominent on the shins (**Fig 17.40**). It has many causes (**Table 17.11**).

Chilblains (perniosis)—This is a recognisable pattern of cold-induced lymphocytic vasculitis, again with involvement of the fat. It may present as lesions on the fingers or toes but is also relatively common on the lateral thighs in patients who spend time outdoors in cold wet weather (e.g. equestrian panniculitis, **Fig 17.41**). The lesions are itchy purple nodules, and the affected region of skin or the digits are often cold or acrocyanotic (p. 304–305).

Table 17.11 Causes of erythema nodosum	
Infections	Streptococci Tuberculosis Yersinia
Drugs	Sulphonamides
Inflammatory	Acute sarcoidosis Inflammatory bowel disease
Neoplastic	Lymphomas

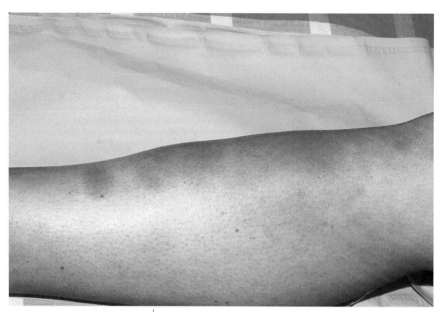

Fig 17.40 Erythema nodosum. Tender red nodules on the shins, not overtly vasculitic

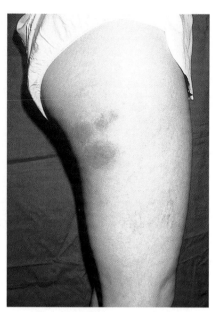

Fig 17.41 Equestrian panniculitis. This is a form of pernio (a cold-induced lymphocytic vasculitis). Lesions typically occur on the lateral thighs in horse riders and may also be seen in this distribution in children

Sweet's disease (acute febrile neutrophilic dermatosis)—This is best considered here as it is characterised histologically by prominent neutrophil polymorph leucocytoclasis, although frank vasculitis is not a feature. It presents as acute nodules and plaques, sometimes triggered by upper respiratory tract infection, although the important association is with haematological malignancies and pre-malignancies (**Fig 17.42**).

Erythema multiforme—This is a lymphocytic vasculitis that may have a specific reaction pattern (target lesions, *see* Fig 2.5 and 13.31) but may cause lesions that appear more acute and overtly vasculitic. Plaques and nodules are the main feature, often with blistering due to epidermal necrosis and prominent upper dermal oedema. Lesions with typical target morphology suggest that the trigger is the herpes simplex virus, but there are numerous other causes (*see* Table 13.3).

Stellate lesions

Acute meningococcal meningitis is the prime cause of vasculitic lesions with a prominent stellate pattern (*see* Fig 2.12).

Livedo

The livedo pattern of vascular damage has been considered separately (*see* earlier in this chapter, **Table 17.6**).

ARTERIAL AND VENOUS DISEASE

Arterial disease due to proximal atheroma or where there is gangrene tends to be the province of surgeons rather than dermatologists and is not discussed in detail here. The features of arterial and venous disease are listed in **Tables 17.12** and **17.13**, respectively. However, it is important (especially with regard to treatment) to be aware that many patients have features of both; similarly, chronic venous disease and lymphoedema (*see* below) often coexist.

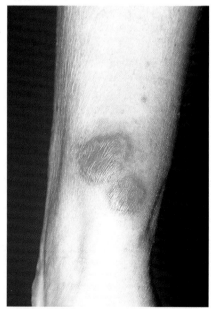

Fig 17.42 Sweet's disease. Acute inflammatory plaques on the arm with a characteristic yellowish-coloured bolstered edge due to intense infiltration with neutrophil polymorphs

Table 17.12 Clinical signs of arterial disease

Pallor, cyanosis, poor capillary refill

Cool skin

Poor peripheral pulses

Atrophic shiny skin, loss of hairs

Dystrophic nails

Ulceration

Gangrene (17.43)

Table 17.13 Clinical signs associated with venous disease

Varicose veins and 'venous flare'

Thrombophlebitis

Signs of deep venous thrombosis

Induration, lipodermatosclerosis

Shape change ('champagne bottle' leg)

Colour change (dusky, brown pigmentation)

Atrophie blanche

Cellulitis

Ulceration (*see* chapter 12)

Dermatitis

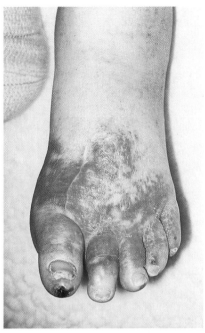

Fig 17.43 Arterial disease. Acute arterial obstruction causing pallor, reticulate dusky erythema and gangrene of the tip of the hallux

VENOUS OBSTRUCTION

Venous obstruction may occur as a result of intravascular causes, e.g. thrombosis, vessel wall inflammation, or external compression, e.g. cervical rib, tumour. The features are distal swelling and pain in acute cases. The most important in dermatological differential diagnosis are deep venous thrombosis of the leg compared with cellulitis, and superior vena cava obstruction compared with angio-oedema of the face. In superior vena cava obstruction, the arms may also be swollen, and chest veins are dilated (**Fig 17.44**). The usual cause is bronchial carcinoma.

LYMPHOEDEMA

Lymphoedema is not caused by an abnormality of blood vessels but of lymphatic vessels. It is appropriate to discuss it here as lymphoedema of the legs commonly occurs with, or is in the differential diagnosis of, chronic venous disease; in some cases, the physical signs of the two conditions may be mixed. Causes and features of lymphoedema are listed in **Tables 17.14** and **17.15**. In the legs, lymphoedema is usually bilateral; asymmetrical lymphoedema of a leg in the absence of an obvious reason (such as surgery to inguinal lymph nodes) is suspicious of proximal obstruction by a pelvic tumour. Unilateral lower leg lymphoedema may also be caused by artefact (**Fig 17.45**).

Although lymphoedema is often said to be non-pitting compared with other causes of oedema, this is not a reliable clinical sign. Absent pitting in chronic oedema is due to the presence of fibrosis preventing fluid displacement. Fibrosis occurs in any type of chronic oedema, and this includes

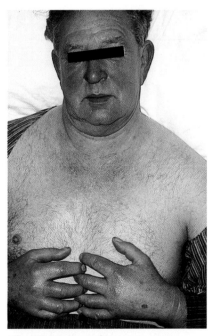

Fig 17.44 Superior vena cava obstruction. Dusky plethoric facies, oedema of the face and hands and dilated veins of the upper chest in superior venal cava obstruction

323

Table 17.14 Causes of lymphoedema

Primary
Familial, congenital, idiopathic
Associated with pleural effusions and yellow nail syndrome (19.63)

Secondary
Infections
   Erysipelas/cellulitis (12.30)
   Other bacterial infections
   Granuloma inguinale
   Filariasis
Iatrogenic
   Surgery
   Radiotherapy
Neoplastic
   Tumour infiltration (e.g. breast, pelvic)
Other causes of fibrosis
   Retroperitoneal fibrosis
   Chronic venous disease/lipodermatosclerosis
Artefactual
Localised
   Pre-tibial myxoedema (11.31, 11.32)
   Rosacea (14.13)
   Tongue/lip (Melkersson–Rosenthal syndrome)

Table 17.15 Features of lymphoedema

Swelling with limited pitting

Deeply bound down clefts between regions of oedema

Inability to pinch skin on toes (Kaposi—Stemmer sign)

Hyperkeratosis with deep fissures and warty changes
('mossy foot' or elephantosis verrucosa nostra*)

Nodules*

Secondary bacterial and dermatophyte infection

Association with yellow nail syndrome (*see* Chapter 19)

*Late changes.

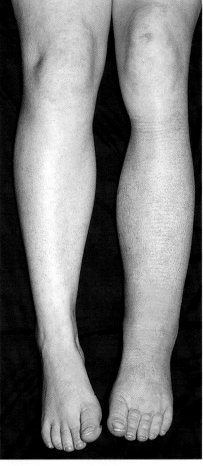

Fig 17.45 Unilateral swollen limb due to self-application of a tourniquet (Secretan's syndrome). Note the sharp demarcation between the thin limb above the site of constriction compared with the distal oedema, which is unlike the pattern seen in idiopathic lymphoedema

chronic venous oedema. Conversely, pitting can be shown in early lymphoedema.

Another physical sign in established disease where there is some fibrotic change is the inability to pick up a pinch of skin on the dorsum of the second toe, the Kaposi–Stemmer sign. The leg may become grossly enlarged with warty nodules and pronounced skin tethering (**Fig 17.46**).

Reticulate lymphoedema

Usually, lymphoedema diffusely affects the relevant limb (most often both lower legs) but with more prominent warty or even nodular changes in the region of the ankle. A recently described new variant, which occurs on the upper part of the lower leg, consists of compressible ridges (**Fig 17.47**) with a distribution and spacing similar to that of erythema ab igne (*see* 6.23). It seems likely that this pattern of lymphoedema is due to protrusion of lymphoedematous tissue through areas of thermally damaged skin (the cause of erythema ab igne), and it might therefore be best termed 'lymphoedema ab igne'.

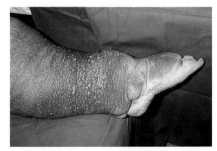

Fig 17.46 Chronic lymphoedema. Massive oedema with typical tethering at the base of the toes and at the ankle (*see also* 7.31)

ANGIOMAS, LOCALISED VASCULAR LESIONS AND VASCULAR MALFORMATIONS

Some angiomas have already been described because they are likely to present as nodules, for example capillary angiomas (**Figs 17.48** and **17.49**, *see also* Fig 9.66), Campbell de Morgan spots (*see* Fig 6.24), pyogenic granuloma (*see* Fig 9.65) and angiokeratomas (*see* p. 176). Others have been discussed in the sections on erythema and telangiectasia.

Four main areas remain:

- Superficial flat or plaque angiomas.
- Kaposi's sarcoma.
- Deep vascular malformations.
- Lymphangioma.

Superficial flat or plaque angiomas

Several benign and malignant vascular tumours may present as flat or plaque-type erythematous lesions but are relatively rare and often not clinically specific. Port-wine angioma is a recognisable pattern of malformation of blood vessels that has a dermatomal distribution on the face. It is typically a broad, flat, purplish red angioma (**Figs 17.50** and **17.51**). Localised angiomatous nodules may develop in these lesions in elderly patients.

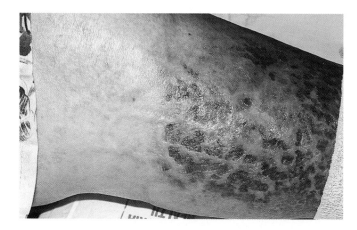

Fig 17.47 Reticulate pattern of lymphoedema, showing the site and pattern similarity to erythema ab igne. In this patient, there is also some hyperkeratosis of the lower leg, a relatively common feature in elderly patients, but accentuating the visibility of the lymphatic ridges in this case

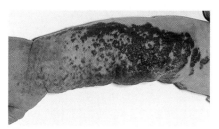

Fig 17.48

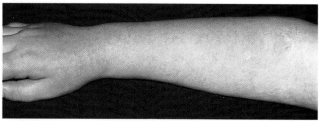

Fig 17.49

Figs 17.48, 17.49 Strawberry naevus. This is a pattern of angioma that presents shortly after birth. Some patients require treatment, but untreated lesions (as in this case) may show remarkable spontaneous resolution (17.49)

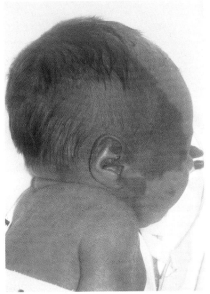

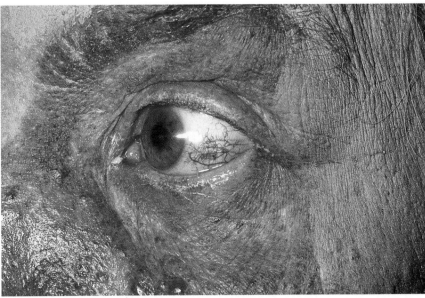

Fig 17.50

Fig 17.51

Figs 17.50, 17.51 Port-wine stain. These are typically flat and red in colour at an early age (17.50) but may become a deeper purple and more palpable with increasing age (17.51). The importance of port-wine angioma is an association with intracranial angioma (Sturge–Weber syndrome) and with conjunctival angiomatous vessels (17.51) and glaucoma (17.50 *courtesy of Dr D W A Milligan*)

Kaposi's sarcoma

Kaposi's sarcoma occurs in a variety of forms, including a 'classic' type, endemic Kaposi's sarcoma and AIDS-associated Kaposi's sarcoma. The classic type causes nodules on the leg or foot that are overtly angiomatous. By comparison, lesions of AIDS-related Kaposi's sarcoma are flatter macules or plaques—they may be subtle and bruise-like or grey in colour (**Figs 17.52** and **17.53**). They are usually multiple and often affect mucosal sites such as the palate or conjunctivae. Hyperkeratotic, nodular or ulcerative lesions may develop. They may be mimicked by infective lesions or other vascular nodules that occur in HIV-positive patients, such as the lesions of bacillary angiomatosis.

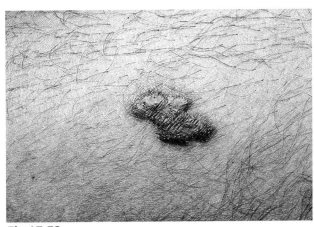

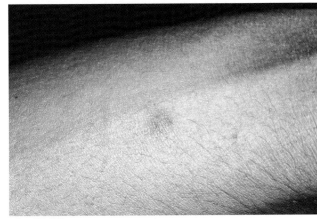

Fig 17.52

Fig 17.53

Figs 17.52, 17.53 Kaposi's sarcoma. Lesions may be varied in appearance, typically rather purple plaques (17.52) but also quite subtle bruise-like lesions (17.53)

Deep vascular malformations

Deep vascular malformations may present because of surface vascular changes or ulceration but may also cause swelling or length asymmetry of limbs, venous dilatation, asymmetrical temperature of skin and other changes. Multiple nodular lesions may be associated with internal angiomas in the liver or gastrointestinal tract.

Lymphangioma

Lymphangiomas may be huge and complex lesions, sometimes with other vessels also involved in a hamartomatous process, but the more common dermatological type is the lymphangioma circumscriptum (*see* Fig 9.70). They are described in Chapter 9 but are also included here since bleeding into the lesions is common, and they may be diagnosed as an abnormality of blood vessels.

18 Hair

NORMAL HAIR MORPHOLOGY AND HAIR CYCLE

Body hair

There are major inherited differences in body hair distribution among normal individuals. The whirling pattern of body hair in dark-skinned children appears to follow the pattern of Blaschko's lines (*see* Fig 2.10).

The lower triangle pubic hair is present in men and women. Pubic hair above this line, sometimes referred to as the escutcheon, is present in men and approximately 10% of healthy females (**Fig 18.1**). Chest hairs are unique to males although periareolar breast hair is common in females.

Hair cycle

A single follicle goes through several cycles of hair growth and rest in its lifetime (**Fig 18.2**). Normally, 85–90% of all scalp hairs are in the anagen or growth phase, 10–15% in the resting or telogen phase and approximately 1% in the catagen or transitional phase. In the catagen phase, cell division in the hair matrix stops. The outer root sheath degenerates and retracts around the widened lower portion of the hair shaft to become a club hair. During the telogen phase, the non-growing hair is shed.

In the early part of the anagen (growth) phase, a new hair is produced, which pushes out any remaining club or telogen hair. Between 50 and 100 of the 100 000 scalp hairs are shed each day.

Close inspection of normal scalp hair reveals that many follicles have more than one hair emerging from a single follicular opening (**Fig 18.3**). On the scalp, hair grows approximately 0.4 mm each day (6 inches a year). The maximum length of the hair is determined partly by the growth rate but more by the duration of the anagen growth phase. On average, on the scalp, this lasts around 1000 days, although anagen is longer in people who can grow their

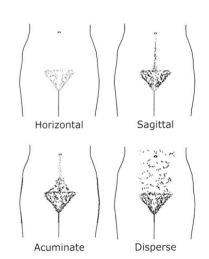

Horizontal   Sagittal

Acuminate   Disperse

Fig 18.1 Normal female pubic hair. Ninety per cent of 227 healthy American women aged 18–40 years had a horizontal pattern of pubic hair distribution, 9% the acuminate, 1% the sagittal and none the disperse pattern. Almost 17% of normal men aged 30–40 years have the horizontal pattern of pubic hair. This distribution may be different in other ethnic groups (from Dupertuis CW, Atkinson WB & Elftman H (1945) *Human Biol*, 17: 137)

329

hair very long and conversely shorter in people whose hair only grows to a relatively short maximum length (short anagen syndrome). The anagen phase is much shorter in body hair, eyebrows and eyelashes.

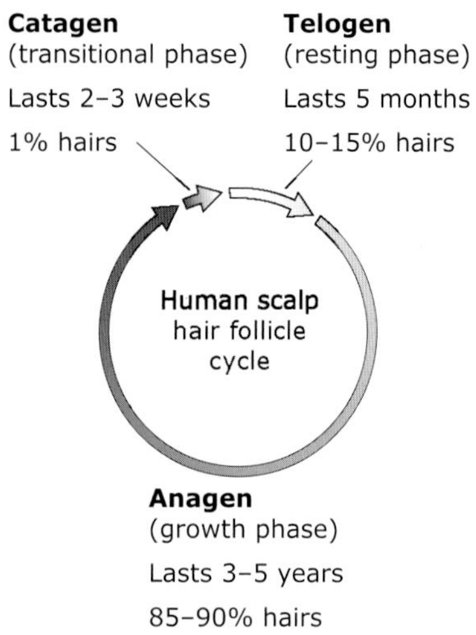

Trichogram or forcible hair pluck

This test is used to determine the proportion of hairs in anagen or telogen but is rarely used in clinical practice and remains an investigational, rather than a diagnostic, test. Using rubber-tipped artery forceps, a group of hairs—somewhere between 10 and 60, depending on the enthusiasm of the operator—are pulled out and looked at under a microscope. The proportion of telogen and anagen hairs (**Fig 18.4**) can be assessed from this sample and hair morphology can be examined at the same time. Artefactual abnormalities, such as extracting anagen hairs without the inner or outer root sheath, and fracture of an anagen hair, can occur.

Hair types

Languo hairs are present only on the fetus *in utero* and disappear at about 8 months. They are visible on premature babies as soft fine non-pigmented hairs (**Fig 18.5**).

Vellus hairs are fine downy hairs that cover the entire body surface except the palms and soles. Under the influence of androgens, vellus hair will convert to terminal hair.

Terminal hairs are the thicker pigmented hairs found on the scalp, eyelash and eyebrow and as secondary sexual hair.

Catagen
(transitional phase)
Lasts 2–3 weeks
1% hairs

Telogen
(resting phase)
Lasts 5 months
10–15% hairs

Human scalp
hair follicle
cycle

Anagen
(growth phase)
Lasts 3–5 years
85–90% hairs

Fig 18.2 Hair cycle.

DIAGNOSTIC TIPS AND PITFALLS

- There are approximately 100 000 hairs on a healthy scalp; between 50 and 100 hairs are shed each day

- A normal scalp hair grows for almost 3 years (i.e. the anagen phase of the follicle cycle lasts 3 years) and then rests (i.e. the follicle goes into telogen), and the hair is shed

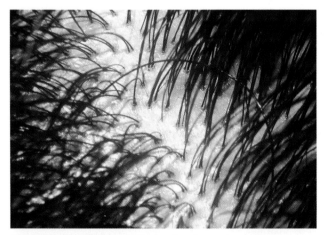

Fig 18.3 Normal scalp hair. On the scalp, a single follicular opening is often shared by several terminal hairs growing from separate follicles. Close inspection of normal scalps reveals that this is common, although most easily seen in people with diffuse alopecia

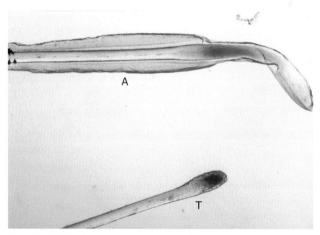

Fig 18.4 Plucked anagen and telogen hairs. Anagen hairs (A) are firmly attached to their surroundings. When forcibly pulled out the normal anatomy is usually distorted and hairs may vary in appearance depending on how much of the outer root and inner root sheath is attached to the hair shaft. The dermal papilla and fibrous sheath usually remain behind. Shed telogen hairs (T) have the classic club hair appearance. Plucked telogen hairs may have an epithelial sac covering the club root

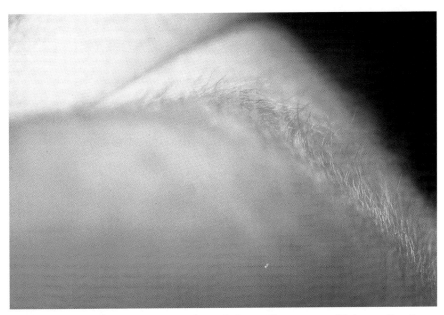

Fig 18.5 Lanugo hairs on a newborn infant. There are multiple small soft downy hairs visible on this baby's skin. This is the second growth of lanugo hair and is shed soon after birth. The first coat of longer lanugo hair is lost *in utero* at 7–8 months

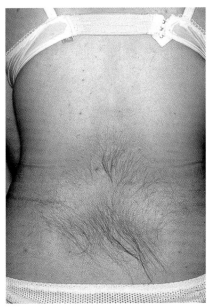

Fig 18.6 Localised hypertrichosis—faun tail. This is commonly associated with occult spina bifida (*see* 12.35)

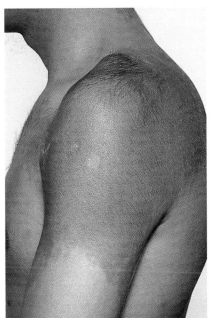

Fig 18.7 Becker's naevus. A common benign type of epidermal naevus with associated increased hair growth, which is more common in men and appears at puberty (*see* 9.37)

Fig 18.8 Hypertrichosis after inflammation. Hypertrichosis may occur at sites of skin inflammation, e.g. around leg ulcers, and in this case after erythema nodosum. Repeated rubbing may also produce hair growth, for example on the shoulder in people who carry heavy weights

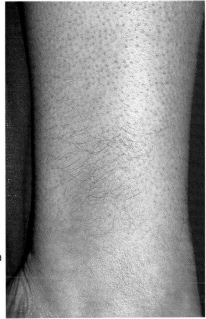

INCREASED HAIR GROWTH

Hypertrichosis

Hypertrichosis is the growth of terminal hair, in a man or woman, at a site not normally hairy (**Fig 18.8**). This increased hair growth is not due to androgen stimulation, so other features of virilisation are not present. Hair growth may be generalised or localised (**Table 18.1** and **Figs 18.6–18.9**).

Table 18.1 Causes of hypertrichosis

Localised	Congenital	Giant congenital naevus, pigmented naevi, Becher's naevus (18.7), naevoid hypertrichosis Spina bifida occulta—faun tail (18.6)
	Acquired	At the sites of constant rubbing or irritation, e.g. around leg ulcers, associated with chronic inflammatory disorders (18.8) Porphyria (18.9)
Generalised	Congenital	Sex-linked and autosomal-dominant generalised Hypertrichosis, hypertrichosis lanuginosa Fetal hypertrichosis occurs in 10% of neonates with fetal alcohol syndrome
	Acquired	Drug-induced—minoxidil, diazoxide, cyclosporin A, phenytoin, systemic corticosteroids Anorexia nervosa and any cause of rapid weight loss Porphyria cutanea tarda (18.9) Paraneoplastic (lanugo type hair)

Table 18.2 Causes of hirsutism

Ovarian: polycystic ovary disease

Adrenal: Cushing's syndrome, virilising tumours, adrenogenital syndromes

Pituitary: acromegaly, hyperprolactinaemia

Iatrogenic: testosterone, stanozolol

Table 18.3 Signs of virilisation

Absent or scanty periods

Acne

Reduction in breast size

Clitoral hypertrophy

Fronto-temporal balding

Deepening of the voice

DIAGNOSTIC TIPS AND PITFALLS

- Scalp hair grows approximately 0.4 mm each day (6 inches a year). The maximum length of the hair is determined mostly by the duration of the anagen or growth phase. People who cannot grow their hair long have a shorter anagen cycle than usual

- Hypertrichosis is the growth of terminal hair at a site not normally hairy, whereas hirsutism is the development of male pattern hair distribution in a female and means that other signs of virilisation may be present

Hirsutism

Hirsutism is the development of male pattern hair distribution in the female, caused by endogenous or exogenous androgens (**Table 18.2**). Coarse terminal hairs appear on the face (**Fig 18.10**), the male escutcheon and the chest. Other signs of androgen-induced virilisation may also be present (**Table 18.3**).

DECREASED SCALP HAIR

Hair loss may occur by several mechanisms, including:

- Increased rate of hair fall, e.g. anagen effluvium, telogen effluvium, alopecia areata.
- Decrease in hair shaft diameter (e.g. fine hair in hyperthyroidism).
- Decrease Sign hair growth rate or in the duration of the anagen phase.
- Gradual loss of active follicles (which leads to a decrease in scalp hair but not an increased rate of hair fall, e.g. male pattern baldness).

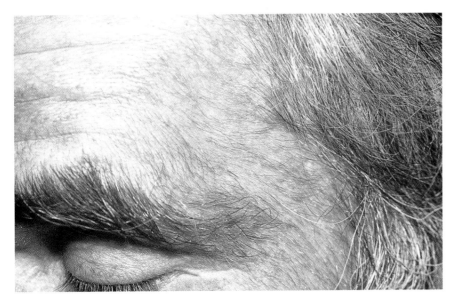

DIAGNOSTIC TIPS AND PITFALLS

- If baldness is identified, the first question to ask is 'is it scarring or non-scarring alopecia?'

- In non-scarring alopecia (e.g. alopecia areata, male pattern alopecia), the follicle is intact but does not produce a viable hair. The follicle opening may be visible but may also be so small that it is virtually invisible to the naked eye

- Increased breakage of hairs, e.g. hair-shaft abnormalities, mechanical damage such as trichotillomania.
- Scarring of hair follicles (e.g. discoid lupus erythematosus).

When examining a patient with hair loss, it is useful to consider whether this is due to a scarring or non-scarring process.

Non-scarring alopecia

In non-scarring alopecia, the follicle is intact but does not produce a viable hair. Non-scarring alopecia can be diffuse, involving all scalp sites equally, or patterned, where hair loss is localised to particular parts of the scalp (**Table 18.4**). Several congenital patterns of non-scarring hair loss have been described, including loss on the vertex, over the cranial sutures and on the temples (triangular alopecia; **Fig 18.11**). These all become apparent in early childhood and are not usually associated with hair fall; for example, in triangular alopecia, the affected area has intact follicles with fine vellus hairs but without terminal scalp hairs (rather than a shedding process). Acute diffuse hair loss may be the result of anagen or telogen effluvium (**Table 18.5**). Both must be distinguished from diffuse alopecia areata by the absence of 'exclamation mark' hairs and other features (*see* pp. 334–338). Gradual diffuse hair loss (**Fig 18.16**) is more common and is usually idiopathic (*see* **Table 18.4**). It is important to distinguish cases where diffuse hair loss is accompanied by inflammation, such as may occur in dermatomyositis (**Fig 18.17**).

Anagen effluvium

Anagen hair loss (**Fig 18.15**) is due to arrest of hair growth in the anagen phase and occurs immediately after the insult, which is usually iatrogenic (e.g. chemotherapy) and recognised by the patient. The anagen hair root appears dystrophic and pale and lacks its root sheath—a similar pattern occurs in a rare congenital disorder known as the loose anagen syndrome. Alopecia areata is also due to anagen hair loss but generally produces a patchy, rather than diffuse, hair loss.

A physical sign of pemphigus vulgaris has rather confusingly been described as 'normal anagen effluvium'—in this entity, hairs are easily plucked out but have apparently normal morphology of anagen roots and an

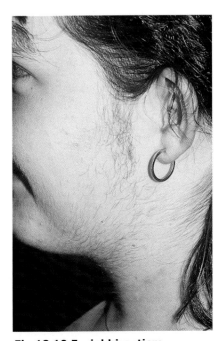

Fig 18.10 Facial hirsutism.
Terminal hair growth is visible on the chin of this 40-year-old woman with idiopathic hirsutism. Increased hairiness at other sites, especially the thighs and abdomen, is usually also present

Table 18.4 Non-scarring alopecia

Diffuse hair loss	Patterned hair loss
Sudden onset with overt hair fall	*Patchy*
Anagen effluvium (18.15)	Tinea capitis (18.42)
Telogen effluvium	Alopecia areata (18.20)
Diffuse alopecia areata	Secondary syphilis
	Psoriasis
Gradual onset	Trichotillomania (18.41) and other mechanical loss (p. 344)
Idiopathic (18.16)	Circumscribed congenital alopecia, e.g. triangular alopecia
Endocrine: myxoedema, hypopituitarism	
Nutritional: iron deficiency	*Crown hair loss alone*
Connective tissue disease: Systemic lupus	Female pattern androgenic alopecia (18.12, 18.13)
erythematosus, dermatomyositis (18.17)	
Infection: AIDS	*Temporal recession with or without crown hair loss*
Drugs: carbimazole, warfarin	Male pattern androgenic alopecia (18.14)
Diffuse alopecia areata	Cutaneous virilisation in a female
Congenital	*Marginal alopecia*
Ectodermal dysplasias	Oophiasic pattern alopecia areata (18.19)
Hair shaft abnormalities (p. 342–344)	Traction alopecia (18.39, 18.40)
Loose anagen syndrome	Frontal fibrosing alopecia

intact root sheath. The mechanism is that there is a split above the basal keratinocytes of the follicle (*see* Chapter 13), so the entire follicular root sheath can be plucked out very easily.

Telogen effluvium

Telogen loss is delayed by up to 3 months, and the precipitating event may not be immediately obvious. It is really a form of moulting in which the hair cycles of many hairs become synchronised rather than random and therefore leads to a phase of synchronised loss of hair. It is particularly common after pregnancy. Up to about 40% of hairs may be lost, although this is often not apparent to anybody except the patient. Women with long hair may find it particularly apparent after a second pregnancy as the process may recur before regrowth from the first episode has reached the length of the original hairs.

Alopecia areata

Body and beard hair are commonly affected in alopecia areata. Complete scalp hair loss is called alopecia totalis (**Fig 18.17**) and complete scalp and body hair loss alopecia universalis. The oophiasic or marginated pattern of alopecia (**Fig 18.19**) is associated with a worse prognosis. Nail changes, including fine pitting, occur in up to 66% of cases (*see* Fig 19.17). White hairs are usually not affected, and this can produce striking colour changes as the pigmented, but not the white, hairs are lost in an individual with greying hair (**Fig 18.20**). Loss of eyebrow and eyelash hairs (**Fig 18.21**) can be disfiguring.

In alopecia areata, a poorly understood type of cell-mediated inflammatory reaction occurs around the hair follicle, damaging hair bulb cells and melanocytes and leading to hair loss and depigmentation. The extent of the inflammation around the follicle determines the type of damage seen in the hair.

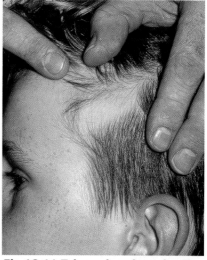

Fig 18.11 Triangular alopecia. The affected area has intact follicles with fine vellus hairs but without terminal scalp hairs. Hair loss occurs because the hairs do not grow, rather than as a result of hair shedding

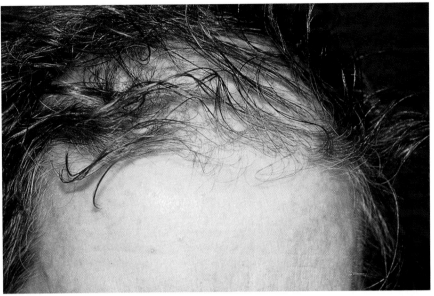

Fig 18.12

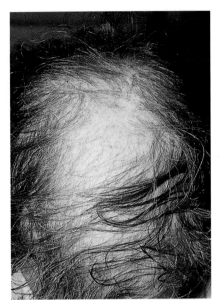

Fig 18.13

Figs 18.12, 18.13 Female pattern androgenic alopecia. There is loss of hair density over the centre of the scalp (18.12) with retention of the normal frontal (18.13) hair line

Severe damage causes the hair to become dystrophic, enter telogen and break off. Hairs break because the keratogenous or hardening zone of the follicle, which is a few millimetres above the hair bulb, is also damaged by the inflammatory reaction, resulting in a weakened hair that breaks off just below the scalp surface. This leaves a dystrophic telogen hair remnant in the follicle. As this remnant is extruded from the follicle, the thin dystrophic and depigmented telogen hair root becomes visible at the follicle opening, with the normal-thickness remnant of the hair shaft above it producing the characteristic exclamation mark hair (**Figs 18.22** and **18.23**). The associated absence of pigment in the tapered portion of the exclamation mark hair adds to the impression of tapering.

The inflammatory reaction on the hair root may result in virtual destruction of the hair remnant, leading to so-called cadaverised hairs (**Fig 18.24**). These black comedone-like plugs are visible in follicle orifices at the active margin and can be expressed from the follicle using a comedone expressor. They are the degeneration products of the pigmented hair matrix, shaft and sheath and are considered to be a sign of aggressive disease with a poor prognosis.

DIAGNOSTIC TIPS AND PITFALLS

- Loss of substance in bald scalp skin compared with adjacent hairy skin does not necessarily indicate scarring alopecia; this loss of substance may simply be caused by loss of the hair roots in the bald areas (e.g. in alopecia areata)

Table 18.5 Comparison of telogen and anagen effluvium

Telogen effluvium	Anagen effluvium
2–4 months after the insult	1–4 weeks after the insult
20–50% of hairs lost	80–90% of hairs lost
Club hairs lost	Anagen hairs lost with a pigmented bulb
No hair shaft abnormalities	Hair shafts may be narrowed or fractured
Causes	**Causes**
Acute, especially febrile, illness	Cancer chemotherapy
Childbirth (hairs are maintained in anagen during pregnancy)	Poisoning by thallium, arsenic, vitamin A toxicity
Radiation therapy	
Dietary	
Drugs: warfarin, heparin, etretinate, carbamazepine, allopurinol	
Physical stress	

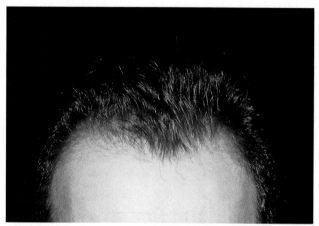

Fig 18.14 Male pattern androgenic alopecia. Initially, there is temporal recession followed by loss of hair from the crown of the head. Hairs at these sites become steadily finer before reverting to vellus hairs

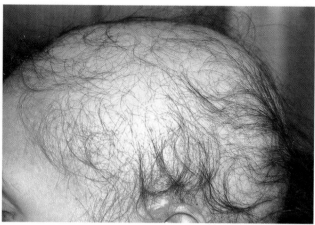

Fig 18.15 Anagen effluvium. This patient took 750 000 IU of vitamin A for acne. She developed weakness, exfoliation, blurred vision and loss of peripheral vision, followed by complete hair loss, and her nails turned white

Less severely affected hairs are also weakened at the keratinous zone, but not so severely that they break. These hairs can be made to kink when bent or pushed inwards, the kink corresponding to the shaft defect produced by the episode of alopecia (**Fig 18.25**). The kink gives the hair the shape of a coude catheter, and the term coudability was coined for this sign in alopecia areata. This sign is either difficult to show or infrequently present. It should be looked for in normal-length hairs at the margin of a patch of alopecia areata where there are also exclamation mark hairs. Other less severely affected hairs are probably temporarily affected but do not break or go into telogen. The important conclusion to draw from this is that exclamation mark hairs are not always present in alopecia areata.

DIAGNOSTIC TIPS AND PITFALLS

- Acute diffuse hair loss may be the result of an anagen or telogen effluvium. The former is usually caused by a toxin, e.g. chemotherapy, and is obvious to the patient. By contrast, telogen hair loss is delayed by up to 3 months, and the precipitating event may not be immediately obvious

- In diffuse alopecia areata, multiple broken 'exclamation mark' hairs can be identified

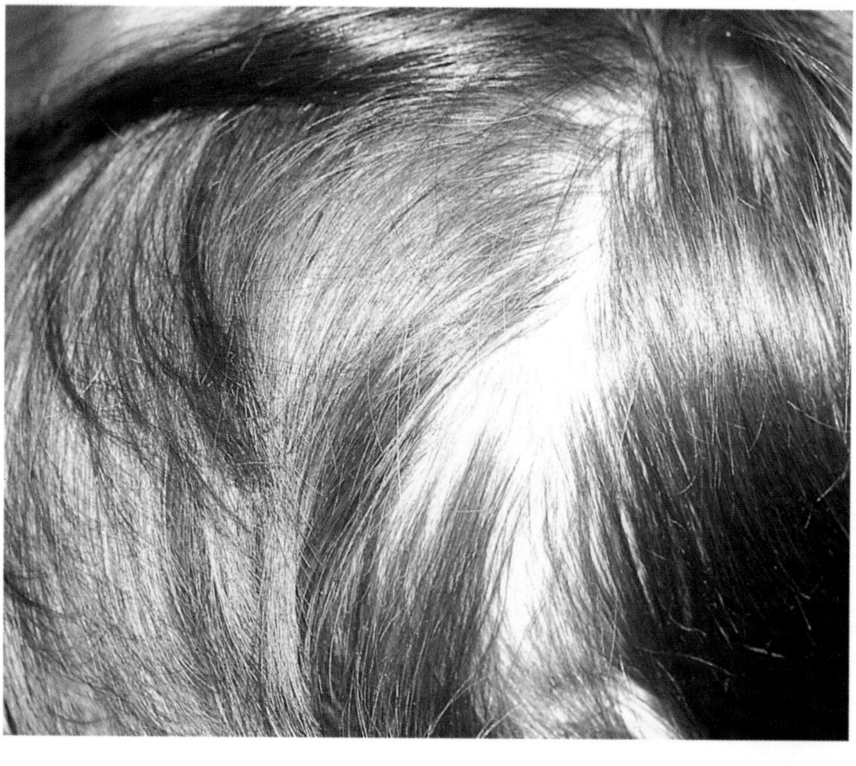

Fig 18.16 Diffuse idiopathic hair loss. There is diffuse hair thinning equally on the top and sides of the scalp. Compare with 18.12 and 18.13, showing female pattern androgenic alopecia. This 22-year-old woman had a low serum iron concentration but did not respond to repletion of her iron stores

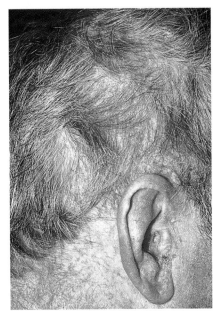

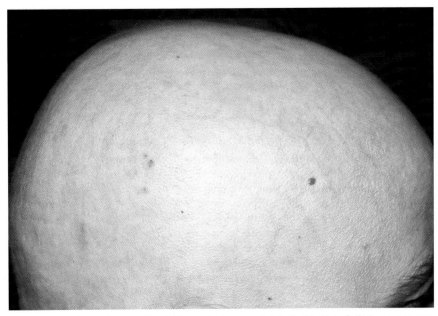

Fig 18.17 Dermatomyositis. It is diagnostically and therapeutically important to distinguish diffuse alopecia with inflammation from other causes of diffuse hair fall. In this man (same as in 5.4), dermatomyositis has caused diffuse scalp redness with generalised hair loss. This occurs in 20% of patients with dermatomyositis. Subsequent poikiloderma developing in affected areas may cause scarring alopecia

Fig 18.18 Alopecia totalis. This scalp is completely bald. Hair follicle remnants are visible as tiny pits regularly spaced across the scalp. This is a type of alopecia areata

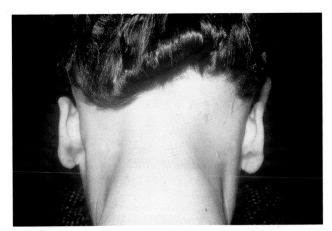

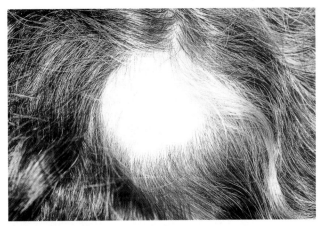

Fig 18.19 Marginal (oophiasic) pattern alopecia areata. Loss of hair at the temple, neck or forehead margins presages a poorer prognosis for regrowth than the patchy variety

Fig 18.20 Alopecia areata patch of white hair regrowing. White hair is less commonly affected than pigmented hair in alopecia areata. Initial regrowth may be white hairs, and in patients with greying hair, the depigmented hairs may be spared

Scarring alopecia

Hair loss resulting from destruction of the hair follicles may occur at any site but is most noticeable in the scalp and beard. The bald skin is smooth and shiny and may be tethered or depressed (atrophic) compared with the

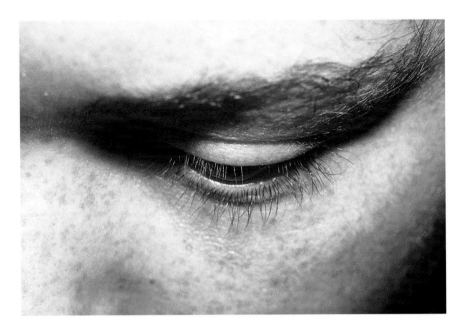

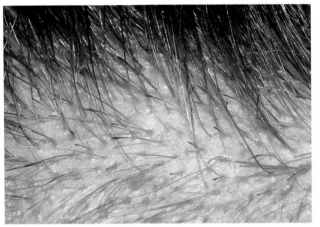

Fig 18.22

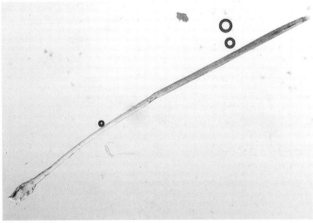

Fig 18.23

Figs 18.22, 18.23 'Exclamation mark' hairs. At the border of the bald area, exclamation mark hairs can usually be seen in active alopecia areata (18.22). The plucked exclamation mark hairs are dystrophic telogen hairs with a tapered and depigmented base (18.23); note also that the broken end is ragged, unlike the sharply cut-off end seen in trichotillomania (p. 344)

surrounding tissues (**Fig 18.26**). Depression of the skin may also be present in alopecia areata; in this case, it is due to loss of hair root substance in the bald areas compared with the surrounding hair-bearing skin. There may be signs of the active underlying disease within the intact hair at the edge of the bald area, for example the redness, scaling and follicular plugging of discoid lupus erythematosus (**Fig 18.27**). In erosive pustular dermatosis of the scalp (**Fig 18.28**), the patient presents with crusted pustules and surface erosion, and scarring only becomes obvious after treatment.

Absence of visible follicles alone is not pathognomonic of scarring alopecia, since follicles may become almost invisible, e.g. in longstanding male pattern baldness. More common causes are listed in **Table 18.6**. Some of these are discussed below.

DIAGNOSTIC TIPS AND PITFALLS

- The skin in scarring alopecia is smooth and shiny and may be tethered or depressed (atrophic) compared with the surrounding tissues. Paradoxically, the bald area will rarely have the appearance of a thickened twisted scar. There may be associated signs of the active underlying disease within the zone of intact hair at the edge of the bald area

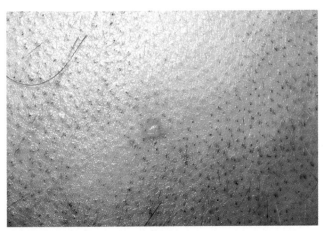

Fig 18.24 Cadaverised hairs in alopecia areata. There are multiple black hair remnants left in the follicles—the degeneration products of the pigmented hair matrix, shaft and sheath. These can be expressed using a comedone expressor, as has been done to a hair at the centre of the picture

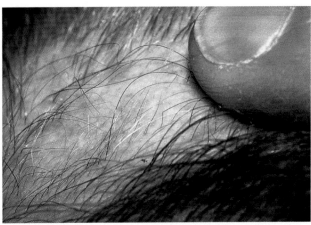

Fig 18.25 Coudability in alopecia areata. Less severely affected hairs are also weakened at the keratinous zone, but not so severely that they break. These hairs can be made to kink when bent or pushed inwards, the kink corresponding to the shaft defect produced by the episode of follicle inflammation

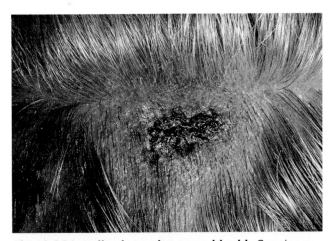

Fig 18.26 Localised scarring pemphigoid. Scarring or bullous skin changes without mucosal lesions may occur—usually on the scalp, forehead or neck. In this case, there is just an erosion in the scalp, which heals with scarring. Milia may also be present (*see* 13.37)

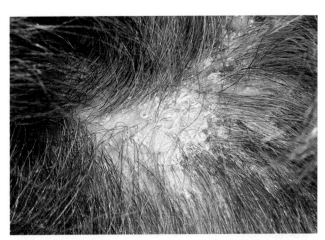

Fig 18.27 Scarring alopecia in discoid lupus erythematosus. Alopecia with loss of follicles and some residual inflammation at the periphery. Active inflammation may cause irreversible hair loss and requires aggressive therapy

Aplasia cutis

Aplasia cutis is a congenital absence of skin and subcutaneous tissue and is present at birth as a sharp marginated wound with a granulating base. Approximately 60% of cases occur on the scalp, at the vertex near the sagittal suture or over the parietal bones (**Fig 18.31**). The area usually measures 1–2 cm in diameter, but areas up to 9 cm in diameter have been recorded. It is important to identify these as not being due to clumsy obstetrics. It can be distinguished from circumscribed congenital alopecias (**Table 18.4**), even when these affect the vertex, as these have normal skin quality apart from the absent appendages.

DIAGNOSTIC TIPS AND PITFALLS

- Neonatal patchy baldness is more likely to be the result of cutis aplasia or circumscribed congenital alopecia rather than due to the obstetrician

Table 18.6 Causes of scarring (cicatricial) alopecia

Infection
Bacterial
  Pyogenic carbuncles, folliculitis, tuberculosis, tertiary syphilis
Fungal
  Kerion, favus, microsporum canis
Viral
  Herpes zoster

External injury
Burns, trauma, radiotherapy (18.30)

Developmental
Naevus sebaceous (9.57)
Aplasia cutis (18.29)

Neoplasms
Squamous and basal cell carcinoma (18.31), etc.
Secondary deposits (9.78), lymphoma

Inflammatory dermatoses
Discoid lupus erythematosus (18.27), lichen planus, dermatomyositis,
scleroderma/morphoea, sarcoidosis, lupus vulgaris, necrobiosis lipoidica
(some of these may result in the appearance of pseudo-pelade when the disease
becomes inactive, and only the damage remains)

Blistering disorders
Cicatricial pemphigoid (18.26), porphyria cutanea tarda, epidermolysis bullosa

Idiopathic
Pseudo-pelade (18.32)
Folliculitis decalvans (18.33)
Folliculitis keloidalis (18.34)
Erosive pustular dermatosis of the scalp (18.28)

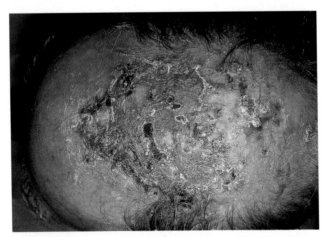

Fig 18.28 Erosive pustular dermatosis of scalp. This odd condition was originally described in women but does occur in men. The patient presents with extensive crusted and pustular areas on the scalp. Healing follows topical steroid therapy, but the area is permanently scarred. It needs to be distinguished from neoplasia and localised blistering disorders

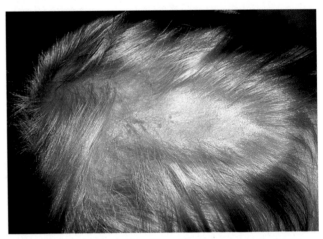

Fig 18.29 Aplasia cutis. Smooth shiny depressed scar tissue, which is present at birth (ulceration may be present initially)

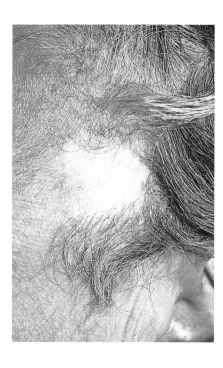

Fig 18.30 Scarring alopecia after radiotherapy. A patch of scarred alopecia remains at the site of radiotherapy for a basal cell carcinoma of the scalp

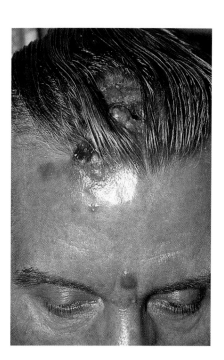

Fig 18.31 Squamous cell carcinoma of scalp. This man had a large and rapidly growing squamous cell carcinoma of the scalp causing hair destruction. The tumour had already metastasised at presentation. A skin metastasis is visible on the glabella

Pseudo-pelade

Pseudo-pelade of Brocq (pelade = alopecia) presents as irregular patches of scarring alopecia usually joined in a haphazard way, with isolated hairs or groups of hairs remaining within the bald areas but no areas of folliculitis (**Fig 18.32**). The lesions may appear hypopigmented and depressed below the skin surface (likened to 'footprints in the snow'). The name was originally chosen because the appearance was considered similar to alopecia areata. Similar features are seen as an end-point of various inflammatory dermatoses (**Table 18.6**). Even when specific dermatoses are not clinically apparent, there may be sporadic development of new lesions without significant overt inflammation.

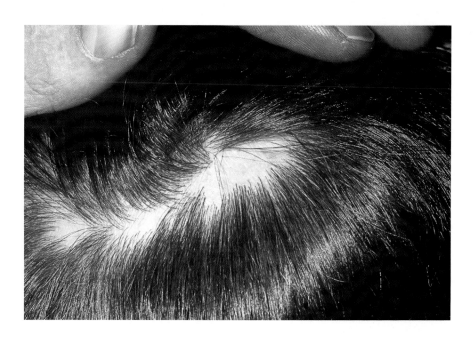

Fig 18.32 Pseudo-pelade. There are several oval or linear-shaped areas of scared alopecia with a very well–defined difference between the involved and uninvolved patches. The overall appearance has been graphically described as 'footprints in the snow'

341

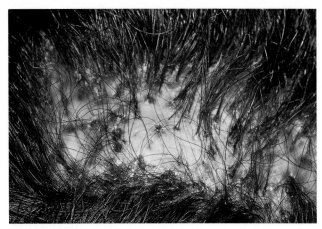

Fig 18.33 Folliculitis decalvans. Patchy scarred alopecia, in which hairs grow in bunches coming from a central follicular opening. There is associated folliculitis of surrounding follicles

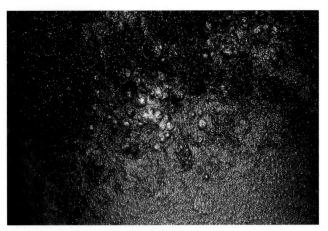

Fig 18.34 Folliculitis keloidalis. Follicular papules or pustules occur on the nape of the neck, particularly in Afro-Carribeans

Folliculitis decalvans

Folliculitis decalvans (calvans = balding) presents as bald areas of scarring alopecia, with follicular pustules at the periphery and bunches of terminal hairs left within the bald areas (**Fig 18.33**), known as 'tufted follicles' or poly-trichia (a feature that can be seen in other inflammatory scarring alopecias, such as that due to some forms of tinea capitis). Folliculitis decalvans is thought to be part of a spectrum referred to as 'central centrifugal scarring alopecia.'

Folliculitis keloidalis (nuchal acne keloid)

Follicular papules or pustules occur on the nape of the neck, particularly in Afro-Carribeans. Early inflammatory pustules give way to hard keloidal papules. These become confluent, and a large keloid is left. Active pustular folliculitis is visible at the periphery (**Fig 18.34**).

Hair shaft abnormalities

Hair shaft abnormalities, resulting in fragile hair that easily breaks, occur in a number of rare congenital anomalies, and only the more common varieties are described here. They are diagnosed by hair shaft microscopy (and may require scanning electron microscopy in some instances). In Netherton's syndrome, one of the congenital disorders with erythroderma and hair shaft defects, the eyebrow hairs are more reliable than scalp hair for microscopy. Hair shaft breaks are also seen after mechanical damage or infection, and these must be distinguished from the exclamation mark hairs of alopecia areata (**Table 18.7**).

Monilethrix

Although inherited as an autosomal dominant trait, monilethrix may not become obvious until adolescence. The hair is thin and breaks easily and usually, only short stubbly hair is apparent (**Figs 18.35–18.37**). Close examination of the hair shaft reveals the characteristic beaded appearance.

DIAGNOSTIC TIPS AND PITFALLS

- Broken scalp hairs can be caused by hair pulling (trichotillomania), alopecia areata or a fungal infection of the hair shaft

- Scalp fungal infections caused by anthropophilic fungi present with bald areas fringed with grey coated broken hairs and associated fine scale and little inflammation

- Some animal ringworm infections, notably from cattle, present with patchy hair loss and painful swelling and pustular discharge (kerion)

- Absent fluorescence under Wood's light examination in areas of hair loss does not exclude fungal infection. For example, human ringworm species and *Trichophyton* species

Table 18.7 Comparison of features of broken hairs

	Alopecia areata	Fungal infection	Mechanical damage	Hair shaft abnormalities
Morphology of the broken hairs	Exclamation mark hairs or coudability	Dull grey or black dots on hairs	Bristly hair, no completely bald patches	Beading, nodes or spangles visible on hair shaft
Plucking individual hairs	Easily removed	Easily removed	Difficult to pull out	Easily broken before removal
Appearance of the plucked hairs	Dystrophic telogen hairs	Fungal hyphae visible on potassium hydroxide preparation	Normal anagen hair	Shaft defect visible
Trichogram of hair adjacent to the bald area	>50% telogen hairs	Normal (i.e. 10–15% telogen hairs)	100% anagen hairs	Variable

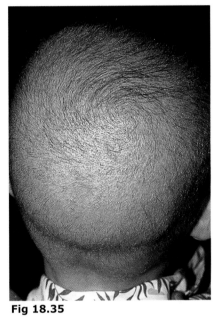

Fig 18.35

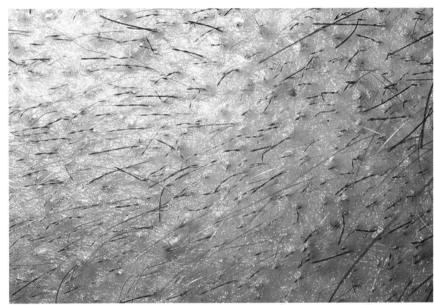

Fig 18.36

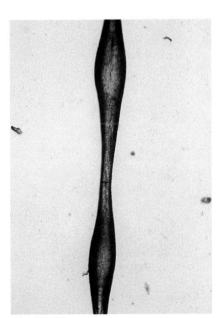

Fig 18.37

Figs 18.35–18.37 Monilethrix. The scalp is covered by multiple short and broken hairs (18.35). Closer inspection shows that the hair shafts are of uneven thickness (18.36), and the regular nodes can be clearly seen when examined under the microscope (18.37)

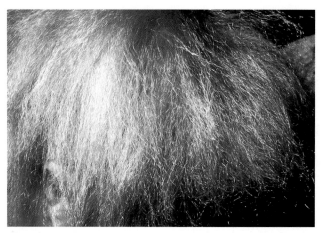

Fig 18.38 Pili torti. The hair is flattened and twisted around the longitudinal axis, resulting in each hair shaft assuming a spiral-like appearance and reflecting light at intervals along its length

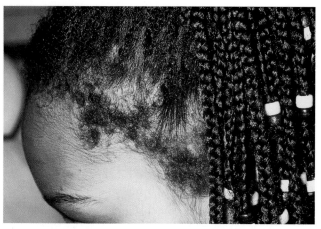

Fig 18.39 Traction alopecia in braided hair. Traction from plaited hair styles or long hair tied back may cause hair loss

Pili torti

In pili torti, the hair shaft is flattened and twisted, giving it a spangled appearance. Light is reflected from the flattened hair shaft surfaces at different endpoints depending on the position of the observer (**Fig 18.38**).

Trichorrhexis nodosa

Trichorrhexis nodosa is a common acquired cause of brittle or split-end hairs. Node-like swellings appear along the hair shaft, with fissuring or fractures at the site of the nodes. The hair cuticle splits due to repeated chemical and physical damage, and the cortical substance ruptures out, producing a swelling or node on the hair shaft that is easily broken.

Mechanical damage

Traction alopecia

Repeated use of tight hair rollers, or a hair style that pulls hairs, such as a long pony tail or tight braiding (**Fig 18.39**) causes a permanent hair loss at the margins of the scalp (**Fig 18.40**). Initially, there is an associated folliculitis around the affected hairs.

Trichotillomania

Trichotillomania, a type of hair loss, occurs when a disturbed patient consciously pulls out his or her own hair. Constant plucking or hair pulling leads to patches of hair loss, in which the remaining hairs are of various lengths but mostly shorter than 3 mm, since hairs shorter than this cannot be picked up with the fingers. There are no completely bald areas, and the hairs feel stubbly when the palm is brushed over the scalp, as the broken ends are not tapered as occurs in normal hair (**Fig 18.41**). The broken hairs are still in the anagen (growth) phase and so are difficult to remove if plucked by the physician. By contrast, the short hairs of diffuse alopecia areata are all dystrophic telogen hairs and come out easily when plucked with forceps. The broken root of the plucked hair can be identified with the naked eye. The area

> **DIAGNOSTIC TIPS AND PITFALLS**
>
> - Repeated use of tight hair rollers, a long pony tail or tight braiding can cause permanent hair loss at the margins of the scalp

> **DIAGNOSTIC TIPS AND PITFALLS**
>
> - 'Split ends' or trichorrhexis nodosa are common and are caused by repeated chemical and physical damage to the hair

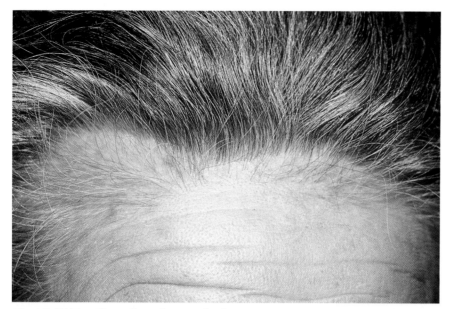

Fig 18.40 Traction alopecia marginal pattern. Repeatedly using tight rollers may lead to this type of marginal alopecia, in which a few straggly hairs have survived

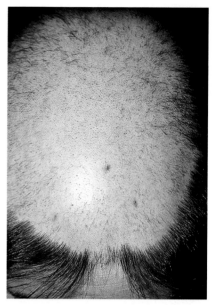

Fig 18.41 Trichotillomania. There is characteristic preservation of the frontal hair line. Hairs are mostly less than 3 mm long, and some scalp excoriations are present. Difficulty arises in cases where alopecia areata and trichotillomania co-exist (*see* pp. 346–347)

involved is usually sharply demarcated on the crown or fronto-parietal region. Although the entire scalp may be affected, the hair margin is commonly retained (**Fig 18.41**). Associated loss of eyebrow and eyelash hair is seen in approximately 25% of cases, so this is not helpful in distinguishing trichotillomania from diffuse alopecia areata. Some patients are said to swallow the plucked hairs, and hairs, and hairs may be found in the mouth, or a hair ball may be palpated in the stomach.

Hair rubbing

Regular hair rubbing causes frictional damage, and hairs break off near the scalp. This is most commonly seen in the lateral half of the eyebrow in children or adults with itchy facial eczema. In small babies who sleep on their back, a patch of hair loss and spangling of the hair shaft, producing a pseudo-pili torti-like appearance, may appear over the occiput. In the first year of life, synchronised loss of telogen hairs from the occiput and parietal areas may result in temporary patterned hair loss at these sites (occipital alopecia of the newborn).

Other causes of broken hairs

Fungal infection (tinea capitis, kerion)—Fungi normally found only in humans, the anthropophilic fungi, e.g. *Trichophyton tonsurans*, *Trichophyton violaceum* and *Microsporum audouinii*, produce little inflammation, as might be expected from a parasite in harmony with its host. These anthropophilic fungal infections may be of endothrix or ectothrix type (**Table 18.8**). Endothrix infections invade the hair shaft within the follicle, so the hair breaks off within the follicle and is seen as a black dot. Ectothrix infections grow on the surface of the hair shaft and invade the shaft only above the scalp surface, so that breakage leaves short (less than 5 mm long) hairs protruding from the follicle. The broken hairs may have a grey appearance due to fungal hyphae growing on the surface of the hair, and these may fluoresce green under Wood's light (**Fig 18.43**), *see also* pp. 63–66.

Table 18.8 Patterns of scalp ringworm

Clinical pattern	Hair appearance	Fungus	Fluorescence
Patchy alopecia, fine scale, little or no inflammation	Broken grey hairs (ectothrix fungi)	*Microsporum audouinii* *Microsporum canis*	Greenish yellow* Greenish yellow
	Black dots (endothrix fungi)	*Trichophyton tonsurans* *Trichophyton violaceum*	None None
Patchy hair loss, swelling and pustular discharge		*Trichophyton mentagrophytes* *Trichophyton verrucosum*	None None

*Although *M. canis* is an animal ringworm, in the UK, it normally presents with non-inflamed scaly alopecia.

By contrast, fungal infections caused by animal ringworm, e.g. *Trichophyton mentagrophtyes* and *Trichophyton verrucosum*, produce inflammatory swelling in association with hair loss (**Table 18.8** and **Table 18.9**). *Microsporum canis* is an exception to this rule; this infection, usually acquired from cats, produces a well-circumscribed patch of non-inflamed hair loss (**Fig 18.42**).

Differential diagnosis of extensive broken hairs

The clinical appearance of diffuse hair loss produced by diffuse alopecia areata and by trichotillomania can be almost indistinguishable, especially when exclamation mark hairs are absent (*see* above). Hair loss at other sites is not helpful, as this occurs in both conditions (*see* above). Furthermore, in some patients, trichotillomania and alopecia areata may co-exist, although it is often difficult to decide which came first.

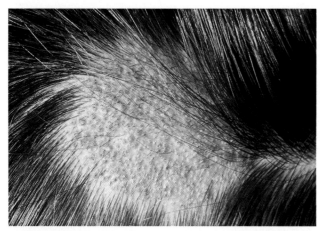

Fig 18.42 Tinea capitis. *Microsporum canis* infection caused a patch of alopecia with multiple broken hairs. There is no inflammation of the adjacent scalp

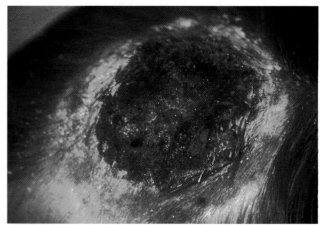

Fig 18.43 Fluorescence in tinea capitis. UV-light examination of a patch of *Microsporum canis* alopecia. Greenish-yellow fluorescence is best seen on a single hair as indicated by the arrow. Only *M. canis* and *Microsponum audouinii* regularly fluoresce with Wood's light. The fluorescence is seen only on the broken hairs, not on the surrounding scale. The trichophyton species, except *Trichophyton schoenleinii*, do not fluoresce, so Wood's light examination cannot be used to exclude fungal infection with these organisms

Table 18.9 Likely animal* source in animal ringworm

Microsporum canis	Cat, dog, horse, monkey
Trichophyton mentagrophytes	Mouse, rat, dog, rabbit, guinea-pig, monkey, cow, horse
Trichophyton verrucosum	Cow, horse

*Human-to-human spread can occur with all these fungi.

In both conditions, and occasionally in extensive fungal infections and congenital hair shaft anomalies, extensive broken hairs can be the principal feature. **Table 18.7** is an attempt to outline the clinical differences that may help in distinguishing these conditions. In general, broken hairs in alopecia areata are dystrophic and can be easily plucked out, and cadaverised hairs and kinkable or coudable hairs may be present. In trichotillomania, the broken hairs are all bristly anagen hairs that are difficult to pluck out, and there is no root depigmentation. Hair shaft abnormalities can be readily identified by careful examination of the individual hairs, although occasionally, microscope examination is required. Fungal infections are normally excluded by fungal culture and potassium hydroxide microscopy, although the features listed in **Table 18.7** may also be helpful. It is important to recognise that absent fluorescence under Wood's light examination does not exclude fungal infection (**Fig 18.43**).

HAIR COLOUR CHANGES

In albinism and piebaldism (**Fig 18.44**), the hair is white from birth.

Acquired pigment change may be seen in pernicious anaemia and vitiligo, where patchy loss of pigmentation occurs. In alopecia areata, white hairs are less likely to be shed than pigmented hairs, thus in patients who previously had both pigmented and white hairs, development of alopecia totalis may lead to loss of pigmented hairs but retention of the white hairs. This creates

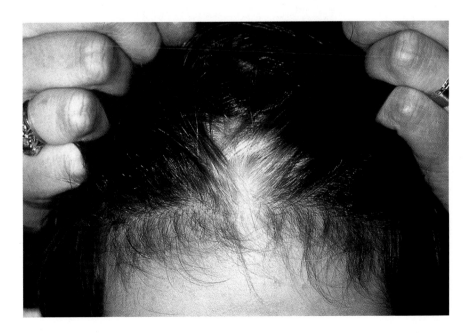

Fig 18.44 Piebaldism. The white forelock is characteristic of piebaldism and a useful distinguishing feature from vitiligo. White patches in piebaldism are present from birth and often have hyperpigmented borders. 3.19 shows other features of the same patient

the impression of having 'gone white' very quickly (**Fig 18.45**). Cases of white hair turning grey have been reported in hypothyroidism. In kwashiorkor, loss of hair colour during periods of protein deficiency produces bands of light reddish-blonde hair and normally pigmented hair—the 'flag sign'; similar changes occur in protein deficiency due to gut disease.

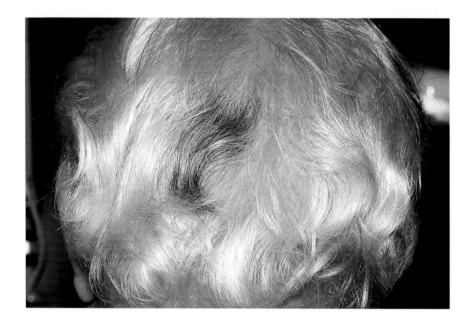

Fig 18.45 Alopecia areata with generalised white hair. This man developed almost total alopecia. The white hairs were unaffected as was a patch of pigmented hairs on the occiput, resulting in this remaining patch of black hair

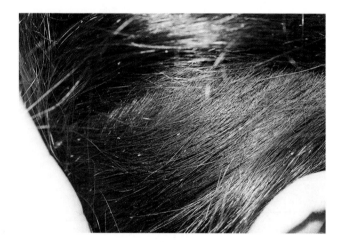

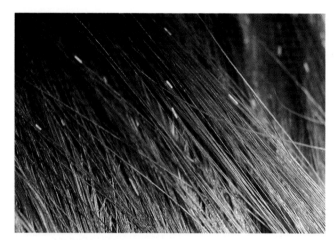

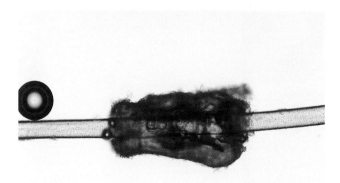

Fig 18.46–18.48 Hair casts. These keratin casts are not a sign of disease but may occur in psoriasis and seborrhoeic eczema. They may initially be confused with nits

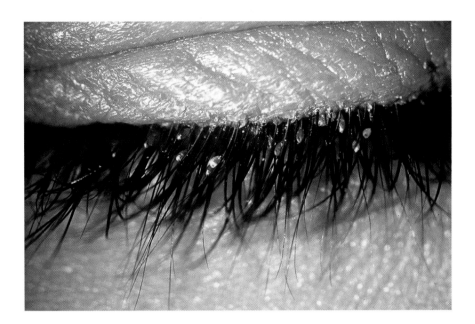

Fig 18.49 Pubic lice on the eyelashes

External pigments also cause colour changes:

- Green—copper from drinking water or industrial sources, copper algicides used in swimming pool water.
- Yellow—vioform medicaments, nicotine staining.
- Orange—dithranol stains (especially in grey or fair hair).

ADDITIONS TO THE HAIR

Small objects attached to the hair may be normal keratin peripilar casts (**Figs 18.46–18.48**) or the egg cases (nits) (**Figs 18.49** and **18.50**) left from parasitic infestations due to scalp, body or pubic lice. Peripilar casts, or scale due to inflammatory dermatoses, can be moved up and down the hair shaft, whereas egg cases are firmly attached to the hair. Adult lice can be identified with the naked eye as tiny insects attached to the hair (**Fig 18.50**).

In the axilla, bacterial concretions collect on the hairs in *Trichomycosis axillaris* (**Figs 18.51** and **18.52**).

SCALING IN THE SCALP

Scaling without associated hair loss occurs in a number of dermatoses. Fine diffuse scaling is due to dandruff or seborrhoeic eczema (**Fig 18.53**). Localised patches of well-defined scale separated by normal scalp are characteristic of psoriasis (**Fig 18.54**), and in pityriasis amiantacea (**Fig 18.55**), small adherent scales are formed through which the hair shafts grow, resulting in the hairs being stuck together by the scale. Because of this, hairs may be shed in clumps; single telogen hairs will not fall out of the adherent scale.

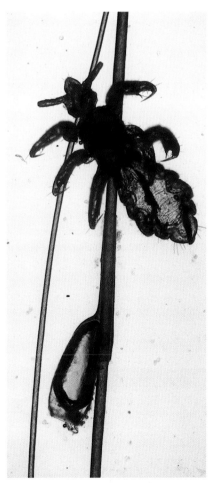

Fig 18.50 Head louse and egg (nit). Not that the egg case is fixed on the side of the hair shaft, rather than forming a cast around it (compare with 18.48)

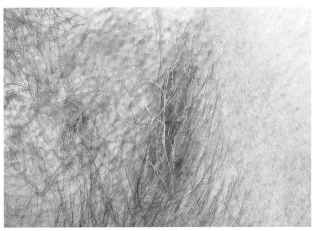

Fig 18.51

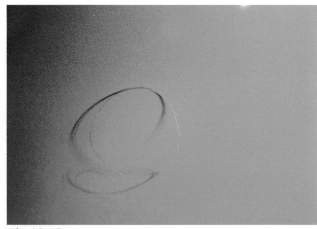

Fig 18.52

Figs 18.51, 18.52 Trichomycosis axillaris. Yellowish concretions of corynebacteria collect on the axillary hairs, producing an amorphous appearance of axillary hair and a thickening around the hair shaft (18.51). The portion of a plucked hair from within the follicle is relatively spared (18.52)

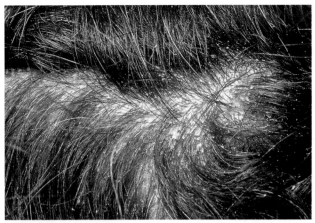

Fig 18.53 Seborrhoeic dermatitis of the scalp. There is a generalised fine scaling of the scalp. This is not raised and there are no spared areas

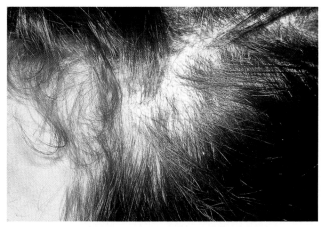

Fig 18.54 Psoriasis of the scalp. There is a well-demarcated patch of hyperkeratotic scale on this young girl's scalp with adjacent areas of uninvolved scalp skin. This is often better appreciated by feeling the scalp, when patchy hyperkeratotic plaques can be readily felt

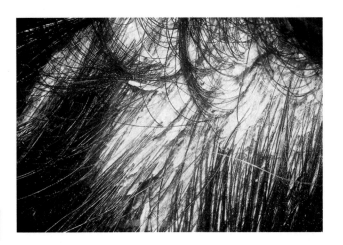

Fig 18.55 Pityriasis amiantacea. This may be the result of psoriasis or eczema. Adherent flakes of scale form on the scalp. The hairs grow through these, but as the scale is not shed the hairs remain joined together at the base by the scale

19 Nails

NAIL PHYSIOLOGY

Fingernails grow approximately 0.5–1 mm per week, toenails approximately 1 mm per month. It takes approximately 6 months for a fingernail to grow from the matrix (proximal) to the free edge, and 18 months for a toenail to be replaced. Nail growth decreases with increasing age and poor circulation. Nail thickness increases distally because the nail bed contributes throughout its length to the thickness of the nail plate, adding a further 25% to the thickness determined by the matrix. The portion of the nail plate that is formed from the nail bed is called the ventral nail and can be left intact as a rather thin and soft nail in some disorders where the nail matrix has been destroyed. The lunula (**Fig 19.1**) corresponds to the nail matrix. There is no adequate explanation for the white colour of the lunula, although this colour difference is apparent in both the nail plate and bed when the nail is removed.

The onychodermal band of Terry is the rim of pale nail, approximately 1 mm wide, visible at the distal end of the nail. It is often separated from the larger main pink zone of the nail plate by a thin white line. The nail bed just proximal to the onychodermal band appears more red than the remainder of the nail bed. Pressing the tip of the finger results in blanching of the onychodermal band and the proximal hyperaemic area more readily than the remainder of the nail plate. One explanation proposed for this observation is that this area has a different blood supply to the rest of the nail. Exaggeration of the colour differences in the onychodermal band has been recorded in cirrhosis, but similar changes are also seen in some normal individuals, and it seems unlikely that this is a useful physical sign.

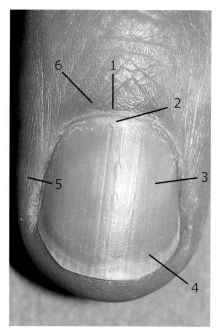

Fig 19.1 Normal nail. The various parts of a normal nail: cuticle (1), lunula (2), nail plate (3), onychodermal band (4), lateral nailfold (5), posterior nailfold (6)

NORMAL VARIATIONS AND COMMON ANOMALIES

White flecks

White flecks (acquired punctate leuconychia) are common normal variants (**Figs 19.2** and **19.3**). They are generally held to be incomplete keratinisation within the nail plate and seem to be the result of repeated minor trauma. They are not due to calcium insufficiency, a popular misconception. White flecks may disappear spontaneously or grow out with the nail.

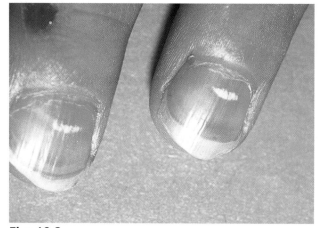

Figs 19.2

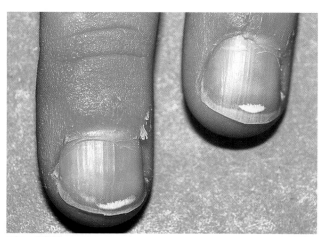

Figs 19.3

Figs 19.2, 19.3 White flecks (acquired punctate leuconychia). These appear to develop spontaneously but are probably due to forgotten mild trauma to the nail matrix. They are commonly curved and appear concurrently on several nails (19.2), usually in young people. Most disappear spontaneously before reaching the distal nail margin, whereas others grow out with the nail (19.3) as shown here 4 weeks later

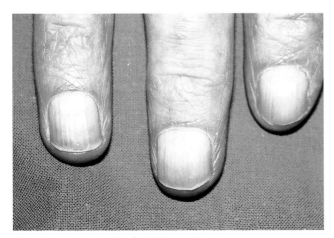

Fig 19.4 Longitudinal ridging. This is very common, but becomes more obvious with increasing age. Beading of the ridges also occurs. Longitudinal ridges in children usually point towards the centre of the nail rather than running parallel

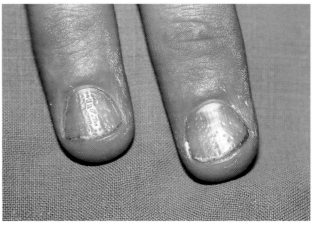

Fig 19.5 Shiny nails and pitting in psoriasis. Nails commonly reflect back light when photographed and thus may appear polished. In these nails from a man with itchy psoriasis, the rims of the deep psoriatic pits have been smoothed off by constant rubbing, producing an appearance similar to well polished brass

Longitudinal ridging

Longitudinal ridging becomes more obvious in old age. The ridges may appear beaded (**Fig 19.4**), with an appearance reminiscent of a string of sausages.

Shiny nails

Shiny nails, due to rubbing, are commonly seen in longstanding itchy skin conditions (**Fig 19.5**). The most common is atopic dermatitis. The free edge of the nail may also become bevelled (with a concave rather than the usual convex shape) due to prolonged scratching.

Pigmented streaks

Longitudinal pigmented bands are found in approximately 90% of Afro-Caribbeans (**Fig 19.6**). The stripes vary in width from 1–7 mm and may be single or multiple. They are absent at birth, and their number increases with age. The extent of pigmentation correlates with depth of skin colour, and in some extremely dark individuals, nail pigmentation may be diffuse rather than linear. Histological examination shows that the streaks and diffuse pigmentation are due to melanin deposition within the nail plate. See also discussion of Hutchinson's sign (pp. 375–376).

CONGENITAL ANOMALIES

There are numerous congenital abnormalities that affect nails, characteristically symmetrically and sometimes affecting the digits as well. The most commonly diagnosed types are those causing altered shape of the nails (e.g. racquet nails, **Fig 19.9**) or altered thickness (e.g. pachyonychia congenita). Small, or even absent, nails may occur as an isolated phenomenon or in conjunction with underlying abnormalities of the distal phalanx. However,

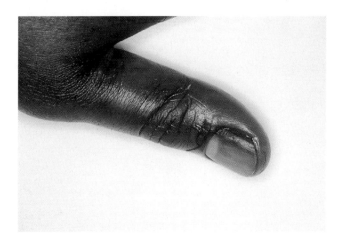

Fig 19.6 Pigmented streaks in black skin. A typical benign pigmented streak in an Afro-Caribbean; although dark, the lesion had uniform width and was of long duration. Almost 90% of Afro-Carribeans have pigment bands, and these are commonly multiple

congenital (sometimes familial) colour changes also occur, e.g. congenital leukonychia (pale white nails). Common congenital abnormalities, such as thickened fifth toenails, should always be considered in children with abnormal nails, as incorrect antifungal treatment is a common pitfall.

Nail patella syndrome

The nail patella syndrome is an autosomal dominant trait. Patients have an absent or small patellae, prominent iliac horns (which can be felt but usually require radiography to confirm their presence) and missing or small altered nails (**Figs 19.7** and **19.8**). The nail changes are best seen on the thumb. A V-shaped lunula is the only feature on some nails and is pathognomonic. The importance of recognising these features is that associated renal anomalies, including glomerulonephritis, occur in approximately 30% of cases. Eye abnormalities, including glaucoma, also occur.

> ### DIAGNOSTIC TIPS AND PITFALLS
>
> - Always consider congenital abnormalities in the differential diagnosis of nail dystrophy in children, especially if changes in nail size or thickness are symmetrical and are not associated with tinea pedis

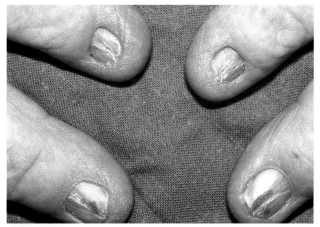

Figs 19.7

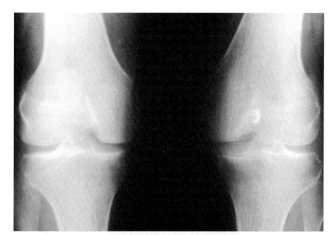

Figs 19.8

Figs 19.7, 19.8 Nail patella syndrome: nails and radiography of knees. Nails may be absent, small or split (19.7). Pterygium formation may occur, and the triangular lunula is said to be pathognomonic and is usually best seen on the thumb. Bony changes include absent or small patellae (19.8), bilateral posterior iliac horns and hypoplasia of the capitulum and head of the radius. The clinically significant features are the associated renal and ocular changes

Racket (racquet) nails

Racket (racquet) nails are shorter than they are wide (hence brachyonychia Greek brachys = short), and the terminal phalanx may also be short (**Fig 19.9**). In isolation, they have no significance. They are usually inherited as an autosomal dominant trait, but seem to be more common in women. They should not be confused with the finger shortening that occurs after reabsorption of the terminal phalanx in hyperparathyroidism.

Congenital malalignment of the toes

Congenital malalignment of the toes results in thickened nails (**Fig 19.10**) in children. These grow slowly, are generally very hard to cut and are usually malaligned so they do not grow straight. All the toenails are affected, but changes are usually noticed on the great toenail only.

NAIL CHANGES DUE TO PHYSICAL INJURIES

Mechanical trauma

Repeated minor trauma to the toenails due to poorly fitting footwear causes black discoloration under the toenails due to subungual haemorrhage. There is associated lateral ridging, splitting, splinter haemorrhages and onycholysis. The hallux is the most commonly affected, and the changes are symmetrical (**Fig 19.11**). In joggers, similar changes on the more lateral toenails have been recorded. Isolated subungual haematomas due to a single episode of trauma lead to discoloration of the nail bed. As the nail grows, the straight transverse margin defined by the cuticle can be distinguished (**Figs 19.12** and **19.13**). Other features that suggest a traumatic haematoma include an arcuate white band arising from the margin of the lunula, the fact that the pigment does not extend the full length of the nail (compare with pigmented streaks discussed on p. 376), associated splinter haemorrhages or any similar lesion in an adjacent toe, or symmetrical involvement of the hallux nails (**Fig 19.11**).

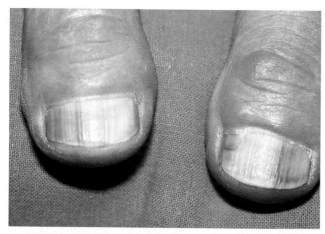

Fig 19.9 Racket (racquet) nails. These short nails are wider than they are long and were originally considered to resemble tennis rackets. The terminal phalanx is usually shorter, and the big toe may be similarly affected. As an isolated finding this appearance is of no clinical importance

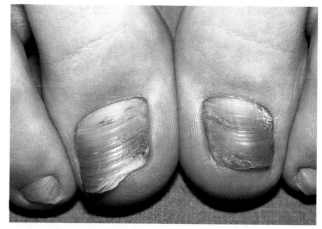

Fig 19.10 Congenital malalignment of the great toenails. The nails are thicker and grow slowly, characteristically curving laterally with ridging of the nail plate. These changes can be readily distinguished from a fungal dystrophy, as the nail plate is formed from very hard keratin that does not crumble

355

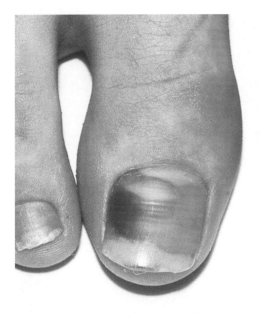

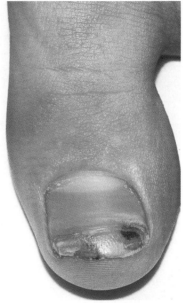

Fig 19.11 Trauma changes in a footballer's great toenails. This condition usually affects the hallux nails and is bilateral in most cases. The nail is slightly thickened and distorted, with grey/green/brown discoloration due to bruising (*photo courtesy of Dr W D Paterson*)

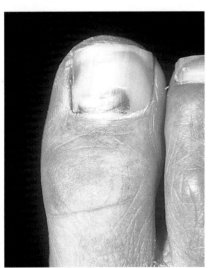

Fig 19.12

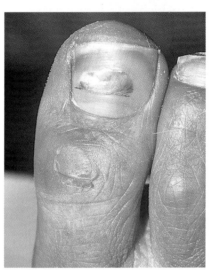

Fig 19.13

Figs 19.12, 19.13 Subungual haematoma in the great toenail. This can be distinguished from subungual melanin pigment because the colour includes red or purple, longitudinal spread of the blood is visible along ridges under the nail, and there is a sharp proximal border (19.12), which is initially just proximal to the cuticle, but becomes apparent as the nail grows (19.13). Small white bands within the pigmented area become more prominent as the area grows out

Chemical and other injuries

Handling solvents or oils can cause koilonychia, onycholysis and roughening of the nail plate (**Fig 19.14**). Acrylic nail polishes and hardeners may cause onycholysis and noticeable damage to the nail plate. Previous radiotherapy (an old treatment for periungual warts) may cause small and dystrophic nails.

DEFECTS OF THE NAIL PLATE

Koilonychia

In koilonychia (hollow nails), the nails are spoon-shaped and, depending on the underlying cause, may be thick, thin or normal (**Figs 19.15** and **19.16**), (**Table 19.1**).

> ### DIAGNOSTIC TIPS AND PITFALLS
>
> - Bilateral/symmetrical subungual pigmentation of hallux nails in children and young adults is highly likely to be due to repetitive minor injuries

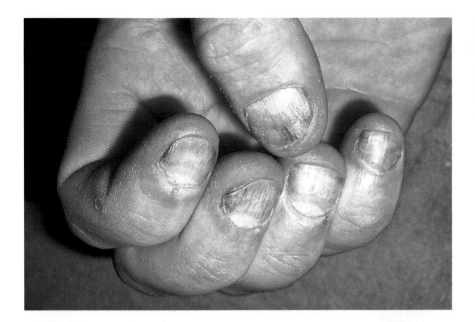

Fig 19.14 Oil-induced koilonychia. Abnormal nails in a motor mechanic. Repeated contact with oil and solvents lead to onycholysis and mild koilonychia, with a roughened and discolored nail

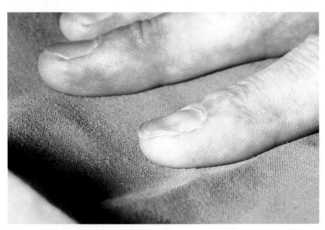

Figs 19.15 Koilonychia (hollow or 'spoon-shaped' nails). A single nail was involved due to trauma. Note the nicotine staining of the finger end.

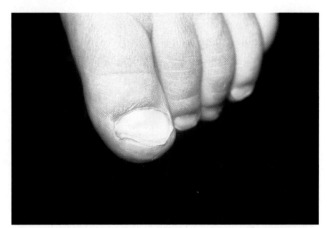

Figs 19.16 Koilonychia in infants. Most babies and small children have koilonychia of their toenails, and this is best seen on the great toenail. It disappears spontaneously after about 4 years of age

---

Table 19.1 Common causes of koilonychia (Greek koilos = hollow)

Systemic
Congenital
Autosomal dominant
Haematological
Iron deficiency with or without anaemia, polycythaemia, haemochromatosis
Others
Syphilis, endocrine disease

Local
Trauma
Solvents, corrosives, thioglycate (acid perms used by hairdressers), acrylic nail polishes

Cutaneous diseases
Raynaud's disease
Lichen planus
Alopecia areata

Physiological
In babies and toddlers, koilonychia of the hallux is common (19.16)

Nail pitting

Pits may be arranged longitudinally or horizontally, but these different patterns do not help with the differential diagnosis of the cause (**Table 19.2**). The morphology of individual pits can be helpful; pitting in psoriasis is well defined and discrete, whereas eczema produces a shallower or rippled pattern of pitting. A very fine pitting occurs in trachyonychia/20 nail dystrophy (p. 363) (Greek trachys = rough). Pitting associated with alopecia areata may resemble that seen in eczema or trachyonychia. In psoriasis, the pitting is due to areas of parakeratosis (retained nucleated keratinocytes) in the dorsal nail plate, which are subsequently shed to leave small pits.

Clubbing

Although listed here as a shape change in the nailplate, this is actually due to hypertrophy of the soft tissues under the nail, which becomes secondarily distorted (**Fig 19.19**). The normal angle between the posterior nailfold and the nail plate becomes flattened, and the nail is overcurved. A simple test for the presence of clubbing is to oppose opposite nails; in clubbing, there is loss of the normal elongated diamond-shaped gap seen between the two nails, and at the proximal end of the nail, there is a V-shaped gap. Some of the more common causes are listed in **Table 19.3**.

Table 19.2 Common causes of nail pitting	
Deep pits	Psoriasis (19.5)
	Reiter's disease
Shallow pits	Alopecia areata (19.17)
	Eczema (19.18)
	Pityriasis rosea
	Syphilis

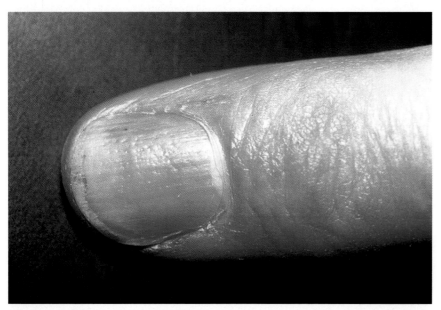

Fig 19.17 Nail pitting in alopecia areata. There are multiple tiny pits on the nail plate surface, producing a roughened appearance

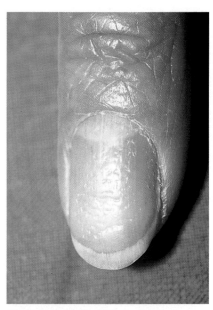

Fig 19.18 Nail pitting—eczema. Nail-plate abnormalities occur as a result of periungual eczema. Here, pits and transverse furrows have been created

Table 19.3 Common causes of clubbing

Respiratory system (80% of cases)
Thoracic tumours: bronchogenic, pleural, lymphoma
Chronic sepsis: bronchiectasis, abscess, empyema
Pulmonary fibrosis: cryptogenic fibrosing alveolitis, asbestosis

Cardiovascular system
Subacute bacterial endocarditis
Cyanotic heart disease

Alimentary tract
Chronic liver disease
Ulcerative colitis
Crohn's disease

Congenital

Endocrine
Thyrotoxicosis ('thyroid acropachy')

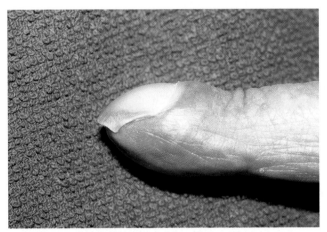

Fig 19.19 Clubbing. There is a swelling of the soft tissues under the nail, which pushes the nail plate upwards causing loss of the normal 180 degree, or less, angle made between the nail plate and the nailfold. The nail can be rocked on the underlying terminal phalanx by the application of gentle pressure

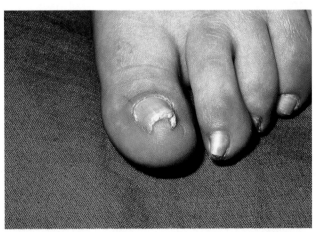

Fig 19.20 Pincer nails. This condition is usually most apparent on the thumb and great toe. The inward curved lateral borders cut into the nail bed, and this is usually greatest at the free margin of the nail

Pincer nails

Pincer nails is usually a hereditary condition, although some cases seem to be due to wearing poorly fitting shoes (**Fig 19.20**). The transverse overcurvature of the nail plate may increase distally, so that the nail becomes cone-shaped or more pointed towards the tip. The residual area of soft tissue left between the distal pincers of the nail may become painful, due to compression of dermis and bone.

Thickened nails

Causes of thickened nails are listed in **Table 19.4**.

Table 19.4 Common causes of thickened nails

Dermatological disease	Psoriasis (19.21), pityriasis rubra pilaris, eczema, fungal infection (onychomycosis), chronic vascular disease
Old age	Thickened toenails are common in elderly people, probably due to impaired peripheral circulation (19.22); onychogryphosis (19.23) is an extreme example
Trauma	
Congenital	Pachyonychia congenita

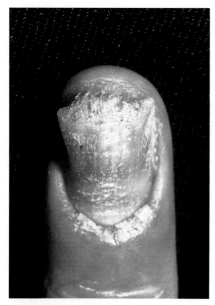

Fig 19.21 Thickened nail—psoriasis

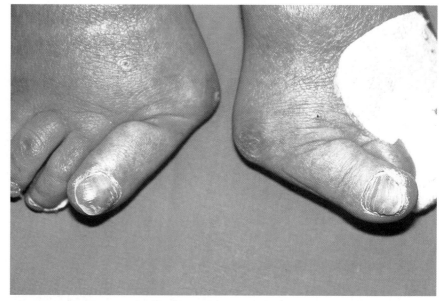

Fig 19.22 Ischaemic dystrophy of elderly people. Toenails are thickened, brittle and hard. Crumbly nails also occur in which case a co-existing fungal infection must be excluded by fungal culture

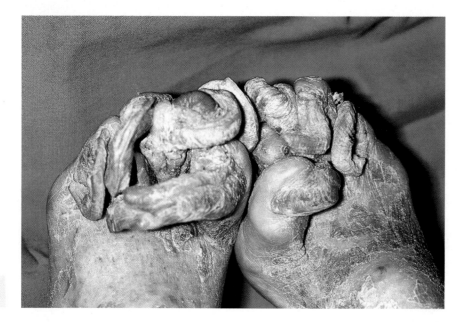

Fig 19.23 Onychogryphosis. There are a range of causes, including trauma, fungal infection and skin disease, causing thickening of the nails. Eventually the nail becomes too hard to cut and is left to grow unchecked, creating further trauma to the nail (*photo courtesy of Dr S Natarajan*)

Nail ridging and Beau's lines

Transverse ridges

Ridges may be transverse or longitudinal; the latter are normal in old age (*see* **Fig 19.4**). Beau's lines are transverse ridges, which occur when nail growth stops temporarily, usually because of acute illness (**Fig 19.24**). In systemic causes, all the nails are affected at the same time, although because of differences in nail growth rates, the changes will be seen first on the fingernails, in particular the middle fingernail—the fastest growing nail—and lastly on the toenails. Multiple Beau's lines (or multiple transverse white bands) may be present in individuals having cyclical chemotherapy. If the nail stops growing for more than 2 weeks, the defect in the nail is usually so great that the distal half is shed (onychomadesis, **Fig 19.31** Greek madesis = loss of hair!). Beau's lines are usually most apparent on the thumb and big toenail, probably because damage to these thicker nails can be greater without the nail being lost.

In habit tic dystrophy (**Fig 19.30**), the actual grooves are transverse, but they are multiple, and in established cases the overall arrangement is longitudinal. In early cases, where the initial habit is picking in the region of the cuticle, a smaller number of proximal transversely oriented grooves are apparent.

Longitudinal ridges

Longitudinal ridging can result from a variety of causes (**Figs 19.25–19.30** and **Table 19.5**).

A more 'grooved' or guttered appearance of the nail plate occurs due to compression of the nail matrix under the proximal nailfold. This may occur due to periungual warts, myxoid (mucous) cysts or by a tumour, which is usually readily identifiable (**19.57, 19.58**).

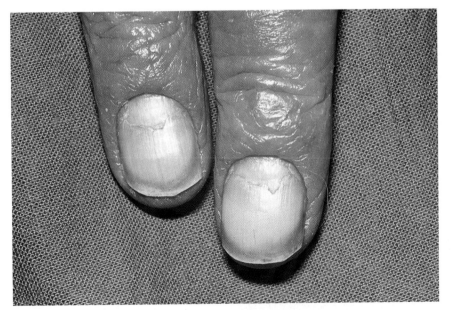

Fig 19.24 Beau's lines in drug-induced erythroderma

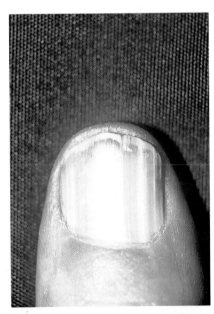

Fig 19.25 Darier's disease. White longitudinal streaks are common in Darier's disease. Where the streak meets the free margin, there is usually a V-shaped notch. Nail splits and subungual keratoses also occur

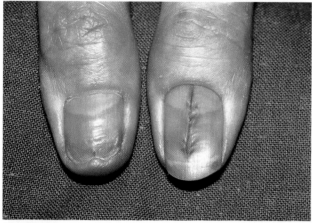

Fig 19.26

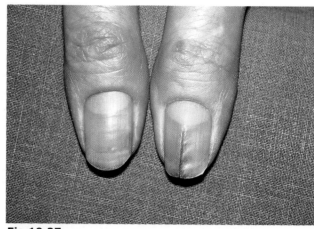

Fig 19.27

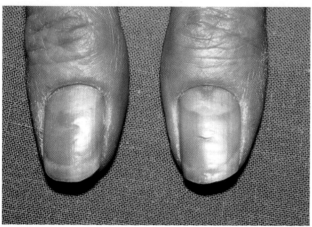

Fig 19.28

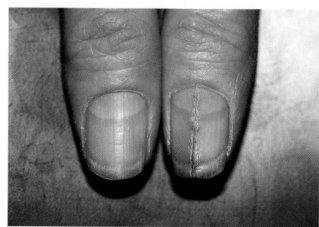

Fig 19.29

Figs 19.26–19.29 Median canaliform dystrophy. There is a central longitudinal fissure starting proximally (19.26). The same nails photographed 7 months (19.27), 20 months (19.28) and 36 months (19.29) later show spontaneous resolution followed by recurrence

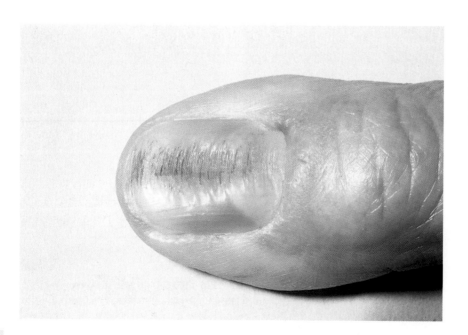

Fig 19.30 Habit tic dystrophy. Constant manipulation of the finger end adjacent to the matrix causes transverse ridges of the nail; as the nail grows, serial ridges occur, and the final result appears as a longitudinal ridge

Table 19.5 Types of nail ridging	
Longitudinal	Darier's disease (19.25)
	Median canaliform dystrophy (19.26–19.29)
	Physiological (19.4)
	Focal damage to nail matrix
	Pterygium
Transverse	Beau's lines (19.24), onychomadesis
	Habit tic (19.30)
	Eczema

Nail shedding

Nail shedding may occur due to trauma, severe acute illness, severe skin disease, drug reactions (**Fig 19.31**), radiotherapy or spontaneously (onychomadesis).

Rough nails

Changes to the nail surface producing roughness and opacity of the nail plate with splitting at the free margin occur in alopecia areata (**Fig 19.17**), psoriasis and lichen planus. The appearance varies from a fine 'sandpapered' morphology to quite pronounced surface roughness. The term '20 nail dystrophy' or trachyonychia was applied to such cases in which all the nails were involved (**Figs 19.32** and **19.33**). However, in childhood at least, histological changes in 20 nail dystrophy seem to be those of lichen planus.

Flaky nails

Distal flaking of the free margin of the nails, or brittle nails (lamella dystrophy), occurs in approximately 20% of the population. It is common in children and adults and is the result of repeated trauma and immersion in hot soapy water or solvents (**Fig 19.34**).

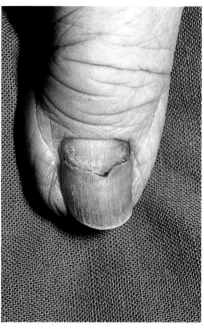

Fig 19.31 Nail shedding. This was associated with an idiosyncratic reaction to azathioprine

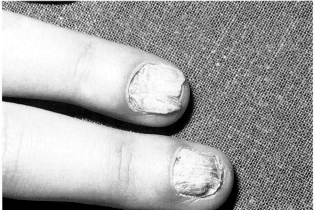

Fig 19.32

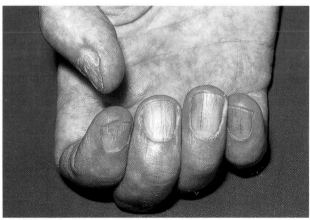

Fig 19.33

Figs 19.32, 19.33 Rough nails due to 20 nail dystrophy. The nails may have prominent surface roughness and splitting (19.32) or may appear white with a mild surface roughness resembling a sandpapered nail plate (19.33)

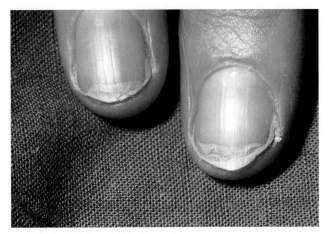

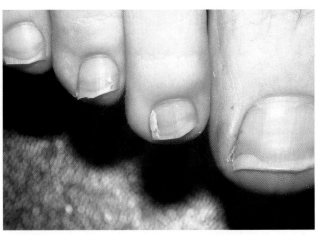

Fig 19.34 Flaky nails. The free margin of the nail is split into several layers. It is common in those who have a lot of contact with water and detergents

Fig 19.35 White superficial onychomycosis. Superficial invasion of the nail plate of the second toe produces a patchy white change visible on the nail surface. The surface is soft, opaque and powdery, and the whiteness can easily be scrapped away. The nail plate is not thickened. *Trichophyton rubrum* was cultured

Fungal infections of the nail

Fungal infections of the nail are usually the result of infection with *Trichophyton rubrum* or *Trichophyton mentagrophytes*. The commonest route of infection is from the free edge of the nail or adjacent lateral nailfold ('distal/lateral subungual onychomycosis'), but direct involvement of the surface of the nail plate may occur ('superficial white onychomycosis'), and less commonly infection may be acquired through the cuticle before spreading under the nail ('proximal subungual onychomycosis'; **Figs 19.35–19.37**). The

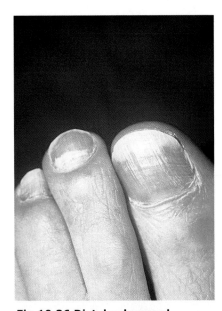

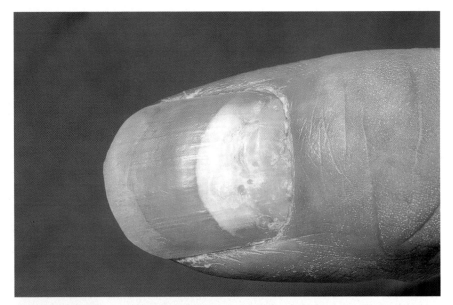

Fig 19.36 Distal subungual onychomycosis. Fungal invasion via the distal or lateral edge of the nail is common. The distal nail turns yellowish-white, thickens and crumbles and starts to separate from the nail bed. *Trichophyton rubrum* was cultured

Fig 19.37 Proximal superficial onychomycosis. Infection occurs via the cuticle area with invasion of the nail plate. Hyperkeratotic debris collects under the normal surface nail plate, causing it to separate from the nail bed. Note the very well-demarcated spreading edge and that the nail plate surface ridges are not interrupted by the subungual process. In this case, the patient was immunocompetent (this pattern of fungal infection may occur in patients with HIV infection). *Trichophyton rubrum* was cultured

Table 19.6 Differential diagnosis of fungal nail infection

Psoriasis	Pitting (19.5) does not occur in fungal nail dystrophy. Salmon patches (19.50) do not present in fungal dystrophies. Asymmetrical involvement may occur in both psoriasis and fungal infections
Chronic paronychia	The cuticle is lost. The nail plate is ridged and damaged on the surface, but without subungual hyperkeratosis
Leuconychia	Spontaneous white flecks can be distinguished from white superficial onychomycosis; the former cannot be scraped away because the whiteness is due to changes deep within the nail plate (19.2, 19.3)
Eczema	Secondary nail damage in eczema may produce horizontal ridging and pitting (19.18), but the nail remains hard and does not crumble
Habit tic damage	The nail is deformed, but the nail plate is normal and does not crumble (19.30)
Congenital anomalies	Pachyonychia congenita and congenital malalignment of the great toe (19.10) are usually symmetrical. Although thickened and deformed, the nail plate is hard
Ischaemic dystrophy of the elderly	Poor peripheral circulation causes thickening, roughness and sometimes onycholysis of the toenail plate (19.22). Secondary infection by candida can occur. The combination is predictably common in diabetics. Exclusion of a co-existing fungal infection requires fungal culture
Trauma	Both big toenails are affected—particularly common in footballers (19.11)

latter is of importance as it is disproportionately common in immuno-suppressed patients or those with AIDS. In advanced disease, the initial morphology may be lost. Physical signs that may help with the differential diagnosis of nail fungal infections are summarised in **Table 19.6**. Candida nail dystrophy may occur secondary to ischaemia as in Raynaud's disease, following chronic paronychia, in chronic mucocutaneous candidiasis or without an obvious cause (**Fig 19.38**). It is particularly important therapeutically to distinguish between dermatophyte fungal nail dystrophy and chronic paronychia (p 370). Factors that predispose to chronic candidal paronychia are listed in **Table 19.7**.

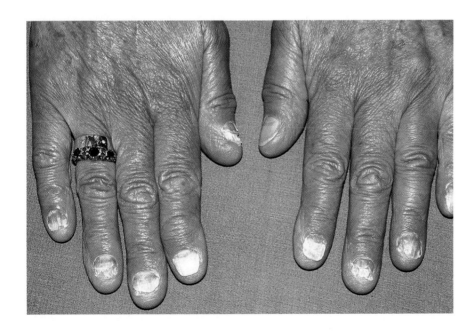

Fig 19.38 Candida nail dystrophy. Nine of this woman's fingernails were affected with koilonychia, thickening, onycholysis and splitting. All her nails returned to normal after a course of itraconazole. No predisposing cause was found

Table 19.7 Causes of acute and chronic paronychia

Acute	
Bacterial	*Staphylococcus aureus*
	Streptococcus pyogenes
Viral	Herpes simplex (nurses and dentists)
Chronic*	
Candida albicans	Occupational: barmaids, cooks, diabetics, dentists. Chronic mucocutaneous candidiasis usually only affects the nail plate
	Hypoparathyroidism
Mycobacterium tuberculosis	Occupational: mortuary attendants and pathologists

*Consider the possibility of melanoma or carcinoma in solitary nail involvement, and pustular psoriasis if several nails are involved.

DEFECTS OF THE NAILFOLDS

Ingrown toenail

In ingrown toenail, painful redness and swelling followed by the development of granulation tissue occur due to a small spicule of nail penetrating the lateral nailfold (**Fig 19.39**). The spicule is formed by a combination of trauma, incorrect cutting of the nail and poor footwear.

Pterygium

Scarring of the posterior nailfold skin and the dorsal matrix results in fusion of the posterior nailfold on to the nail plate (**Fig 19.40** and **Table 19.8**). The nail may be completely eroded at the point of attachment and divided into two portions. The commonest cause in single or adjacent nails is old trauma.

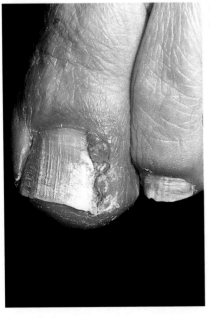

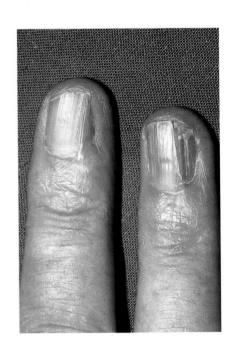

Fig 19.39 Ingrown toenail with associated nail plate fungal infection

Fig 19.40 Pterygium. Fusion of the posterior nailfold and nail plate due to lichen planus

Table 19.8 Causes of pterygium

Trauma
Lichen planus
Chronic ischaemia
Radiotherapy to nails
Nail patella syndrome
Dystrophic epidermolysis bullosa
Other bullous disorders affecting the proximal nailfold

Nailfold telangiectasia

The blood supply to the posterior nailfolds is essentially the same as that at other skin sites except that within the tongue of skin that forms the posterior nailfold, the capillary loops run parallel rather than vertical to the surface. Capillaries in the thin skin of the posterior nailfold are thus easily visible and can be inspected using an ophthalmoscope. The nailfold capillaries are most evident in the ring finger. Normal nailfold capillaries can usually just be seen as uniform loops of similar thickness capillaries, arranged in rows (**Fig 19.41**). Alterations to this pattern occur in connective tissue diseases, in which there is also elongation and a ragged shape of the cuticle. Some loss of nailfold capillary vasculature occurs in patients with psoriatic arthritis.

The capillary changes seen in dermatomyositis (**Figs 19.42** and **19.43**) and systemic sclerosis (scleroderma) (**Figs 19.44** and **19.45**) are morphologically similar to each other, although they are usually most obvious in dermatomyositis. Capillaries disappear, leaving gaps in the normally uniform rows of regular loops. Some remaining capillary loops become dilated and deformed, producing 'giant capillary loops' (**Fig 19.42**). In dermatomyositis, changes also occur on the cuticles, which become ragged, and the posterior nailfolds become red and thickened (**Fig 19.43**). It is these changes that seem to be most helpful in making a diagnosis, rather than the shape of the nailfold capillaries.

In lupus erythematosus, the capillaries lose the normal tight loop shape and become irregular or tortuous but are not dilated.

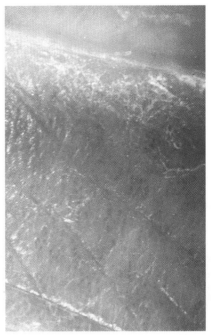

Fig 19.41 Normal nailfold capillaries. These are just visible as tiny capillary loops, uniformly distributed across the posterior nailfold

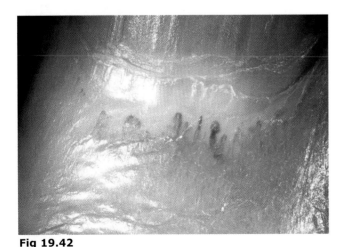

Fig 19.42

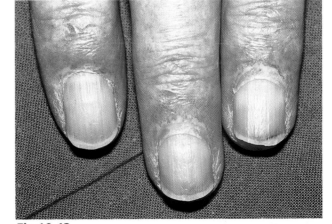

Fig 19.43

Figs 19.42, 19.43 Nailfold capillary changes in dermatomyositis. There are several giant capillary loops and segments without capillaries (19.42). The posterior nailfolds are swollen and erythematous, and the cuticles long and ragged (19.43) (19.42 *courtesy of Dr Colin Munro*)

367

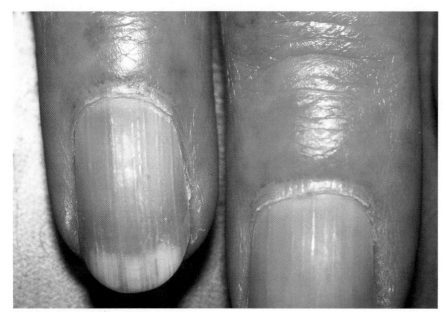

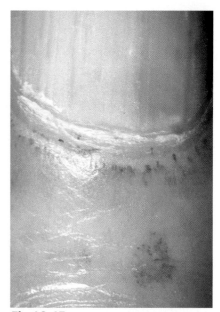

Fig 19.44   Fig 19.45

Figs 19.44, 19.45 Nailfold capillary changes in systemic sclerosis. The capillaries are dilated and irregularly distributed along the posterior nailfold (19.44). Remnants of old nailfold capillaries appear as linear fragments of altered blood visible in the cuticles. Note also the mat telangiectasis on the terminal phalanx (19.45). Same patient as shown in 11.39

Paronychia

The term paronychia is used to describe inflammation of the nailfolds. Acute paronychia results in redness, swelling, tenderness and pustules of the lateral and posterior nailfold (**Fig 19.46**). Infection of the soft tissue, usually by *Staphylococcus aureus*, is the commonest cause. Secondary nail dystrophy with transverse ridging is common.

Herpes simplex infection of the nailfolds can also appear rapidly but is characterised by grouped vesicles, which may be pustular (herpetic whitlow). Acute paronychia rarely progresses to chronic paronychia.

Chronic paronychia (**Table 19.8**) is insidious in onset. The nailfold is red and swollen but not particularly painful. The cuticle is lost, the proximal nailfold is often thickened and has a rolled or 'bolstered' appearance, and there is gap between the nail plate and nailfold (**Fig 19.47**). In some cases, cheesy white material can be squeezed from the posterior nailfold, from which *Candida* species (*C. albicans, C. parapsilosis*) or, less commonly, *Klebsiella* species or *Proteus* organisms (usually thought to be commensal organisms taking advantage of a damaged nailfold rather than primary pathogens) can be cultured. The nail plate may be irregularly transversely ridged but does not have the subungual hyperkeratosis that is characteristic of dermatophyte fungal infection.

Scaling and hyperkeratosis of the nailfolds

Scaling and hyperkeratosis of the nailfolds are usually caused by psoriasis. Redness and peeling of the nailfold skin are also a feature of zinc deficiency (**Fig 19.48**) and acrokeratosis paraneoplastica (**Fig 19.49**). The latter is a cutaneous manifestation of internal malignancy seen in men with solid tumours of the upper gastrointestinal or respiratory tract. In this rare condition, there is hyperkeratosis and flaking of the nail plate and ultimately

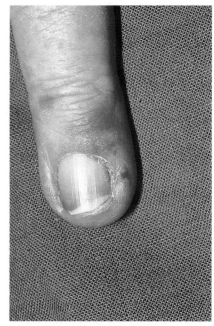

Fig 19.46 Acute paronychia. There is swelling and redness of the nailfold. Note that the cuticle is intact

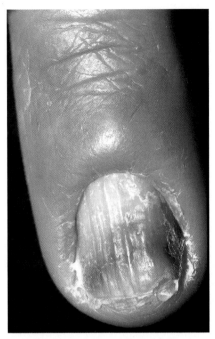

Fig 19.47 Chronic paronychia.
There is swelling and redness of the posterior and lateral nailfold, loss of cuticles and associated mild dystrophy of the nail plate. Thick cheesy white material may be squeezed from the junction between the nail plate and nail bed. The lesion is usually surprisingly pain free

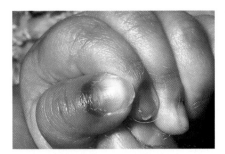

Fig 19.48 Zinc deficiency in a breast-fed premature infant.
There was erythema and scaling of the nailfolds of the thumb, index and middle fingers of both hands. Other features are shown in 5.28 and 5.29. The clinical features are the same as for acrodermatitis enteropathica, although the zinc deficiency is due to inadequate intake rather than malabsorption. Premature infants are zinc deficient, and breast milk does not contain sufficient excess of zinc to compensate (from Munro CS *et al.* (1989) *Brit J Dermatol* 121: 773, with permission)

DIAGNOSTIC TIPS AND PITFALLS

- Distinction between dermatophyte infection of the nail (onychomycosis, which requires systemic therapy) and chronic candidal paronychia (which is best treated topically) is therapeutically important, but the two are often confused

- In onychomycosis, the features are distal subungual hyperkeratosis, with normal surface of the nail plate in the common types, whereas in chronic paronychia, there is loss of the cuticle, a bolstered proximal nailfold, transverse ridging of the nail plate and no subungual hyperkeratosis

complete nail loss with only fragments of crumbling nail plate attached to the red nail bed.

Discoloration of the nailfolds, Hutchinson's sign

Uneven macular pigmentation of posterior and lateral nailfolds occurs in acral lentiginous melanoma (**Figs 19.68** and **19.69**). If the tumour is situated in the nail matrix, an associated pigmented band will also be present (Hutchinson's sign, *see also* pp. 376–378). However, there are benign causes of Hutchinson's sign, including Peutz–Jegher's syndrome, Laugier–Hunziker syndrome (**Figs 19.73** and **19.74**), AIDS and drugs (zidovudine, minocycline). Non-melanoma skin cancers of the nail may be pigmented (especially Bowen's disease at this site, which may also be multiple). Also, the colour of subungual haematomas or benign pigmented bands can sometimes be visualised through a thin cuticle (pseudo-Hutchinson's sign).

DEFECTS OF THE NAIL BED

Onycholysis

Detachment of the nail from the nail bed is common, and there are a variety of causes (**Table 19.9**).

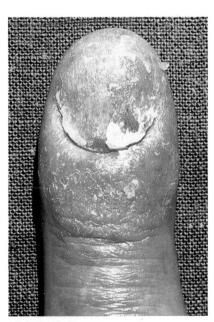

Fig 19.49 Acrokeratosis paraneoplastica (Basex syndrome). There is virtually a complete loss of the nail plate, with only remnants attached to the nail bed, in this elderly man with a carcinoma of the larynx

Table 19.9 Common causes of onycholysis

Dermatological	Psoriasis (19.50), Reiter's disease, contact dermatitis
Systemic	Thyrotoxicosis, chronic ischaemia (19.22) Yellow nail syndrome (19.63), pregnancy
Trauma	Direct injury, excessive manicuring
Drug-induced	Retinoids, cytotoxics
Photo-onycholysis	Usually fingernails only—tetracyclines, thiazides, benoxaprofen, chlorpromazine
Infection	Dermatophyte, candida (19.38), viral warts
Chemical irritants	Hot soapy water immersion, false nails, nail varnish remover, solvents and oils (19.14)
Idiopathic	Usually women with long nails (? traumatic)

Salmon patches (oil drop sign)

Salmon pink patches on the nail bed visible through the nail plate are due to psoriasis in the nail bed (**Fig 19.50**). This can be a helpful diagnostic feature, sometimes called the oil drop sign, because it enables psoriatic and fungal nail dystrophy to be distinguished clinically. The appearance may be seen in isolation but usually occurs just proximal to an area of psoriatic onycholysis. It is due to areas of parakeratosis (retention of nucleated keratinocytes) that grow distally with the nail—when these grow as far as the onychodermal band, they are shed, leading to onycholysis (hence the frequency of this appearance proximal to psoriatic onycholysis). Attempts to remove debris and keratinous scale from the onycholytic psoriatic nail may result in trauma of the nail bed and further extension of the nail-bed psoriasis. Psoriatic nails should be kept short and only cleaned with a soft nail brush.

Splinter haemorrhages

Splinter haemorrhages are purpuric lesions, which develop a linear shape because the nail bed capillaries run along the well-defined folds that exist in the nail bed. The most common cause of splinter haemorrhages is trauma (**Fig 19.51**), but the most important causes are related to embolic and vasculitic disorders, such as subacute bacterial endocarditis (**Fig 19.52**). In this disorder, there may be evidence of vasculitis elsewhere, especially in the finger pulps (Osler's nodes, **Fig 19.53**) and the palms and soles (Janeway's lesions).

TUMOURS ASSOCIATED WITH THE NAIL

Subungual heloma or corn

A subungual heloma or corn appears as a painful dark spot under the nail and may produce splitting or elevation of the nail tip. It must be distinguished from a subungual melanoma.

Subungual exostosis

Subungual exostoses are out-growths of normal bone or calcified cartilage from the terminal phalanx of any digit. They may be confused with subungual solitary warts but can be distinguished by characteristic changes on radiographs (**Figs 19.54** and **19.55**).

DIAGNOSTIC TIPS AND PITFALLS

- A salmon pink or waxy yellowish colour proximal to onycholysis is strongly suggestive of psoriatic nail dystrophy

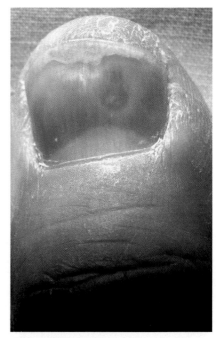

Fig 19.50 Onycholysis and salmon patches (*photo courtesy of Dr David de Berker*)

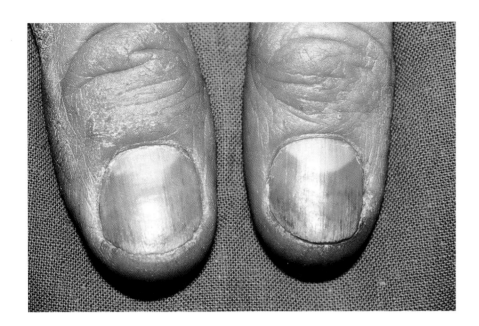

Fig 19.51 Traumatic splinter haemorrhages

Koenen's tumours

Periungual fibrokeratoma occurs in 50% of patients with tuberous sclerosis (**Fig 19.56**), but it also occurs as solitary sporadic lesions (**Fig 19.57**). It may cause longitudinal ridging or guttering of the nail plate due to pressure on the matrix.

Acquired periungual fibrokeratoma presents as a solitary benign nodule with a hyperkeratotic tip arising out of the posterior nailfold, and it virtually always causes guttering of the nail plate (**Fig 19.57**). By contrast, the periungal fibromas in tuberous sclerosis are multiple and fleshy.

Pyogenic granuloma

Pyogenic granuloma of the finger presents as an extremely vascular tumour of recent onset (*see* Fig 9.65), usually arising after minor trauma, and may have a well-defined collar of normal skin resembling an acorn cup (*see* Fig 9.11).

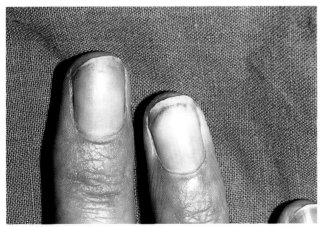

Fig 19.52

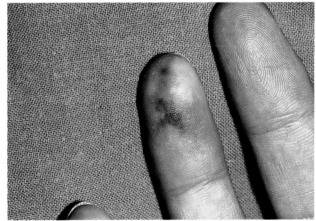

Fig 19.53

Figs 19.52, 19.53 Splinter haemorrhages and Osler's nodes. The patient presented with embolic cerebrovascular disease. The splinter haemorrhages are visible along the distal margin of the nail plate (19.52). The Osler node occurred as a circumscribed indurated tender red area of the finger pulp (19.53)

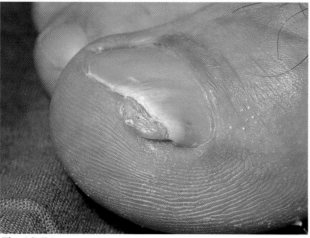

Fig 19.54

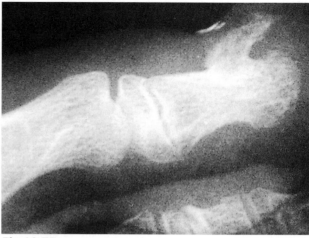

Fig 19.55

Figs 19.54, 19.55 Subungual exostosis. There is a small bony spicule protruding from the terminal phalanx, which can be shown by radiography. Unlike subungual warts, they are solitary, hard and painful

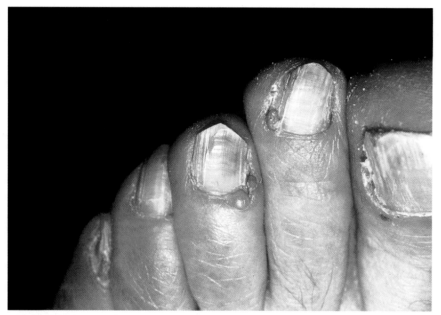

Fig 19.56 Koenen's tumours in tuberous sclerosis. Multiple fleshy periungual fibrokeratomas in a patient with tuberous sclerosis, who was the mother of the patient shown in 3.26. Approximately 30% of patients with tuberous sclerosis have fibrokeratomas

Fig 19.57 Acquired periungual fibrokeratoma. There is obvious nail guttering produced by this solitary fibrokeratoma, which arises in otherwise healthy individuals. Tuberous sclerosis must be excluded by the absence of other features. Acquired fibrokeratoma is usually solitary, produces a well-formed nail gutter and is surmounted by a little hyperkeratotic tip

Pyogenic granulomas may arise on the proximal nailfold (**Fig 19.58**). When they arise on the nail bed, they perforate the nail plate and must be distinguished histologically from amelanotic melanomas.

Glomus tumour

Glomus bodies are neurovascular arteriovenous anastomoses, of which there are many on the finger ends. In response to cold, glomus bodies dilate, whereas arterioles constrict, so that blood supply to digits is preserved in cold weather. Benign tumours of glomus bodies may appear under the nail plate, where they produce intolerable pulsating or spontaneous pain, made worse

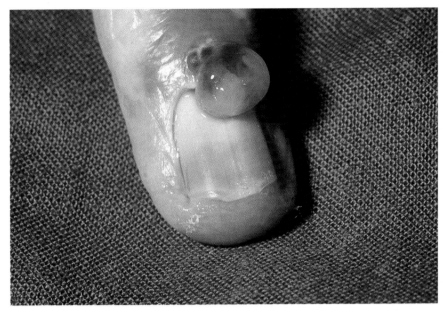

Fig 19.58 Pyogenic granuloma. There is a fleshy vascular tumour on the posterior nailfold, producing a groove in the nail plate

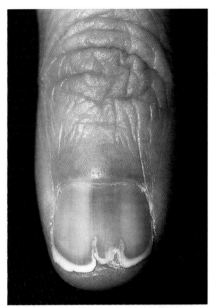

Fig 19.59 Glomus tumour of the nail bed. The red colour is typical and, especially if the tumour is proximal, there may be damage to the overlying nail plate (as in this case)

by minor trauma. The tumour can be seen through the nail plate as a red or bluish patch up to 10 mm in diameter, but the changes are usually unimpressive until an attempt is made to squeeze the nail plate. Nail-plate ridging or splitting may be present (**Fig 19.59**).

Myxoid cysts

Myxoid cysts (digital mucous cysts) are soft cystic dome-shaped skin-covered papules, usually found on the posterior nailfold of the finger or toe (*see* Fig 13.34); pressure on the underlying nail plate may cause guttering. Puncture of the cyst results in release of a gelatinous material. When Methylene Blue dye is injected into the distal interphalangeal joint, it also enters the cyst, showing that virtually all myxoid cysts are connected to the joint. This supports the theory that myxoid cysts are derived from extruded joint fluid.

Periungual warts

Periungual warts (**Fig 19.60**) are common. Posterior nailfold warts occur in children who bite or chew their fingers, in which case the virus is often spread to the lips. Subungual warts can become impossible to treat without removal of the nail plate and extensive diathermy or carbon dioxide laser destruction of the affected area.

Carcinoma of the fingertip

Bowen's disease or squamous carcinoma (**Fig 19.61** and **19.62**) of a digit may present as chronic paronychia, isolated nail dystrophy, destruction of the nail or subungual keratosis. A biopsy should be performed if doubt exists.

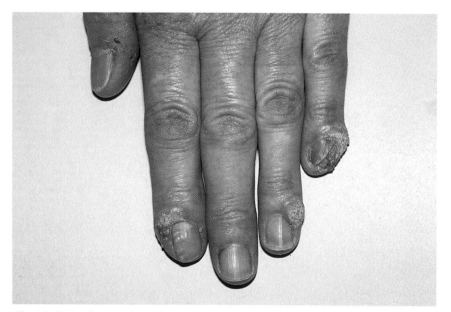

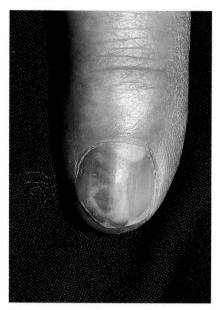

Fig 19.60 Periungual warts. This shows multiple warts on the fingertips. On the little finger, the nail plate is becoming lifted up by warts growing into the nail bed. Notice the changes produced by chewing the nailfolds present on the thumb. Persistent finger tip warts usually occur only in nail biters and finger chewers who constantly damage their finger ends, providing more sites for the virus to penetrate

Fig 19.61 Squamous cell carcinoma of the nail bed. In this case, a relatively subtle lesion presented as colour change without significant damage to the nail plate (compare with 19.62)

NAIL COLOUR CHANGES AND PIGMENTED STREAKS

There are multiple causes of nail colour change. Most are incidental features and rarely present diagnostic difficulty. Complete lists are included in specialist textbooks. Some of the common types of colour change are given in Tables 19.10 and 19.11.

Pigmented streaks

Eighty per cent of African–Carribeans have pigmented streaks in the fingernails (**Fig 19.6**). The appearance of pigmented streaks in whites suggests the

Table 19.10 Common causes of pigmented streaks (longitudinal melanonychia)

Benign naevus of the matrix

Physiological in black skin (19.6)

Traumatic

Laugier–Hunziker syndrome
With lentigines of the lips, mouth and hands (19.72, 19.73)

Systemic disease
Addison's disease, post-adrenalectomy for Cushing's syndrome, AIDS

Drugs
Mepacrine (19.69), zidovudine, chemotherapeutic drugs, including busulphan, cyclophosphamide

Melanoma (19.65–19.68)

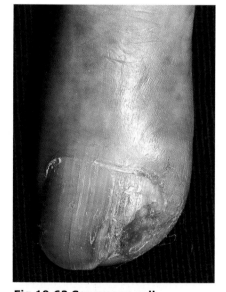

Fig 19.62 Squamous cell carcinoma of the right index finger. This 60-year-old woman had had recurrent 'infections' with a pustular discharge from under her nail for many years. On examination, there was an area of nail-bed discoloration visible through the intact nail plate, minimal onycholysis and a pustular discharge. The nail plate had to be removed to enable a biopsy to be taken of the nail bed. This confirmed the presence of a moderately differentiated squamous cell carcinoma

Table 19.11 Causes of other nail colour changes

Generalised whitening	Cirrhosis, chronic hypoalbuminaemia, renal failure, etc. (19.70) of the nail
Proximal half white	Half and half nails occur in 10% of patients with chronic renal failure—it does not correspond to the degree of renal impairment (19.71)
Other colours	Blue—drugs, e.g. antimalarials (19.69), minocycline (*see* 3.13) Yellow—yellow nail syndrome (19.63) Green—pseudomonas infections (19.64) Tan—scopulariopsis infection Brown—exogenous agents (nicotine, dithranol/anthralin, hydroquinone), drugs (psoralens, chlorpromazine, mepacrine) Red—polycythaemia, carbon monoxide poisoning, systemic lupus erythematosus (especially red lunulae)

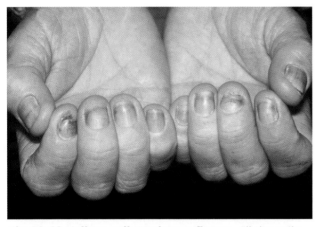

Fig 19.63 Yellow nail syndrome finger. All the nails are yellowish and thickened. There were identical changes in the toenails

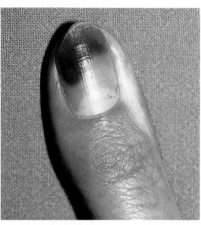

Fig 19.64 Pseudomonas infection. There is onycholysis and a green colour to the nail plate. Pseudomonas was cultured from nail clippings

development of a subungual melanoma, but there are many other causes (*see* Table 19.10). Features that suggest a benign aetiology include Afro-Caribbean racial origin, multiple bands and thin or unchanging bands.

Features that are suggestive of melanoma include:

- Pigmented streaks more than 3 mm wide, changing in morphology or wider proximally than distally—the latter occurs if the tumour width expands faster than the time taken for the nail to grow from the tumour to the free nail edge.
- Pigment spread from the nail plate on to the posterior nailfold—Hutchinson's sign (**Figs 19.65** and **19.66**). However, there are also benign causes of Hutchinson's sign and other potential causes of confusion (*see* p. 369).
- Nail destruction, although this also occurs in subungual corn, pyogenic granuloma and fungal infections, etc.
- Age 50–70 years.
- Digit affected (thumb > hallux > index finger).

Note that the origin of a pigmented streak may be obscured by the nail plate and can only be shown surgically (**Figs 19.67** and **19.68**).

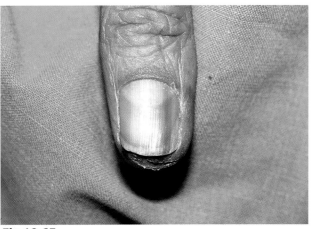

Fig 19.65

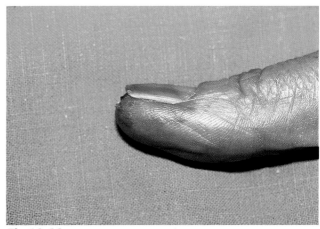

Fig 19.66

Figs 19.65, 19.66 Acral lentiginous melanoma *in situ* There is a faint pigment band on the nail plate (19.65); pigment spread on to the lateral nailfold and finger end (Hutchinson's sign) is most evident in the lateral view (19.66)

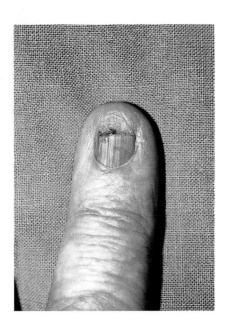

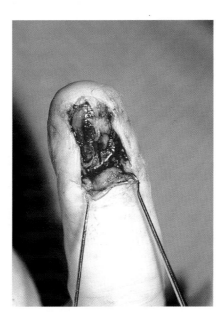

Figs 19.67, 19.68 Acral lentiginous melanoma. The nail is slightly pigmented (19.67), although a previous biopsy has obscured this. The nail plate was thickened and smaller than the equivalent nail on the other hand. After the nail plate had been removed, pigmentation of the nail bed could be clearly seen (19.68)

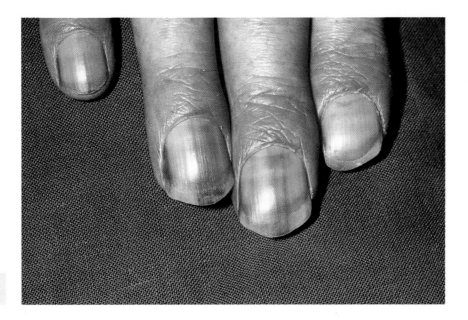

Fig 19.69 Nail pigmentation due to mepacrine. These are grey–brown pigmented bands associated with mepacrine treatment for discoid lupus erythematosus

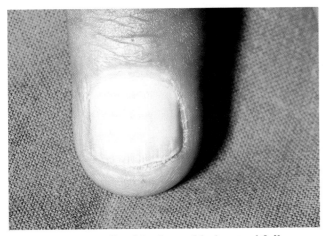

Fig 19.70 Generalised leukonychia in renal failure.
This shows loss of lunula and sparing of the onychodermal band of Terry

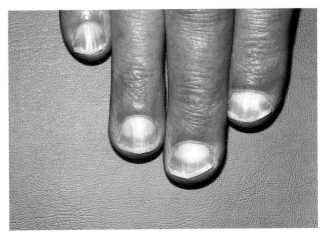

Fig 19.71 Half and half nails in a patient with rheumatoid disease and chronic renal failure. The proximal portion is white and the distal red, pink or brown. This condition occurs in approximately 10% of patients with chronic renal failure. The level and extent of colour change are not related to the severity of the uraemia

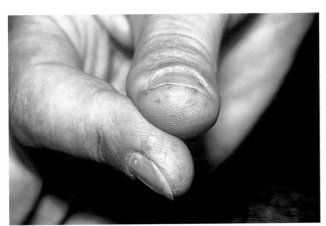

Fig 19.72

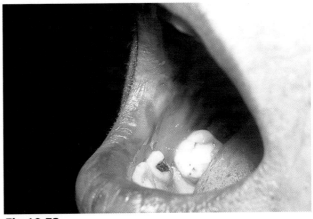

Fig 19.73

Figs 19.72, 19.73 Laugier–Hunziker syndrome. This is a benign cause of isolated pigmented streaks in the nail bed; they are just visible on the nail (19.72). Pigment spread on to the nailfolds may occur. Other characteristic features include brown macules on the lips and buccal mucosa (19.73) and pigmented macules on the fingertips (19.72)

Bibliography

Further reading references by chapter

General reading

Fitzpatrick TB, Eisen AZ, Wolff K, Freedburg IM & Austen KF (1987) *Dermatology in General Medicine*, 3rd edn. McGraw-Hill, New York.

Champion RH, Burton JL, Burns DA & Breathnach SM (eds) (1996) *Rook, Wilkinson & Ebling Textbook of Dermatology*, 6th edn. Blackwell Scientific Publications, Oxford.

Habif TP (1990) *Clinical Dermatology. A Color Guide to Diagnosis and Therapy*, 2nd edn. Mosby, St Louis.

Harper J, Oranje A & Prose N (2000) *Textbook of Pediatric Dermatology*. Blackwell Science, Oxford.

Braun-Falco O, Plewig G, Wolff HH & Winkelmann RK (1991) *Dermatology*, 3rd revised edn. Springer-Verlag, Berlin.

2. Shapes and patterns of lesions

Happle R (1985) Lyonisation and the lines of Blaschko. *Hum Genet* 70: 200–206.

Farthing CF, Staughton RCD, Harper JI *et al.* (1986) Papuloerythroderma: a further case with the deck chair sign. *Dermatologica* 172: 65–66.

3. Colours, hyperpigmentation, hypopigmentation

Ortonne J-P, Mosher DB & Fitzpatrick TB (1983) *Vitiligo and Other Hypomelanoses of Hair and Skin*. Plenum Medical Book, New York.

Fulk CS (1984) Primary disorders of hyperpigmentation. *J Am Acad Dermatol* 10: 1–16.

Colver GB, Mortimer PS, Millard PR, Dawber RPR & Ryan TJ (1987) The 'dirty neck' a reticulate pigmentation in atopics. *Clin Exp Dermatol* 12: 1–4.

Hud JA, Cohen JB, Wagner JM & Crus PD (1992) Prevalence and significance of acanthosis nigricans in an adult obese population. *Arch Dermatol* 128: 941–944.

Reisfeld PL (2000) Blue in the skin. *J Am Acad Dermatol* 42: 597–605.

4. Elicitation of physical signs

Clarke A & Burn J (1991) Sweat testing to identify female carriers of X-linked hypohidrotic ectodermal dysplasia. *J Med Genet* 28: 330–333.

Gupta R & Perry M (1999) Digital examination for oral cancer. *BMJ* 319: 1113–1114.

Knight JM, Hayduk MJ, Summerlin D-J & Mirowski GW (2000) 'Strawberry' gingival hyperplasia. A pathognomonic mucocutaneous finding in Wegener granulomatosis. *Arch Dermatol* 136: 171–173.

Pride HB (1999) Child abuse and mimickers of child abuse. *Adv. Dermatol.* 14: 417–455.

6. Normal variants and common anomalies

Selmanowitz VJ & Krivo JM (1975) Pigmentary demarcation lines. *Br J Dermatol* 93: 371–377.

Nürnberger F & Müller G (1978) So called cellulite: an inventive disease. *J Dermatol Surg Oncol* 4: 221–229.

Lewis T (1927) *The Blood Vessels of the Human Skin and their Responses*. Shaw & Sons, London.

Kirkham N *et al.* (1989) Diagonal ear lobe creases and fatal cardiovascular disease: a necropsy study. *Br Heart J* 61: 361–364.

Cunliffe WJ *et al.* (2000) Comedogenesis. *Br J Dermatol* 142: 1084–1091.

7. Scale and crust

Paramsothy Y & Lawrence CM (1987) Tin tack sign in localised pemphigus foliaceus. *Br J Dermatol* 116: 127–129.

Caro MR & Senear FE (1947) Psoriasis of the hands: non-pustular type. *Arch Dermatol Syphilol* 56: 629–632.

Buno IJ, Morelli JG & Weston WL (1998) The enamel paint sign in the dermatologic diagnosis of early-onset kwashiorkor [letter]. *Arch Dermatol* 134: 107–108.

8. Plaques

Bernhard JD (1990) Auspitz sign is not sensitive or specific for psoriasis. *J Am Acad Dermatol* 22: 1079–1081.

10. Macular and maculopapular rashes

Goodyear HM *et al.* (1991) Acute infectious erythemas in children: a clinico-microbiological study. *Br J Dermatol* 124: 433–438.

Bialecki C, Feder HM & Grant-Kels JM (1989) The six classic childhood exanthems; a review and update. *J Am Acad Dermatol* 21: 891–903.

Grilli R, Izquierdo, Farina MC *et al.* (1999) Papular-purpuric 'gloves and socks' syndrome: polymerase chain reaction demonstration of parvovirus B19 DNA in cutaneous lesions and sera. *J Am Acad Dermatol* 41: 793–796.

11. Textural changes in skin

Burton JL (1982) Thick skin and stiff joints in insulin dependent diabetes mellitus. *Br J Dermatol* 106: 369–371.

Hartley AC (1986) Finger pebbles: a common finding in diabetes mellitus. *J Am Acad Dermatol* 14: 612–617.

12. Ulcers

Moss C & Ince P (1987) Anhidrotic and achromians lesions in incontinentia pigmenti. *Br J Dermatol* 116: 839–849.

Asboe-Hansen G (1960) Blister spread induced by finger pressure, a diagnostic sign in pemphigus. *J Invest Dermatol* 34: 5–9.

Feingold DS (1982) Gangrenous and crepitant cellulitis. *J Am Acad Dermatol* 6: 289–299.

16. Weals

Czarnetzki BM (1986) *Urticaria*. Springer-Verlag, Berlin.

17. Erythema and vascular disorders

Piette WW & Stone MS (1989) A cutaneous sign of IgA-associated small dermal vessel leukocytoclastic vasculitis in adults (Henoch–Schönlein purpura). *Arch Dermatol* 125: 53–56.

Cox NH & Paterson WD (1991) Angioma serpiginosum: a simulator of purpura. *Postgrad Med J* 67: 1065–1066.

Hirschmann JV & Raugi GJ (1992) Dermatologic features of the superior vena cava syndrome. *Arch Dermatol* 128: 953–956.

Cox NH, Paterson WD & Popple AW (1996) A reticulate vascular abnormality in patients with lymphoedema—observations in eight patients. *Br J Dermatol* 135: 92–97.

18. Hair

Shuster S (1984) 'Coudability': a new physical sign of alopecia areata. *Br J Dermatol* 111: 629.

Sperling LC (1991) Hair anatomy for the clinician. *J Am Acad Dermatol* 25: 1–17.

Rook A & Dawber PR (eds) (1991) *Diseases of the hair and Scalp*, 2nd edn. Blackwell Scientific Publications, Oxford.

Sperling LC (2000) A new look at scarring alopecia. *Arch Dermatol* 136: 235–242.

19. Nails

Baran R & Dawber RPR (eds) (1984) *Diseases of the Nail and their Management*. Blackwell Scientific Publications, Oxford.

Minkin W & Rabhan NB (1982) Office nailfold capillary microscopy using an ophthalmoscope. *J Am Acad Dermatol* 7: 190–193.

Baran R (1979) Longitudinal melanotic streaks as a clue to Laugier–Hunziker syndrome. *Arch Dermatol* 115: 1448–1449.

Index

*Numbers in **bold** refer to figure legends and tabular material. Where there is a textual reference to the topic on the same page, bold is not used.*

Index

Index

Index

Index